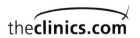
theclinics.com

CLINICS IN LABORATORY MEDICINE

Clinical Toxicology

GUEST EDITORS
Christopher P. Holstege, MD
Daniel E. Rusyniak, MD

March 2006 • Volume 26 • Number 1

An Imprint of Elsevier, Inc.
PHILADELPHIA   LONDON   TORONTO   MONTREAL   SYDNEY   TOKYO

W.B. SAUNDERS COMPANY
A Division of Elsevier Inc.

Elsevier, Inc. • 1600 John F. Kennedy Blvd., Suite 1800 • Philadelphia, Pennsylvania 19103-2899

http://www.theclinics.com

CLINICS IN LABORATORY MEDICINE
March 2006
Editor: Patrick Manley

Volume 26, Number 1
ISSN 0272-2712
ISBN 1-4160-3733-X

Reprints: For copies of 100 or more, of articles in this publication, please contact the Commercial Reprints Department, Elsevier Inc., 360 Park Avenue South, New York, New York 10010-1710. Tel. (212) 633-3813. Fax: (212) 462-1935, e-mail: reprints@elsevier.com.

The ideas and opinions expressed in *Clinics in Laboratory Medicine* do not necessarily reflect those of the Publisher. The Publisher does not assume any responsibility for any injury and/or damage to persons or property arising out of or related to any use of the material contained in this periodical. The reader is advised to check the appropriate medical literature and the product information currently provided by the manufacturer of each drug to be administered to verify the dosage, the method and duration of administration, or contraindications. It is the responsibility of the treating physician or other health care professional, relying on independent experience and knowledge of the patient, to determine drug dosages and the best treatment for the patient. Mention of any product in this issue should not be construed as endorsement by the contributors, editors, or the Publisher of the product or manufacturers' claims.

Clinics in Laboratory Medicine (ISSN 0272-2712) is published quarterly by W.B Saunders, 360 Park Avenue South, New York, NY 10010-1710. Months of publication are March, June, September, and December. Business and editorial offices: 1600 John F. Kennedy Blvd., Suite 1800, Philadelphia, PA 19103-2899. Accounting and Circulation Offices: 6277 Sea Harbor Drive, Orlando, FL 32887-4800. Periodicals postage paid at New York, NY and additional mailing offices. Subscription prices are $165.00 per year (US individuals), $255.00 per year (US institutions), $85.00 (US students), $190.00 per year (Canadian individuals), $315.00 per year (foreign institutions), $110.00 (foreign students). Foreign air speed delivery is included in all *Clinics* subscription prices. All prices are subject to change without notice. POSTMASTER: Send address changes to *Clinics in Laboratory Medicine*, Elsevier Periodicals Customer Service, 6277 Sea Harbor Drive, Orlando, FL 32887-4800. **Customer Service: 1-800-654-2452 (US). From outside of the US, call 1-407-345-4000.** E-mail: hhspcs@harcout.com.

Clinics in Laboratory Medicine is covered in *EMBASE/Exerpta Medica, Index Medicus, Cinahl, Current Contents/ Clinical Medicine, BIOSIS* and *ISI/BIOMED*.

Printed in the United States of America.

GUEST EDITORS

CHRISTOPHER P. HOLSTEGE, MD, Director, Division of Medical Toxicology, University of Virginia, Charlottesville; Medical Director, Blue Ridge Poison Center, University of Virginia Health System, Charlottesville; and Associate Professor, Departments of Emergency Medicine & Pediatrics, University of Virginia Charlottesville, Virginia

DANIEL E. RUSYNIAK, MD, Fellowship Director, Medical Toxicology; Assistant Professor, Department of Emergency Medicine, Indiana University School of Medicine, Indianapolis, Indiana

CONTRIBUTORS

MELROSE KANKU ALLEN, MD, Emergency Medicine Resident, Department of Emergency Medicine, University of Virginia, Charlottesville, Virginia

KEVIN S. BARLOTTA, MD, Emergency Medicine Resident, Department of Emergency Medicine, University of Virginia, Charlottesville, Virginia

STEPHEN G. DOBMEIER, RN, BSN, CSPI, Director, Blue Ridge Poison Center, University of Virginia Health System, Charlottesville, Virginia

DAVID L. ELDRIDGE, MD, MA, Assistant Professor (Pediatrics), Department of Pediatrics, Brody School of Medicine, East Carolina University, Greenville, North Carolina

TIMOTHY ERICKSON, MD, FACEP, FACMT, FAACT, Professor, Department of Emergency Medicine; Director, Section of Clinical Toxicology; and Director, Emergency Medicine Residency Program, University of Illinois, Chicago, Illinois

BLAKE FROBERG, MD, Medical Toxicology Fellow, Department of Emergency Medicine, Division of Medical Toxicology, Indiana University School of Medicine, Indianapolis, Indiana

R. BRENT FURBEE, MD, FACMT, Medical Director, Indiana Poison Center, Department of Emergency Medicine, Indiana University School of Medicine, Indianapolis, Indiana

MICHAEL I. GREENBERG, MD, MPh, Professor (Emergency Medicine), Department of Emergency Medicine, Drexel University College of Medicine, Medical College of Pennsylvania Hospital, Philadelphia, Pennsylvania

RACHEL HAROZ, MD, Toxicology Fellow, Department of Emergency Medicine, Drexel University College of Medicine, Medical College of Pennsylvania Hospital, Philadelphia, Pennsylvania

KENNON HEARD, MD, Assistant Professor (Surgery), Division of Emergency Medicine; Section Chief, Medical Toxicology, University of Colorado School of Medicine; and Attending Physician, Rocky Mountain Poison and Drug Center, Denver, Colorado

CHRISTOPHER P. HOLSTEGE, MD, Director, Division of Medical Toxicology, University of Virginia, Charlottesville; Medical Director, Blue Ridge Poison Center, University of Virginia Health System, Charlottesville; and Associate Professor, Departments of Emergency Medicine & Pediatrics, University of Virginia Charlottesville, Virginia

DANYAL IBRAHIM, MD, Medical Toxicology Fellow, Department of Emergency Medicine, Division of Medical Toxicology, Indiana University School of Medicine, Indianapolis, Indiana

JAMES H. JONES, MD, Vice-Chair; and Associate Professor (Clinical Emergency Medicine), Department of Emergency Medicine, Indiana University School of Medicine, Indianapolis, Indiana

BRYAN S. JUDGE, MD, Associate Medical Director, DeVos Children's Hospital Regional Poison Center; and Assistant Clinical Professor, Grand Rapids MERC/Michigan State University Program in Emergency Medicine, Grand Rapids, Michigan

LOUISE W. KAO, MD, Associate Fellowship Director, Medical Toxicology Fellowship Program, Clinical Assistant Professor, Department of Emergency Medicine, Indiana University School of Medicine Indianapolis, Indiana

MARK A. KIRK, MD, Assistant Professor (Emergency Medicine and Pediatrics); and Fellowship Director, Division of Medical Toxicology, Department of Emergency

KRISTINE A. NAÑAGAS, MD, Adjunct Clinical Assistant Professor, Division of Medical Toxicology, Department of Emergency Medicine, Indiana University School of Medicine; and Medical Toxicology of Indiana, Indiana Poison Center, Indianapolis, Indiana

JEFFREY NORVELL, MD, Assistant Professor (Emergency Medicine), University of Missouri–Kansas City Truman Medical Center, Kansas City, Missouri

ADAM K. ROWDEN, DO, Fellow, Division of Medical Toxicology, Department of Emergency Medicine, University of Virginia, Charlottesville, Virginia

DANIEL E. RUSYNIAK, MD, Fellowship Director, Medical Toxicology; Assistant Professor, Department of Emergency Medicine, Indiana University School of Medicine, Indianapolis, Indiana

JON E. SPRAGUE, PhD, Chair; Professor (Pharmacology), Virginia College of Osteopathic Medicine; and Department of Biomedical Sciences and Pathobiology, Virginia Polytechnic Institute and State University, Blacksburg, Virginia

WILLIAM B. WEIR, MD, Resident, Department of Emergency Medicine, Indiana University School of Medicine, Indianapolis, Indiana

BRANDON WILLS, DO, MS, Clinical Instructor, Department of Emergency Medicine, University of Illinois; and Fellow, Clinical Toxicology, Toxikon Consortium of Cook County, Chicago, Illinois

ANDREA WOLF, MD, Emergency Medicine Resident, Department of Emergency Medicine, Indiana University School of Medicine, Indianapolis, Indiana

CONTENTS

the spider has never been seen. A review of medical literature reveals that most current concepts regarding brown recluse spider envenomation are based on supposition. In this article, we attempt to review critically our present understanding of brown recluse bites with a focus on the published evidence.

FORTHCOMING ISSUES

RECENT ISSUES

ELSEVIER
SAUNDERS

Clin Lab Med 26 (2006) xiii–xiv

CLINICS IN
LABORATORY
MEDICINE

Preface

Clinical Toxicology

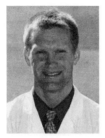 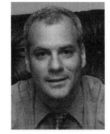

Christopher P. Holstege, MD   Daniel E. Rusyniak, MD
Guest Editors

After the publication of the "Medical Toxicology" issue of the *Medical Clinics of North America* in November 2005, we were asked by Elsevier to adapt and publish those articles deemed suitable for the *Clinics in Laboratory Medicine*. In considering this, we sought advice from many colleagues and friends regarding what aspects of the previous work would be appropriate for this publication's audience. The culmination of this discussion has resulted in this issue. Several of the articles are unchanged from the previous publication, several have been modified, and several are completely new articles.

Medical toxicology is a subspecialty recognized by the American Board of Medical Specialties. Physicians who have trained in this area focus their practice on the prevention, diagnosis, and management of poisoning. Over the past decade, the field of medical toxicology has grown in conjunction with the emergence of new pharmaceuticals, abused drugs, chemicals within the workplace, and weapons of mass destruction. For this issue, we invited authors from many of the outstanding medical toxicology training programs to address a variety of pertinent topics. A detailed discussion on gross and microscopic pathology was purposely omitted, because the emphasis is on clinical presentation, pathophysiology, appropriate diagnostic testing, and management of acute and chronic poisoning. It is our hope that clinicians from all backgrounds will glean some information from this issue that will help them to provide exceptional care for individuals who have been poisoned.

Christopher P. Holstege, MD
Division of Medical Toxicology
Departments of Emergency Medicine & Pediatrics
University of Virginia
P.O. Box 800774
Charlottesville, VA 22908-0774, USA

E-mail address: ch2xf@virginia.edu

Daniel E. Rusyniak, MD
Department of Emergency Medicine
Indiana University School of Medicine
1050 Wishard Boulevard, R2200
Indianapolis, IN 46202-2859, USA

E-mail address: drusynia@iupui.edu

CLINICS IN
LABORATORY
MEDICINE

ELSEVIER
SAUNDERS

Clin Lab Med 26 (2006) 1–12

The Changing Indications of Gastrointestinal Decontamination in Poisonings

Kennon Heard, MD[a,b,c,*]

[a]Division of Emergency Medicine, University of Colorado School of Medicine,
Denver, CO, USA
[b]Medical Toxicology, University of Colorado School of Medicine, Denver, CO, USA
[c]Rocky Mountain Poison and Drug Center, Denver, CO, USA

Gastrointestinal (GI) decontamination is the therapy that is most commonly administered to patients who have had acute oral exposure to poisons. These techniques were used in almost 200,000 poisoning cases reported to North American Poison Centers in 2001 [1]. The theory behind GI decontamination is simple: poisons that are not absorbed into the blood cannot cause systemic toxicity. This principle has been recognized since the fifth century BC [2]; hence decontamination has become accepted without rigorous scientific data. Over the past several years, as practitioners demand quality data to guide treatment decisions, we have observed a deconstruction of "standard" poisoning management. The purpose of this article is to describe the commonly used techniques of decontamination, review the literature that describes their efficacy, and, finally, provide summary recommendations for the use of GI decontamination in the treatment of poisoned patients.

Emesis

Syrup of ipecac is currently available in many countries as a non-prescription product. It is prepared from the *Cephaelis* plant, which contains the alkaloids emetine and cephaeline. These alkaloids are potent emetics,

Portions of this article were previously published in Holstege CP, Rusyniak DE: Medical Toxicology. 89:6, Med Clin North Am, 2005; with permission.

Dr. Heard is supported by a Jahnigen Career Scholars Award from the American Geriatric Society and the Hartford Foundation.

* Division of Emergency Medicine, University of Colorado School of Medicine, 4200 East 9th Avenue, B215, Denver, CO 80262.

E-mail address: kennon.heard@uchsc.edu

inducing vomiting by both direct local GI effects and central nervous system actions. Syrup of ipecac is administered at a dose of 30 mL followed by 240 mL of water. Emesis following syrup of ipecac ingestion typically occurs within 20 minutes and persists for 30 to 120 minutes [3].

The use of syrup of ipecac in the management of poisoned patients has declined [1]. A recent position paper lists several studies that describe the efficacy of ipecac-induced vomiting in reducing systemic absorption of many drugs [3]. This effect is highly time dependent and is unlikely to be clinically relevant beyond 30 minutes post-ingestion. One study of adult patients that compared ipecac-induced vomiting to ipecac plus activated charcoal (AC) reported a longer emergency department (ED) stay and more complications in the ipecac-treated group. Outcomes (admission rate and ICU admission) were not different between the groups [4]. In this study, aspiration pneumonitis occurred in 3 of 93 patients who received ipecac and none of 107 patients treated with AC alone.

Two additional studies have compared ipecac plus AC to ipecac alone as one arm of a study to evaluate gastric emptying [5,6]. Both studies assigned asymptomatic patients to either an AC group or an ipecac-induced vomiting group followed by AC group using an alternate-day protocol. Neither study reported any advantage of ipecac therapy over AC alone. One study patient became obtunded after receiving ipecac. This patient vomited and went on to develop an aspiration pneumonitis.

In summary, no studies demonstrate that the use of ipecac in the treatment of acute poisoning changes clinical outcome. Several studies have shown that ipecac use may result in complications and prolonged ED course. The US Food and Drug Administration has considered removing ipecac from over-the-counter status, and the American Academy of Pediatrics no longer recommends home stocking of ipecac [7]. These positions reflect an established movement to eliminate ipecac as an acceptable therapy, and this author believes that ipecac has no role in the routine management of acutely poisoned patients.

Gastric lavage

Reports of the use of gastric lavage (GL) in the poisoned patient date as far back as the early nineteenth century. GL is not the same as nasogastric aspiration. GL is performed by placing a large-bore (36–40 French) orogastric tube and instilling, then removing several liters of water to wash out stomach contents [8]. In contrast, for gastric aspiration, a smaller nasogastric tube is placed and gastric contents are aspirated without instilling any water. Nasogastric aspiration may be effective in cases of liquid poison ingestion [9], but it is not adequate for ingestion of pills.

In order for GL to be performed, patients must be able to maintain their airways or be intubated. Additionally, lavage should not be performed on patients who have ingested medications that may cause seizures or abrupt central nervous system deterioration unless the patient has been intubated. Patients should be on a cardiac monitor and pulse oximetry. Emergent airway equipment and suction should be immediately available. Before one inserts the tube, it should be used to estimate the distance from the lips to the epigastrium. The patient is placed in the left-lateral decubitus position, the tube is placed in the mouth, and the patient is asked to swallow. The tube is then gently advanced until the estimated length from lips to epigastrium has been inserted. The patient should then be asked to phonate to assure that the tube has not been placed in the trachea. At this point, 200 to 300 mL aliquots of warm saline or tap water are instilled in the tube and allowed to drain by gravity. The endpoint of GL is poorly defined. Most recommend that the procedure be continued as long as pill fragments are observed in the drainage. However, there is no clear definition of when to end the procedure if pill fragments are not observed [8].

A recent position statement concisely summarizes several volunteer studies demonstrating that significant amounts of poison may be removed from the stomach [8]. As with vomiting, the effect is clearly time dependent, and little effect is expected when treatment is delayed beyond 60 minutes. One study using radiographic markers suggested that GL may actually propel gastric contents past the pylorus, moving the poison into the small intestine, where most of the drug will be absorbed [10].

Although the preclinical studies show that GL may decrease drug absorption, three clinical trials have failed to demonstrate improved outcomes when GL is added to AC for the management of undifferentiated symptomatic poisoning patients. Two of these studies used a similar design [5,6]. Symptomatic patients who presented with a history of self-poisoning were assigned on an alternating-day basis to either AC by nasogastric tube or GL followed by AC. The main outcome was the proportion of patients in each group who deteriorated following the treatment.

The similar design and outcome of these study arms permit some general criticisms. First, the use of undifferentiated poisoned patients results in a low power to detect a difference between groups. It is possible that some subgroups would benefit from gastric emptying, even though the overall results of the study were negative. Second, the use of alternate-day assignment results in nonblinded treatment allocation. This process could lead to selection bias, and therefore the two treatment groups would have dissimilar baseline characteristics. Third, the outcome in these studies was highly subjective, and no measure of reliability is provided for any measure. This limitation is further exacerbated by the unblinded assessment of outcome. However, the main limitation to this analysis is the interpretation of the outcomes. Although the proportions of clinical manifestations that resulted in patients being classified as "symptomatic" are not reported, it is likely that most of the patients in this group were classified as "symptomatic" because they had decreased levels of consciousness. The act of GL would certainly be expected to result in an increase in "alertness" more than would the administration of AC. Although this "improvement" is attributable to the treatment, it is unlikely to have been of any clinical significance.

The specific results for these two studies were similar. Kulig and colleagues [5] reported that 22% of patients assigned to GL deteriorated, compared with 27% treated with AC alone. Pond and colleagues [6] reported that 7% of patients assigned to lavage deteriorated, compared with 13% in the AC-alone group. Kulig also performed a post-hoc subanalysis on patients who presented within 60 minutes of ingestion. This analysis found that more patients treated with GL within 60 minutes of ingestion improved when compared with those treated with AC alone. However, the authors relied on a χ^2 analysis rather than a Fischer's exact test (the appropriate test given the results). Applying the more appropriate statistical test results in a non-significant outcome. Because Kulig had identified this potentially important subgroup, Pond and colleagues included a planned subanalysis of patients presenting within 1 hour in their study design. Pond's study also reported a statistically significant difference between the treatment groups (this time using the appropriate statistical analysis). The authors attributed this effect to a baseline difference between the treatment groups in severity of symptoms. They then performed a stratified analysis and suggested that, after adjustment for severity, the beneficial effect of GL is not significant. However, the authors of neither paper discuss a more striking limitation. Patients assessed on days when the protocol resulted in an emptying procedure were statistically less likely to be classified as alert than patients assessed on days when the protocol called for AC alone (RR 0.87 for Kulig and 0.79 for Pond; $P < .01$ for both studies). Given that the assessors were not blinded to treatment assignment, this finding demonstrates selection bias. Such bias would result in patients with milder symptoms being assigned to receive GL and could dilute any treatment effect.

Merigian and colleagues [11] performed the third major study of gastric emptying. This study used a similar treatment protocol to those of Pond and Kulig. However, the authors' outcomes in this study were proportions of patients (1) admitted to the hospital, (2) requiring intubation, and (3) admitted to the ICU. They also compared the rates of aspiration pneumonia. This study found that patients who received gastric emptying (the authors did not analyze ipecac and GL separately) had a similar rate of hospital admission to those who received AC alone (58% in both groups). However, patients who received gastric emptying were more likely to be admitted to the ICU (74/163 versus 40/194) and more likely to be intubated (55% versus 14%) than patients assigned to the AC-alone group. Because the baseline vital signs and mental status scores for these groups were similar, the increased rate of intubation (and subsequent ICU admission) probably reflects aggressive airway management before GL that was not thought to be required when AC was administered without lavage.

Although the three studies just described evaluated GL for the treatment of undifferentiated poisoning, one smaller study has evaluated the role of lavage for treatment of a tricyclic antidepressant (TCA) poisoning. This method overcomes some limitations of the larger studies, because it evaluates a more homogeneous group and because TCA poisoning often produces life-threatening effects. This study compared (1) AC alone with (2) AC plus GL and (3) AC followed by GL, followed by AC. Its basis was the theory that GL could push pills past the pylorus and that prelavage administration of AC could adsorb this poison before systemic absorption. This study found no difference between the three groups in length of hospitalization, ICU stay, intubation, or duration of tachycardia. The small study size resulted in little statistical power. However, the data do not even suggest a trend toward decreased incidence of cardiac or neurologic effects in either GL group.

Complications associated with GL include GI tract perforation, hypoxia, and aspiration. GI tract perforation is a catastrophic but uncommon complication of GL. Although the exact incidence is unknown, one case of esophageal perforation was reported in the 363 patients who received GL in the three major trials discussed here [5,6,11]. Arterial oxygen tension dropped 17% during GL in one prospective study [12]. Although the clinical implications of this phenomenon are unclear, two patients in this series developed transient ST segment elevation during the GL procedure.

Aspiration is a common complication for all poisoning patients. Identifying the marginal risk associated with GL is difficult. In the largest study of gastric emptying, 5% of patients were thought to have aspirated *before* the gastric emptying procedure [6]. However, it is logical to believe that placement of a large-bore tube might impair airway protection and increase the risk for aspiration. Merigian and colleagues [11] reported that patients assigned to gastric emptying were more likely to develop aspiration pneumonia than patients treated without gastric emptying. Interestingly, all the patients who developed aspiration were intubated, and half of them "had an uncomplicated orotracheal intubation" before GL, suggesting that the aspiration occurred despite adequate airway management.

In summary, these studies report no benefit when GL is added to AC in the management of undifferentiated acute poisoning patients. Less conclusive data show no clear effect in TCA poisoning. Despite their many limitations, the studies suggest that this procedure may increase the risk of ICU admission, and the incidence of complications was higher for GL patients than for patients managed without GL in all studies.

Activated charcoal

The theory behind the use of AC is that poisons dissolved in the intestine will be adsorbed to the charcoal particles; hence the poison will remain in the gut rather than moving into the bloodstream. Several common poisons are not well adsorbed by charcoal. Most notable among these are the toxic alcohols, iron, lithium, and most other metals. However, the vast majority of medications are well bound by charcoal.

Charcoal binding is a saturable process. Ideally, the dose of charcoal should provide a large excess of binding to capture as much of the poison as possible. In reality, the dose of charcoal administered tends to be determined by the size of the bottle stocked by the pharmacy. Few studies have been performed to attempt to determine the dose of charcoal. One human study found the optimum ratio of charcoal to drug to be 10:1 (weight:weight) for para-aminosalicylate [13]. Obviously, this study is limited, because it was a volunteer study using only one drug. Current consensus recommendations are that adult overdose patients receive 25 to 100 g [14].

The efficacy of charcoal is time dependent [14,15]. Therefore, charcoal should be administered as soon as possible after the ingestion. A recent consensus statement suggests that charcoal should be administered within 60 minutes of ingestion [16]. One study demonstrated that charcoal decreased acetaminophen absorption by 22% when given 2 hours after the ingestion [17]. The effect may be even greater for sustained-release products [16] or in the setting of anticholinergic effects [18]. Although these are only volunteer studies, they suggest that charcoal may be effective for selected poisoning patients beyond the 60-minute window.

Superactivated charcoal

The property of AC to adsorb a poison is related to the surface area of the charcoal particles. Superactivated charcoal products with increased surface area have been available for more than 20 years. These products decreased systemic medication absorption when compared with standard AC in two volunteer studies [19,20]. They are also considered to be more palatable than standard charcoal products. However, no study has demonstrated a clinical benefit for these products.

Clinical efficacy of activated charcoal

Three of the four major studies described earlier compared gastric emptying plus AC to AC alone in all patients [4–6]. However, the fourth study evaluated AC versus supportive care alone in asymptomatic patients [11]. In this study, 231 patients were assigned to observation and 220 were assigned to AC. The patients were observed in the ED for a minimum of 4 hours and then for an additional 4 hours during the psychiatric evaluation. No patient in either group deteriorated, suggesting that AC provided no benefit in the management of asymptomatic poisoning patients.

Recently, a large study was published comparing AC with supportive care for symptomatic and asymptomatic overdose patients [21]. This study is described as a randomized controlled trial (RCT) where 1479 patients were assigned on an alternating-day basis to either AC or supportive care. The patients were observed for a minimum of 4 hours in the ED, and the major outcomes were the proportion of patients who deteriorated, the number of patients admitted to the hospital or ICU, and the length of stay. The study used predetermined criteria for deterioration. No difference was found in the proportion of patients deteriorating or requiring admission to either the hospital or ICU. The mean ED stay was approximately 1 hour shorter for patients treated without AC, and there was no difference in the length of stay for admitted patients. Although the results of this study are intriguing, some limitations must be recognized. The "randomization" resulted in 399 patients receiving charcoal, whereas 1080 patients were treated with supportive care. The authors do not directly discuss the reason for this imbalance, but their description suggests that, rather than an intent-to-treat analysis, the authors performed a treatment-received analysis. This type of experiment design is subject to bias, because "less sick" patients could be allowed to forgo charcoal, whereas "more sick" patients would receive charcoal. Still, this study reported that no patients deteriorated in a large cohort (1080) of poisoning patients treated with only supportive care.

One additional RCT that has only been reported in abstract form also found that AC offers no benefit over supportive care. This study has limited numbers and is ongoing. Preliminary results suggest that the patients who were given AC had a trend toward longer ED stay and no change in mortality [22].

Several studies have also evaluated charcoal for specific poisonings. Crome and colleagues [23] reported a study of 48 patients with TCA ingestion who were treated with either AC or supportive care. This study found no difference in the duration of coma or drug levels between the two groups. However, its power was severely limited by the sample size. A carefully designed retrospective study of patients evaluated for acetaminophen ingestion reported that administration of AC to patients who ingested more than 10 g and presented within 24 hours was associated with a 64% decrease in the risk for having a toxic acetaminophen level [24]. This effect was largest in patients receiving charcoal within 2 hours of ingestion and diminished markedly after 2 hours. This finding is consistent with the expected course of acetaminophen absorption, suggesting a true effect. Although these data are based only on observation rather than on experimental results, they strongly suggest that AC may decrease the need for antidotal therapy in the setting of acetaminophen overdose.

The major complications of AC are vomiting, intestinal obstruction, and aspiration. Prospective studies have reported the prevalence of vomiting for untreated overdose patients at approximately 10% [21], whereas the prevalence in patients treated with AC is approximately 25% [6,11]. Another study has reported that the incidence of vomiting is similar between AC-treated patients and patients treated only with supportive care [22]. Given the high prevalence of vomiting, some have advocated pretreatment with antiemetics when AC is administered. Intestinal obstruction is a theoretic concern, but it has been reported when multiple-dose AC is used to enhance elimination of drugs, rather than when single doses are used for decontamination [25].

The most serious complication is aspiration. One animal model of AC aspiration demonstrated increased microvascular permeability, a fall in systemic oxygenation, and development of a metabolic acidosis [26]. This study did not show a dramatic increase in lung inflammation, and the charcoal was primarily deposited in the small airways. The authors suggest that the injury due to charcoal may have been caused by subsequent barotrauma from overdistention of the airways due to charcoal plugging. However, in practice, AC aspiration is only rarely unaccompanied by aspiration of gastric contents, so the clinical meaning of this model is limited.

Numerous reports exist of acute lung injury following aspiration of AC. In a recent review, Seger [25] discussed seven cases where charcoal aspiration was implicated as at least a contributing factor in a patient's death. This report included four additional cases where charcoal was implicated as a contributing factor in a life-threatening pulmonary complication and three cases where charcoal was instilled directly into the lung following unrecognized placement of an nasogastric (NG) tube into the trachea. A retrospective study of 50 intubated overdose patients who received charcoal reported a 2% incidence of radiographically proven aspiration pneumonia. Three additional patients in this study were treated for aspiration pneumonia despite normal chest radiographs. The only death reported in the study was unrelated to aspiration [27]. Another retrospective study of 257 patients reported a 28% incidence of aspiration. This study reported that early intubation was protective, and administration of GL and AC to nonintubated patients was associated with an increased risk for aspiration [28].

No treatment for charcoal aspiration has been used routinely. Patients are usually treated with antibiotics for aspiration pneumonia. Patients with charcoal in their sputum are treated with additional pulmonary toilet; bronchial lavage has been used to clear the airways of charcoal deposits [29].

In summary, AC limits the systemic absorption of many drugs in a time-dependent manner and may decrease the need for antidotal therapy for patients who present within 2 hours of acetaminophen ingestion. However, AC has not been shown to improve the outcomes of nonselected poisoning patients. Although serious side effects are uncommon, charcoal does appear to increase the number of patients who vomit, and rare cases of life-threatening aspiration have been reported.

Other binding agents

Two recent studies evaluated the use of magnesium hydroxide to limit the bioavailability of iron [30,31]. Both studies used subtoxic doses of iron and a 5:1 ratio of magnesium hydroxide to elemental iron. The first study administered the antidote 60 minutes after a 5 mg/kg iron dose and used a cross-over design. This study reported that magnesium hydroxide decreased the 12-hour area under the curve for serum iron concentrations by approximately 45% [30]. The second was a randomized, two-arm study.

The magnesium hydroxide was given 30 minutes after a 10 mg/kg iron dose. This study did not report a significant reduction in iron levels, although the mean peak iron level was approximately 10% lower in the treatment group [31]. The authors note that, to achieve a 5:1 ratio of magnesium hydroxide in a 60-kg adult taking 60 mg/kg of elemental iron, a dose of 225 mL of milk of magnesia would be required. This amount is similar to the volume of fluid given when a patient takes 50 g of AC.

Sodium polystyrene sulfate (SPS) is a resin that is most commonly used to treat hyperkalemia. However, SPS also effectively binds lithium. Two volunteer studies have shown that SPS administration decreases the bioavailability of lithium in subtoxic doses [32,33]. Although this technique may be of some use in selected cases, most isolated acute lithium ingestions do well with hydration alone. The increased use of sustained-release lithium products also limits the generalizability of these results in clinical practice. Cholestyramine, a steroid-binding resin, has been used to adsorb digoxin [34], and Fuller's earth has been used to bind paraquat [35]. However, the limited availability of these therapies would likely result in a delay in treatment and negate any clinical benefit over the readily available charcoal.

Whole bowel irrigation

Whole bowel irrigation (WBI) is an extension of the use of cathartics to decrease systemic availability of toxins. The use of cathartics decreases time in the GI tract, theoretically decreasing the time for the poison to be systemically absorbed [36]. The development of isotonic polyethylene glycol (PEG) solutions allows the use of cathartics without the concern of causing fluid or electrolyte alterations [37].

Effective WBI requires the administration of large volumes of PEG. The dosage used in bowel preparation is 2 to 4 L over 12 to 24 hours. The recommended dosage for WBI is 1.5 to 2 L/h. This dose is best administered through a 12-Fr feeding tube. To prevent aspiration, the patient should have the head of the bed elevated to at least 45°. If emesis occurs, the infusion should be discontinued for 30 minutes and restarted at half the previous rate. The rate is then increased as tolerated. Metoclopramide has been advocated as an antiemetic, because it increases GI motility. Patients who are awake should be provided with a bedside commode once the solution begins to pass [38].

Current recommendations are that the PEG be administered until the rectal effluent is clear. However, this endpoint probably does not completely clear the bowel of pill fragments. One study that evaluated the effect of WBI on the evacuation of coffee beans from the bowel found that, at the time of clear rectal effluent, an average of only 2.3 of 10 markers were recovered in the stool [39]. Another study found that WBI (until clear effluent) resulted in more radio-opaque markers moving into the colon at 24 hours than did standard treatment [40]. Although the clinical implications of these studies are unclear, they demonstrate that WBI until clear rectal effluent is not likely to remove all pills from the GI tract.

Volunteer studies have shown that WBI may lower the bioavailability of lithium and ampicillin [41,42]. Although these studies suggest that this treatment may be valuable, volunteer studies use much lower doses of medications, and initiation of WBI is not always clinically feasible in the timeframe they use. No controlled evaluations of WBI for poisoning patients exist. Case reports suggest that it may be useful in the treatment of iron ingestion and sustained-release verapamil ingestion and in the treatment of body packers [43–45].

The common complications of WBI are bloating, cramping, and vomiting. As with charcoal, the main concern is aspiration. No reports exist of aspiration complicating WBI; pulmonary edema and respiratory failure have been reported as complications during bowel preparation [46].

WBI is difficult to perform effectively under most circumstances, and its clinical efficacy is unproved. A recent position paper states that WBI may be considered for ingestion of sustained-release drugs and for iron and lithium poisoning [38]. This option appears best suited for cases where there is evidence of prolonged absorption of the drug (ie, the serum levels continue to rise several hours into the ingestion or there is radiographic evidence of unabsorbed drug in the GI tract).

Summary

Overall, no conclusive data support the use of gastric decontamination in the routine management of the poisoned patient. Studies of asymptomatic patients suggest that no treatment is required, and, given the complications that have been reported, this may be a reasonable approach to most patients. Even in symptomatic patients, the only demonstrable benefit was found in a post-hoc subgroup analysis and involved an outcome of questionable clinical importance.

Given these data, it would be easy to conclude that GI decontamination has no role in the management of the poisoned patient. This conclusion is valid when considering poisoned patients as a group, but all poisoned patients are not the same. Patients with trivial ingestion do well without treatment, and their greatest risk is an iatrogenic complication. Even patients with more serious ingestions usually have good outcomes with supportive care alone. It is no longer sufficient to justify GL or forced administration of AC with the supposition that "the patient could have taken something bad." However, there are some overdoses where limiting the systemic absorption of the poison may limit the toxic effects and prevent serious toxicity. After careful consideration of the risks, GI decontamination should be targeted at patients who, in the opinion of the treating physician, have a potentially life-threatening exposure.

References

[1] Watson WA, Litovitz TL, Klein-Schwartz W, et al. 2003 annual report of the American Association of Poison Control Centers Toxic Exposure Surveillance System. Am J Emerg Med 2004;22:335–404.

[2] Wax P. Historical principles and perspectives. In: Goldfrank LS, Flomenbaum NE, Lewin NA, et al, editors. Goldfrank's toxicologic emergencies. New York: McGraw-Hill; 2003. p. 1–22.

[3] Anonymous. Position paper: ipecac syrup. J Toxicol Clin Toxicol 2004;42:133–43.

[4] Albertson TE, Derlet RW, Foulke GE, et al. Superiority of activated charcoal alone compared with ipecac and activated charcoal in the treatment of acute toxic ingestions. Ann Emerg Med 1989;18:56–9.

[5] Kulig K, Bar-Or D, Cantrill SV, et al. Management of acutely poisoned patients without gastric emptying. Ann Emerg Med 1985;14:562–7.

[6] Pond SM, Lewis-Driver DJ, Williams GM, et al. Gastric emptying in acute overdose: a prospective randomised trial. Med J Aust 1995;163:345–9.

[7] Anonymous. Poison treatment in the home. American Academy of Pediatrics Committee on Injury, Violence, and Poison Prevention. Pediatrics 2003;112:1182–5.

[8] Vale JA. Position statement: gastric lavage. American Academy of Clinical Toxicology; European Association of Poisons Centres and Clinical Toxicologists. J Toxicol Clin Toxicol 1997;35:711–9.

[9] Grierson R, Green R, Sitar DS, et al. Gastric lavage for liquid poisons. Ann Emerg Med 2000;35:435–9.

[10] Saetta JP, March S, Gaunt ME, et al. Gastric emptying procedures in the self-poisoned patient: are we forcing contents beyond the pylorus? J R Soc Med 1991;84:274–6.

[11] Merigian KS, Woodard M, Hedges JR, et al. Prospective evaluation of gastric emptying in the self-poisoned patient. Am J Emerg Med 1990;8:479–83.

[12] Thompson AM, Robins JB, Prescott LF. Changes in cardiorespiratory function during gastric lavage for drug overdose. Hum Toxicol 1987;6:215–8.

[13] Olkkola KT. Effect of charcoal–drug ratio on antidotal therapy efficacy of oral activated charcoal in man. Br J Clin Pharmacol 1985;19(6):767–73.

[14] Chyka PA, Seger D. Position statement: single-dose activated charcoal. American Academy of Clinical Toxicology; European Association of Poisons Centres and Clinical Toxicologists. J Toxicol Clin Toxicol 1997;35:721–41.

[15] Green R, Grierson R, Sitar DS, et al. How long after drug ingestion is activated charcoal still effective? J Toxicol Clin Toxicol 2001;39:601–5.

[16] Laine K, Kivisto KT, Neuvonen PJ. Effect of delayed administration of activated charcoal on the absorption of conventional and slow-release verapamil. J Toxicol Clin Toxicol 1997; 35:263–8.

[17] Yeates PJ, Thomas SH. Effectiveness of delayed activated charcoal administration in simulated paracetamol (acetaminophen) overdose. Br J Clin Pharmacol 2000;49:11–4.

[18] Green R, Sitar DS, Tenenbein M. Effect of anticholinergic drugs on the efficacy of activated charcoal. J Toxicol Clin Toxicol 2004;42:267–72.

[19] Roberts JR, Gracely EJ, Schoffstall JM. Advantage of high-surface-area charcoal for gastrointestinal decontamination in a human acetaminophen ingestion model. Acad Emerg Med 1997;4:167–74.

[20] Krenzelok EP, Heller MB. Effectiveness of commercially available aqueous activated charcoal products. Ann Emerg Med 1987;16:1340–3.

[21] Merigian KS, Blaho KE. Single-dose oral activated charcoal in the treatment of the self-poisoned patient: a prospective, randomized, controlled trial. Am J Ther 2002;9:301–8.

[22] Cooper GM, Le Couteur DG, Richardson D, et al. A randomised controlled trial of activated charcoal for the routine management of oral drug overdose [abstract]. J Toxicol Clin Toxicol 2002;40:313.

[23] Crome P, Adams R, Ali C, et al. Activated charcoal in tricyclic antidepressant poisoning: pilot controlled clinical trial. Hum Toxicol 1983;2:205–9.

[24] Buckley NA, Whyte IM, O'Connell DL, et al. Activated charcoal reduces the need for N-acetylcysteinetreatment after acetaminophen (paracetamol) overdose. J Toxicol Clin Toxicol 1999;37:753–7.

[25] Seger D. Single-dose activated charcoal—back up and reassess. J Toxicol Clin Toxicol 2004; 42:101–10.

[26] Arnold TC, Willis BH, Xiao F, et al. Aspiration of activated charcoal elicits an increase in lung microvascular permeability. J Toxicol Clin Toxicol 1999;37:9–16.

[27] Moll J, Kerns W II, Tomaszewski C, et al. Incidence of aspiration pneumonia in intubated patients receiving activated charcoal. J Emerg Med 1999;17:279–83.

[28] Liisanantti J, Kaukoranta P, Martikainen M, et al. Aspiration pneumonia following severe self-poisoning. Resuscitation 2003;56:49–53.

[29] Pollack MM, Dunbar BS, Holbrook PR, et al. Aspiration of activated charcoal and gastric contents. Ann Emerg Med 1981;10:528–9.

[30] Wallace KL, Curry SC, LoVecchio F, et al. Effect of magnesium hydroxide in iron absoption following simulated mild overdose in human subjects. Acad Emerg Med 1998;5:961–5.

[31] Snyder BK, Clark RF. Effect of magnesium hydroxide administration on iron absorption after a supratherapeutic dose of ferrous sulfate in human volunteers: a randomized controlled trial. Ann Emerg Med 1999;33:400–5.

[32] Belanger DR, Tierney MG, Dickinson G. Effect of sodium polystyrene sulfonate on lithium bioavailability. Ann Emerg Med 1992;21:1312–5.

[33] Tomaszewski C, Musso C, Pearson JR, et al. Lithium absorption prevented by sodium polystyrene sulfonate in volunteers. Ann Emerg Med 1992;21:1308–11.

[34] Henderson RP, Solomon CP. Use of cholestyramine in the treatment of digoxin intoxication. Arch Intern Med 1988;148:745–6.

[35] Idid SZ, Lee CY. Effects of Fuller's Earth and activated charcoal on oral absorption of paraquat in rabbits. Clin Exp Pharmacol Physiol 1996;23:679–81.

[36] Barceloux D, McGuigan M, Hartigan-Go K. Position statement: cathartics. American Academy of Clinical Toxicology; European Association of Poisons Centres and Clinical Toxicologists. J Toxicol Clin Toxicol 1997;35:743–52.

[37] Ambrose NS, Johnson M, Burdon DW, et al. A physiological appraisal of polyethylene glycol and a balanced electrolyte solution as bowel preparation. Br J Surg 1983;70:428–30.

[38] Anonymous. Position paper: whole bowel irrigation. J Toxicol Clin Toxicol 2004;42:844–54.

[39] Scharman EJ, Lembersky R, Krenzelok EP. Efficiency of whole bowel irrigation with and without metoclopramide pretreatment. Am J Emerg Med 1994;12:302–5.

[40] Ly BT, Schneir AB, Clark RF. Effect of whole bowel irrigation on the pharmacokinetics of an acetaminophen formulation and progression of radio-opaque markers through the gastrointestinal tract. Ann Emerg Med 2004;43:189–95.

[41] Smith SW, Ling LJ, Halstenson CE. Whole-bowel irrigation as a treatment for acute lithium overdose. Ann Emerg Med 1991;20:536–9.

[42] Tenenbein M, Cohen S, Sitar DS. Whole bowel irrigation as a decontamination procedure after acute drug overdose. Arch Intern Med 1987;147:905–7.

[43] Tenenbein M. Whole bowel irrigation as a gastrointestinal decontamination procedure after acute poisoning. Med Toxicol 1988;3:77–84.

[44] Buckley N, Dawson AH, Howarth D, et al. Slow-release verapimil poisoning. Use of polyethylene glycol whole-bowel lavage and high-dose calcium. Med J Aust 1993;158:202–4.

[45] Hoffman RS, Smilkstein MJ, Goldfrank LR. Whole bowel irrigation and the cocaine body packer: a new approach to a common problem. Am J Emerg Med 1990;8:523–7.

[46] Marschall HU, Bartels F. Life-threatening complications of nasogastric administration of polyethylene glycol-electrolyte solutions (Golytely) for bowel cleansing. Gastrointest Endosc 1998;47:408–10.

ELSEVIER
SAUNDERS

CLINICS IN
LABORATORY
MEDICINE

Clin Lab Med 26 (2006) 13–30

Utilizing the Laboratory in the Poisoned Patient

David L. Eldridge, MD, MA[a],
Christopher P. Holstege, MD[b],*

[a]Department of Pediatrics, Brody School of Medicine,
East Carolina University, Greenville, NC, USA
[b]Division of Medical Toxicology, Departments of Emergency Medicine and Pediatrics,
University of Virginia, Charlottesville, VA, USA

When evaluating an intoxicated patient, there is no substitute for a thorough history and physical examination. Numerous medical shows on television depict a universal *toxicology screen* that automatically determines the agent causing a patient's symptoms. Samples cannot be simply "sent to the lab," however, with the correct diagnosis to a clinical mystery returning on a computer printout. Clues from a patient's physical examination are generally more likely to be helpful than a "shotgun" laboratory approach that involves indiscriminate testing of blood or urine for multiple agents.

When used appropriately, diagnostic tests may be helpful in the management of an intoxicated patient. When a specific toxin or class of toxins is suspected, requesting qualitative or quantitative levels may be appropriate. The National Academy of Clinical Biochemistry published recommendations for the use of laboratory tests in the evaluation of poisoned patients [1]. Among their recommendations was a list of diagnostic serum tests described as necessary to support a hospital's emergency department (Box 1). This is an excellent list of diagnostic studies that are generally widely available for application in the emergency department.

In a suicidal patient, whose history is generally unreliable, or in an unresponsive patient, for whom no history is available, the clinician may gain further clues as to the cause of a poisoning by responsible diagnostic

Portions of this article were previously published in Holstege CP, Rusyniak DE: Medical Toxicology. 89:6, Med Clin North Am, 2005; with permission.

* Corresponding author. University of Virginia Health System, PO Box 800774, Charlottesville, VA 22908-0774.

E-mail address: ch2xf@virginia.edu (C.P. Holstege).

Box 1. Stat quantitative serum toxicology assays to support an emergency department

Acetaminophen
Lithium
Salicylate
Co-oximetry (carboxyhemoglobin, methemoglobin)
Theophylline
Valproic acid
Carbamazepine
Digoxin
Phenobarbital
Iron
Ethanol
Methanol
Ethylene glycol

Data from Wu AH, McKay C, Broussard LA, et al. National Academy of Clinical Biochemistry Laboratory Medicine practice guidelines: recommendations for the use of laboratory tests to support poisoned patients who present to the emergency department. Clin Chem 2003;49:357–79.

---

testing. This article examines the role of common diagnostic tests in the evaluation of a poisoned patient.

Salicylates

Salicylates are readily available in numerous over-the-counter products. In any patient with history of salicylate ingestion or possessing characteristic signs or symptoms of salicylate poisoning, a serum salicylate level should be obtained. Early identification of salicylate toxicity can be life saving.

After acute salicylate overdose, patients may develop nausea, vomiting, abdominal pain, tinnitus, tachypnea, oliguria, and altered mental status ranging from lethargy to coma [2]. Chronic intoxication can manifest in a similar fashion as acute intoxication, but chronic intoxication typically is more insidious and often misdiagnosed [3]. In all overdoses, a thorough review of the patient's medications is vital.

Several medications have been documented to cause false-positive salicylate levels in commonly used salicylate assays. The most well documented of these is the nonsteroidal anti-inflammatory drug diflunisal (Dolobid) [4,5]. In toxic and therapeutic doses, the presence of diflunisal has caused false-positive serum salicylate levels [6–8]. Another possible important consideration in the interpretation of salicylate levels is the presence of hyperbilirubinemia. Hyperbilirubinemia in term and preterm infants may lead to positive serum salicylate levels in certain fluorescence assays [9].

Interpretation of salicylate levels as a guide for clinical management decisions can be difficult. Perhaps the most well-known attempt at using salicylate levels to predict the severity of salicylate toxicity was the nomogram developed by Done [10]. After examining the clinical symptoms and the salicylate levels in patients who had a single acute overdose, Done created a nomogram that predicted severity of poisoning based on the salicylate level drawn at a given time from ingestion. This tool, however well intentioned, had significant limitations. Because the original development of this nomogram was based on only 38 pediatric patients, its utility for acute adult overdoses is unknown. One of the assumptions allowing the creation of this nomogram was that salicylates are eliminated by first-order kinetics. It since has been well established that some of the pathways for the elimination of salicylates become saturated in overdose and follow zero order kinetics [11]. One study showed that there was significant disagreement between the clinical severity predicted by the nomogram and the severity judged by physicians [12]. The authors no longer recommend its use in the management of a salicylate-poisoned patient.

Using salicylate levels to guide management must be done cautiously and only in conjunction with careful evaluation of a patient's clinical status. One group of investigators examined 97 patients who experienced significant exposures to salicylate. In this study, patients who did not survive the ingestion and patients with reasonably high serum levels (≥ 70 mg/dL) were included [13]. Although toxic levels alone were of poor prognostic value, the investigators identified certain clinical findings that predicted a poor prognosis, including pulmonary edema, fever, coma, and acidosis.

The absorptive phase of salicylates can be unpredictable (either delayed or erratic) owing to bezoar formation, enteric-coated product, gastric outlet obstruction, and pylorospasm [3]. A level drawn soon after the original ingestion may not reflect the potential peak concentration. Initial serial levels should be performed every 2 hours while monitoring the patient clinically. When the levels begin to decline, and the patient's clinical status is improved, levels can be performed less frequently.

The units reported with each level should be documented before management decisions are made. Laboratories alternatively may report levels in terms of milligrams per deciliter and milligrams per liter. This is an important distinction that involves a 10-fold difference in concentration and is infamous for causing confusion. In the extreme cases of these miscommunications, hemodialysis has been ordered for patients thought to have astronomically high salicylate levels that are later proved to be nontoxic [14].

The need to screen all intentional overdose patients for salicylates also is debated. One case review of 737 toxicology screening tests in a year revealed only 31 positive for salicylates (4.2%) [15]. There was no mention in this study of clinical symptoms in any of the patients. Two studies by a group in

Hong Kong further examined the role of salicylate screenings in acutely poisoned patients. In a retrospective study by Chan and colleagues [16], charts were reviewed on 347 patients who had a salicylate level performed. In 264 of these patients (76%), there was no clinical suspicion of salicylate poisoning. Only 3 of the 264 patients (1%) had elevated serum salicylate levels. This study gave no specific details of the clinical presentation of these three patients, only that they did not have typical symptoms of salicylism. The authors concluded that routine screening was unnecessary and should be restricted to only patients truly suspected of having salicylate toxicity. In a follow-up study [17], the same group looked at the practice of serum salicylate screening at their institution after educating their colleagues to their previous study's findings. In this study, they reviewed the discharge summaries of all acutely poisoned patients in a 6-month period who had received a serum salicylate level (total 196 patients). In 88% (172 patients) of the cases, there was no clinical suspicion of salicylate toxicity; only 3 of these patients (1.7%) had an elevated level. None of the three patients had symptoms clearly indicating salicylate toxicity. Their conclusion was that "indiscriminate" measurements of plasma salicylate levels in acutely poisoned patients were unjustified. In the United States, investigators in San Francisco performed a retrospective 2-year chart review ($n = 1820$) to question the necessity of universal screening for salicylates in patients with suicidal ingestion or altered mental status [18]. The authors found 155 patients (8.5%) with detectable levels (> 1 mg/dL). Of these, 111 (6%) had histories negative for salicylate ingestion. Only three of these patients had a significant degree of toxicity. The three patients all presented with significant altered mental status and large anion gaps. These three patients represented only 0.16% of the 1820 patients of whom salicylate levels had been obtained. The authors concluded that universal screening for salicylate poisoning in this population was neither cost-effective nor indicated.

The diagnosis of salicylate poisoning based solely on clinical examination is not without pitfalls. Although large, acute ingestions usually can be detected through history and clinical symptoms, chronic salicylate toxicity can be more difficult to diagnose. Numerous cases have been reported pertaining to a delayed or mistaken diagnosis in the face of significant salicylate toxicity. In these cases, patients presented with nonspecific symptoms, such as fever, abdominal pain, and encephalopathy, and subsequently were misdiagnosed with surgical abdomen, myocardial infarction, sepsis, encephalitis, and alcoholic ketoacidosis [3,19–21]. One study revealed that a delayed diagnosis (at times 72 hours) of chronic salicylate poisoning is associated with higher morbidity and mortality rates compared with poisoning diagnosed on admission [22]. Another study looking at salicylate-related fatalities in Ontario revealed that symptoms and signs of salicylate poisoning apparently were missed even in patients who were alert on presentation [23]. The "classic" finding of ototoxicity was found by one group of investigators to be neither sensitive nor specific for serum salicylate concentration [24]. Characteristic laboratory findings also may not be reliable. Although a wide anion gap metabolic acidosis with respiratory alkalosis often is encountered in association with salicylate poisoning, one case series of 20 elderly patients with chronic salicylate poisoning revealed that 35% of these patients presented with a normal anion gap and P_{CO_2} [25]. In another study performed by Baer and colleagues [26], 52.8% of patients with history of acute salicylate toxicity and a serum bicarbonate > 20 mEq/L had salicylate levels > 30 mg/dL. Because products containing salicylates are readily available, clinical effects of salicylate toxicity are nonspecific, and a lack of metabolic acidosis does not rule out the potential for salicylate toxicity, clinicians should have a low threshold for obtaining serum salicylate levels.

Acetaminophen

An acetaminophen level drawn after a single, acute overdose is one of the few examples where a diagnostic laboratory result, by itself and independent of clinical findings, can be used to make treatment decisions. An area of some controversy is whether acetaminophen screening should be performed on all intentional overdose patients. One of the most worrisome aspects of acetaminophen poisoning is that initial clinical symptoms may be vague (eg, nausea, vomiting, abdominal pain) or even absent in the first 24 hours [27]. This possible delay in diagnosis is particularly problematic because the antidote, N-acetyl cysteine, has been shown to be most effective when initiated within the first 8 hours [28]. Ashbourne and colleagues [29] performed one of the first formal studies looking at the issue of universal acetaminophen screening. This prospective study examined acetaminophen levels in 486 patients with intentional drug ingestion. In this study population, only 7 of 486 patients (1.4%) had no history or clinical symptoms suggesting acetaminophen overdose and had a clinically significant acetaminophen level (> 10 mg/L within 8 hours of ingestion). Only one of these patients had a potentially hepatotoxic level. In their study group overall, Ashbourne and colleagues [29] found that about 1 in 70 patients with an intentional drug overdose who presented to their urban emergency department had an unrecognized acetaminophen overdose, and about 1 in 500 of these patients had a potentially hepatotoxic acetaminophen level. These authors further concluded that, even considering this relatively low yield, the low cost of serum acetaminophen levels might justify screening patients with a history of overdose, considering that acetaminophen has a vague clinical presentation and an effective antidote.

Chan and colleagues [30] sought to assess the value of acetaminophen screening by retrospectively examining the records of 294 patients admitted to their general wards for a variety of acute poisonings. Only 86 of these patients were truly suspected of ingesting acetaminophen, and 8 of them did have plasma levels that were toxic. The remaining 208 patients were screened for acetaminophen, but had no history of acetaminophen ingestion. In this group, 60 had no detectable level, and the remaining 148 had levels that were nontoxic. No potentially serious acetaminophen ingestion was missed by clinical suspicion alone. The authors concluded that a thorough history and physical examination were vital, and that routine plasma acetaminophen screening was not indicated.

Sporer and Khayam-Bashi [18] in San Francisco retrospectively looked at 1820 patients presenting to their emergency department with either altered mental status or suicidal ingestion. At their facility, it was protocol to obtain acetaminophen levels in all patients with this presentation. They found 175 patients (9.6%) with detectable serum acetaminophen levels > 1 µg/mL. Most of these patients ($n = 120$) had given a history of acetaminophen ingestion. Of the remaining patients ($n = 55$), only 5 (0.3%) had what was regarded by the investigators to be a "potentially toxic level" (levels > 50 µg/mL). Even with these relatively high levels, none of the patients required N-acetyl cysteine when their levels were compared with the Rumack-Matthew nomogram, and all did well. Still, the authors noted these cases missed by history alone. Considering even this relatively small number, Sporer and Khayam-Bashi [18] recommended screening all patients with suicidal ingestion and patients with altered mental status in whom ingestion was suspected.

Another retrospective study done by Dargan and colleagues [31] examined acetaminophen screening in 411 patients presenting to the emergency department with either a history of drug overdose ($n = 296$) or loss of consciousness ($n = 115$). In the overdose group, 136 patients denied acetaminophen ingestion. All 136 of these patients had negative acetaminophen levels. In the 115 patients who presented with a loss of consciousness, 4 (3.5%) later proved to have ingested acetaminophen. All four received N-acetyl cysteine and recovered. The authors concluded that universal screening of patients who denied acetaminophen use was of little value, but that, in patients who were found with loss of consciousness, there was potential for missing significant acetaminophen toxicity.

More recently, in the United Kingdom, Hartington and colleagues [32] attempted to validate a clinical decision rule consisting of risk factors to help select out which overdose patients needed serum acetaminophen screening. They used risk factors that had been identified as potentially predictive of such exposure from the literature. Briefly, if the overdose patient denied ingestion of acetaminophen or acetaminophen-containing compounds, had a Glasgow Coma Scale score of 15, understood English well, and had not ingested excessive alcohol, the patient would not need an acetaminophen level drawn. With these parameters, 307 consecutive patients were evaluated in the emergency department. Clinicians obtained levels regardless, but recorded the risk factors that applied. Only 46 of the patients examined with this clinical decision rule in mind would have been excluded from having an acetaminophen level drawn. Of the total patients studied, 155 denied acetaminophen ingestion and were followed through the entire study. Only 13 of these patients had detectable acetaminophen levels, and none required antidotal therapy. Seven of these 13 had normal Glasgow Coma Scale scores and would have been missed with the authors' clinical decision rule and with Dargan and colleagues's recommendations to check only in patients with altered mental status. A second part of the study was to test, through a questionnaire, the level of confidence physicians would require before they would use such an acetaminophen toxicity screening tool. Most physicians (83%) required a false-negative rate of 0.1% before considering using such a decision-making tool. Considering they were able to exclude only 46 of 307 patients with their clinical decision rule, Hartington and colleagues [32] estimated that the sample size of a potential study population would require more than 20,000 subjects to prove its clinical value conclusively. Considering numerous factors (no universal acetaminophen screening study possesses such statistical power, acetaminophen screen is inexpensive, and the potentially severe natural history of ingestion), the authors recommended to continue universal screening.

Osmol gap

The serum osmol gap is a common laboratory test that may be useful when evaluating poisoned patients. This test is discussed most often in the context of evaluating a patient suspected of toxic alcohol (eg, ethylene glycol, methanol, and isopropanol) intoxication. Although this test may have utility in such situations, it has many pitfalls and limitations that limit its effectiveness.

Osmotic concentrations are expressed in terms of osmolality (milliosmoles/kg of solvent [mOsm/kg]) and osmolarity (milliosmoles/liter of solution [mOsm/L]) [33,34]. This concentration can be measured by use of an osmometer, a tool that most often uses the technique of freezing point depression and is expressed in osmolality (Osm_M) [35]. A calculated serum osmolarity (Osm_C) may be obtained by numerous equations [36], involving the patient's glucose, sodium, and urea, which contribute to almost all of the normally measured osmolality [37]. One of the most commonly used of these calculations is as follows [38]:

$$Osm_C = 2[Na^+] + [BUN]/2.8 + [glucose]/18$$

The correction factors in the equation are based on the relative osmotic activity of the substance in question [33]. Assuming serum neutrality, sodium as the predominant serum cation is doubled to account for the corresponding anions. Finding the osmolarity contribution of any other osmotically active substance that is reported in mg/dL (eg, blood urea nitrogen [BUN] and glucose) is accomplished by dividing by one tenth its molecular weight in daltons [33]. For BUN, this conversion factor is 2.8, and for glucose it is 18. Similar conversion factors may be added to this equation in an attempt to account for ethanol and the various toxic alcohols as follows:

$$Osm_C = 2[Na^+] + [BUN]/2.8 + [glucose]/18 + [ethanol]/4.6$$
$$+ [methanol]/3.2 + [ethylene\ glycol]/6.2 + [isopropanol]/6$$

The difference between the measured (Osm_M) and calculated (Osm_C) is the osmol gap (OG) and depicted by the following equation [33]:

$$OG = Osm_M - Osm_C$$

One problem with this calculation is that the units are different because the measured form is in mOsm/kg, and the calculated form is in mOsm/L. This unit difference is generally not considered significant because human serum is a dilute aqueous solution with a specific gravity of 1.01, making these numbers roughly equivalent [35].

If a significant osmol gap is discovered, the difference in the two values may represent presence of foreign substances in the blood [35]. Possible causes of an elevated osmol gap are listed in Box 2. What constitutes a normal osmol gap is widely debated. Traditionally a normal gap has been defined as 10 mOsm/kg or less. The original source of this value is an article by Smithline and Gardner [39], which declared that this number was pure convention. Further clinical study has not shown this assumption to be correct. Glasser and colleagues [40] studied 56 healthy adults and reported that they found the normal osmol gap to range from -9 to $+5$ mOsm/kg H_2O. A study examining a pediatric emergency department population ($n = 192$) found a range from -13.5 to $+8.9$ [41]. Another study by Aabakken and colleagues [42] looked at the osmol gaps of 177 patients admitted to the emergency department and reported their range to be from -10 to $+20$ mOsm/kg H_2O. A vital point brought forth by the authors of this study is that the day-to-day coefficient of variance for their laboratory in regards to sodium was 1%. They believed this variance translated to a calculated analytical standard deviation of 9.1 mOsm in regards to osmol gap. This analytical variance alone may account for the variation found in patients' osmol gaps. Other researchers have voiced this concern that even small errors in the measurement of sodium can result in large variations of the osmol gap [41,43]. Overall, the clinician should recognize that there is likely a wide range of variability in a patient's baseline osmol gap.

There are several concerns in regard to using the osmol gap as a screening tool in the evaluation of the potentially toxic alcohol–poisoned patient. The lack of a well-established normal range is particularly problematic. A patient may present with an osmol gap of 9 mOsm—a value considered normal by the traditionally accepted normal maximum gap of 10 mOsm. If this patient had an osmol gap of -5 just before ingestion of a toxic alcohol,

Box 2. Possible causes of an elevated osmol gap

Toxic alcohols
  Ethanol
  Isopropanol
  Methanol
  Ethylene glycol
Drugs/additives
  Isoniazide
  Mannitol
  Propylene glycol
  Glycerol
  Osmotic contrast dyes
Other chemicals
  Ethyl ether
  Acetone
  Trichloroethane
Disease/illness
  Chronic renal failure
  Lactic acidosis
  Diabetic ketoacidosis
  Alcoholic ketoacidosis
  Hyperlipidemia
  Hyperproteinemia

Data from Refs. [33,34,40,63–66].

however, the patient's osmol gap would have to have been increased by 14 mOsm to reach the new gap of 9 mOsm. If this increase was due to ethylene glycol, it would correspond to a toxic level of 86.8 mg/dL [38]. In addition, if a patient's ingestion of a toxic alcohol occurred at a time distant from the actual blood sampling, the osmotically active parent compound will have been metabolized to the acidic metabolites. The subsequent metabolites have no osmotic activity of their own, and no osmol gap would be detected [36]. Steinhart [44] reported a patient with ethylene glycol toxicity who presented with an osmol gap of 7.2 mOsm owing to delay in presentation. Darchy and colleagues [43] presented two other cases of significant ethylene glycol toxicity with osmol gaps of 4 and 7. The lack of an abnormal osmol gap in these cases was speculated to be due to either metabolism of the parent alcohol or a low baseline osmol gap that masked the toxin's presence.

The osmol gap should be used with caution as an adjunct to clinical decision making and not as a primary determinant to rule out toxic alcohol ingestion. If the osmol gap obtained is particularly large, it suggests an agent or condition from Box 2 may be present. A "normal" osmol should be interpreted with caution; a negative study may not rule out the presence of such an ingestion—the test result must be interpreted within the context of the clinical presentation. If such a poisoning is suspected, appropriate therapy should be initiated presumptively (ie, ethanol infusion, 4-methyl-1H-pyrazole, hemodialysis) while confirmation from serum levels of the suspected toxin is pending.

Anion gap

Obtaining a basic metabolic panel in all poisoned patients is generally recommended. When a low serum bicarbonate is discovered on a metabolic panel, the clinician should determine if an elevated anion gap exists. The formula most commonly used for the anion gap calculation is the following [45]:

$$[Na^+] - [Cl^- + HCO_3]$$

This equation allows one to determine if serum electroneutrality is being maintained. The primary cation (sodium) and anions (chloride and bicarbonate) are represented in the equation [46]. There are other contributors to this equation that are "unmeasured" [47]. Other serum cations are not commonly included in this calculation because either their concentrations are relatively low (ie, potassium) or assigning a number to represent their respective contribution is difficult (ie, magnesium, calcium) [47]. Similarly, there are a multitude of other serum anions (ie, sulfate, phosphate, organic anions) that also are difficult to measure and quantify in an equation [46,47]. These "unmeasured" ions represent the anion gap calculated using the previous equation. The normal range for this anion gap is accepted to be 8 to 16 mEq/L [47], but some authors have suggested that owing to changes in the technique for measuring chloride, the range should be lowered to 6 to 14 mEq/L [46]. Practically speaking, an increase in the anion gap beyond an accepted normal range, accompanied by a metabolic acidosis, represents an increase in unmeasured endogenous (eg, lactate) or exogenous (eg, salicylates) anions [45]. A list of causes of this phenomenon is organized in the classic *MUDILES* mneumonic (Box 3). The "P" has been removed from the older acronym of *MUDPILES* because paraldehyde is no longer available.

It is imperative that clinicians who admit poisoned patients initially presenting with an increased anion gap metabolic acidosis investigate the etiology of that acidosis. Many symptomatic poisoned patients may have an initial mild metabolic acidosis on presentation as a result of the processes resulting in the elevation of serum lactate. With adequate supportive care, including hydration and oxygenation, the anion gap acidosis should

---

Box 3. Potential toxic causes of increased anion gap metabolic acidosis

Methanol
Uremia
Diabetic ketoacidosis
Iron, **I**nhalants (carbon monoxide, cyanide, hydrogen sulfide, toluene), **I**soniazid, **I**buprofen
Lactic acidosis
Ethylene glycol, **E**thanol ketoacidosis
Salicylates, **S**olvents (benzene, toluene), **S**tarvation ketoacidosis, **S**ympathomimetics (eg, amphetamines)

Data from Refs. [45,47,67].

---

improve. If, despite adequate supportive care, an anion gap metabolic acidosis worsens in a poisoned patient, the clinician should consider continued absorption of exogenous acids (ie, salicylate), formation of acidic metabolites (ie, ethylene glycol, methanol, toluene metabolites), or cellular ischemia with worsening lactic acidosis (ie, cyanide) as potential causes.

Bedside testing

A few simple, rapid bedside diagnostic tests have been suggested to aid in the confirmation of toxic ingestion. Favorable characteristics of the "perfect" test include the following points: inexpensive, readily available, and highly sensitive. The first two qualifications are easily obtained, but the last is not consistently present with some of these proposed tests.

Ferric chloride and Trinder spot test

Two bedside tests have been proposed for the rapid identification of a patient with salicylate toxicity. Both tests involve applying a few drops of a prepared reagent to a small sample of a patient's urine and watching for a characteristic color change. The first reagent is ferric chloride. Applying a few drops of a 10% solution of ferric chloride to 1 mL of urine containing even very small amounts of salicylate produces a characteristic purple color caused by the formation of an iron-salicylate complex [48]. This color change also occurs if the urine in question contains acetoacetic acid and phenylpyruvic acid [3]. The urine Trinder spot test uses a reagent composed of mercuric chloride, ferric nitrate, concentrated hydrochloric acid, and deionized water [49]. Applying 1 mL of this solution to 1 mL of urine with salicylates present also leads to a purple color change [3].

One study [50] examined the use of the ferric chloride test in 187 patients presenting to the emergency department. The urine of each of these patients was tested with ferric chloride, and a color change of purple or dark brown was considered positive. These ferric chloride tests subsequently were followed with serum salicylate levels. The sensitivity of the ferric chloride test was 93.2% for salicylate levels 3 mg/dL or greater and 93.8% for levels 30 mg/dL or greater. Specificity was 88.8% and 75.4%, respectively. There were three false-negative results, one of which did have a toxic salicylate level of 34 mg/dL. Another study used ferric chloride in an attempt to test unknown substances (tablets, liquids, and creams) for salicylate content [48]. The expected color change was seen consistently when the product in question contained salicylate and was missing when salicylate was not present. King and colleagues [49] evaluated the clinical utility of the Trinder reagent. The investigators enlisted 12 volunteers who ingested 975 mg of aspirin. Urine samples collected from these individuals at 2 and 4 hours after ingestion produced the characteristic purple color when added to Trinder reagent. The sensitivity of the test in this study was 100% with two false-positive results from controls.

Weiner and colleagues [51] examined the application of these two bedside tests in patients presenting to the emergency department with suspected drug overdose with or without unexplained metabolic acidosis. Both reagents were added to urine samples from all 180 patients enrolled, and confirmatory serum salicylate levels were drawn. Different from the previous studies, however, any darkening of color was regarded as a positive test. Twenty of these patients (11%) had salicylate levels 5 mg/dL or greater. Both tests were 100% sensitive for recognizing these patients. There were several false-positive results (44 with Trinder and 47 with ferric chloride), and the specificities for both tests were relatively low (Trinder 73% and ferric chloride 71%).

Overall, both of these tests could be used for rapid bedside testing. Each is relatively inexpensive, and, when interpretation of color change is performed as suggested by Weiner and colleagues [51], very sensitive. Positive tests indicate the possible presence of salicylate and not toxicity. Both tests should be followed with serum salicylate levels to confirm toxicity and quantitate the salicylate level.

Urine fluorescence

Serum ethylene glycol levels are not readily obtained at many hospitals. A good bedside screening test would be extremely useful in these cases to help prevent morbidity and mortality and avoid expensive (4-methylpyrazole) and labor-intensive (ethanol drip) interventions that are often performed presumptively until definitive diagnosis is possible. Automotive antifreeze is a major source of ethylene glycol exposure. Sodium fluorescein is added to the antifreeze to aid in identifying cooling system leaks. Some sources have suggested that fluorescein excreted in the urine of a patient who has ingested antifreeze would fluoresce with the aid of a Wood's lamp [52].

One of the first studies to look at the possibilities of this test was done by Winter and colleagues [53]. This study had six volunteers ingest the amount of sodium fluorescein found in 1 oz of antifreeze (an approximate ethylene glycol toxic dose). Urine samples were collected at 2-hour intervals for 10 hours. Controls also were obtained from the same volunteers. Samples obtained after fluorescein ingestion and controls were placed in glass nonfluorescent test tubes and examined, seven test tubes at a time, by three evaluators. Fluorescence was reliably identified 100% of the time in the samples collected in the first 2 hours after ingestion. This reliability decreased with time to 60% by 2 to 4 hours and 20% by 4 to 6 hours. Fluorescence was not detected after 6 hours. Controls were identified consistently as negative. As a second part of the study, another group of volunteers ingested fluorescein and had their urine collected during a 6-hour period. These samples were analyzed with a fluorometer. Fluorescence was detected by the fluorometer in all of these samples except the zero time point controls. By Wood's lamp, urine fluorescence could be identified reliably only within 2 hours after ingestion, however. The authors concluded that use of a Wood's lamp in this fashion could be a useful adjunctive test for ethylene glycol poisoning while waiting for serum levels.

Another research group later performed a similar, larger study that resulted in a different conclusion [52]. The volunteers ($n = 28$) provided control urine samples, ingested sodium fluorescein, and provided urine specimens at 1 to 2 and 4 to 6 hours after ingestion. Investigators evaluating the urine samples for fluorescence examined all the samples with a Wood's lamp in two different formats. First each sample was viewed singly in a random temporal sequence. After a break, the samples were presented again in groups of 27 to 30 at a time. With sequential presentation of urine for analysis, the mean sensitivity (35%), specificity (75%), and accuracy (48%) were poor. Grouped presentation of samples for comparison made little difference, and the sensitivity (42%), specificity (66%), and accuracy (50%) also were poor. These values were not significantly better if only the samples within the initial 2-hour period after ingestion (the ideal period reported by Winter and colleagues [53]) were considered. The authors of this study concluded that using this technique had limited diagnostic utility.

In another study, investigators collected convenience urine samples from an inpatient pediatric population (30 samples total) and from a group of healthy children (16 samples total) [54]. None of these children had a history of a suspected poisoning. All samples were examined by Wood's lamp. These samples were placed in containers and compared with a negative control (tap water in a similar container) and a positive control (fluorescein in tap water). Twenty-one of the 30 inpatient samples and 11 of the 16 healthy children's samples were reported as fluorescent by two of the three investigators. Considering this apparent baseline fluorescence, the authors gave serious challenge to using this technique to screen for ethylene glycol toxicity because their data suggested the false-positive rate would likely be high.

There seems to be little advantage to checking for urinary fluorescence by Wood's lamp in individuals suspected of ethylene glycol poisoning. Follow-up studies since the work done by Winter and colleagues [53] so far suggest that such a diagnostic approach lacks the clinical reliability necessary to guide management. The authors see no advantage to performing this proposed bedside test.

Urine drug screening

Many clinicians regularly obtain urine drug screening on altered patients or on patients suspected of ingestion. Such routine urine drug testing is of questionable benefit, however. Kellermann and colleagues [55] found little impact of urine drug screening on patient management in an urban emergency setting, and Mahoney and colleagues [56] similarly concluded that toxic screening added little to treatment or disposition of overdose patients in their emergency department. In a study of more than 200 overdose patients, Brett [57] showed that although unsuspected drugs were detected routinely, the results rarely led to changes in management and likely never affected outcome. In a similar large study of trauma patients, Bast and colleagues [58] noted that a positive drug screen had minimal impact on patient treatment.

Some authors argue in favor of routine testing. Fabbri and colleagues [59] argued that comprehensive screening may aid decisions on patient disposition, resulting in fewer admissions to the hospital and less demand on critical care units. The screen used in their retrospective study tested for more than 900 drugs, however, and is not available to most clinicians. Milzman and colleagues [60] argued in favor of screening trauma victims, stating that the prognosis of intoxicated patients is unduly poor secondary to low Glasgow Coma Scale scores, although patient treatment and disposition did not seem to be affected [60].

The effect of such routine screening in management changes is low because most of the therapy is supportive and directed at the clinical scenario (ie, mental status, cardiovascular function, respiratory condition). Interpretation of the results can be difficult even when the objective for ordering a comprehensive urine screen is adequately defined. Most assays rely on the antibody identification of drug metabolites; some drugs remain positive days after use and may not be related to the patient's current clinical picture. The positive identification of drug metabolites likewise is influenced by chronicity of ingestion, fat solubility, and coingestions. In one example, Perrone and colleagues [61] showed a cocaine retention time of 72 hours after its use. Conversely, many drugs of abuse are not detected on most urine drug screens, including gamma hydroxybutyrate, fentanyl, and ketamine.

Interpretation is confounded further by false-positive and false-negative results. George and Braithwaite [62] evaluated five popular rapid urine screening kits and found all lacked significant sensitivity and specificity. Additionally, cross-reactivity of prescription and over-the-counter medications used in therapeutic amounts for true illness may elicit positive screens. Codeine would give a positive opioid screen, which may be attributed incorrectly to morphine or heroin use.

The utility of ordering urine drug screens is fraught with significant testing limitations, including false-positive and false-negative results. Many authors have shown that the test results rarely affect management decisions. Routine drug screening of patients with altered mental status, abnormal vital signs, or suspected ingestion is not warranted and rarely guides patient treatment or disposition.

Summary

Numerous diagnostic tests may be useful to clinicians caring for poisoned patients. Clinicians should not order a broad range of tests indiscriminately, but rather thoughtfully consider appropriate tests. The results of the tests should be reviewed in the context of the clinical scenario.

References

[1] Wu AH, McKay C, Broussard LA, et al. National Academy of Clinical Biochemistry Laboratory Medicine practice guidelines: recommendations for the use of laboratory tests to support poisoned patients who present to the emergency department. Clin Chem 2003;49: 357–79.

[2] Temple AR. Acute and chronic effects of aspirin toxicity and their treatment. Arch Intern Med 1981;141(3 Spec No):364–9.

[3] Flomenbaum NE. Salicylates. In: Goldfrank LR, Flomenbaum NE, Lewin NA, et al, editors. Goldfrank's toxicologic emergencies. 7th ed. New York: McGraw-Hill; 2002. p. 507–27.

[4] Nordt SP. Diflunisal cross-reactivity with the Trinder method for salicylate determination. Ann Pharmacother 1996;30:1041–2.

[5] Dalrymple RW, Stearns FM. Diflunisal interference with determination of salicylate by the Trinder, Abbott TDx, and Du Pont aca methods. Clin Chem 1986;32(1 Pt 1):230.

[6] Adelman HM, Wallach PM, Flannery MT. Inability to interpret toxic salicylate levels in patients taking aspirin and diflunisal. J Rheumatol 1991;18:522–3.

[7] Szucs PA, Shih RD, Marcus SM, et al. Pseudosalicylate poisoning: falsely elevated salicylate levels in an overdose of diflunisal. Am J Emerg Med 2000;18:641–2.

[8] Duffens KR, Smilkstein MJ, Bessen HA, Rumack BH. Falsely elevated salicylate levels due to diflunisal overdose. J Emerg Med 1987;5:499–503.

[9] Berkovitch M, Uziel Y, Greenberg R, et al. False-high blood salicylate levels in neonates with hyperbilirubinemia. Ther Drug Monit 2000;22:757–61.

[10] Done AK. Salicylate intoxication: significance of measurements of salicylate in blood in cases of acute ingestion. Pediatrics 1960;26:800–7.

[11] Needs CJ, Brooks PM. Clinical pharmacokinetics of the salicylates. Clin Pharmacokinet 1985;10:164–77.

[12] Dugandzic RM, Tierney MG, Dickinson GE, et al. Evaluation of the validity of the Done nomogram in the management of acute salicylate intoxication. Ann Emerg Med 1989;18: 1186–90.

[13] Chapman BJ, Proudfoot AT. Adult salicylate poisoning: deaths and outcome in patients with high plasma salicylate concentrations. QJM 1989;72:699–707.

[14] Hahn IH, Chu J, Hoffman RS, Nelson LS. Errors in reporting salicylate levels. Acad Emerg Med 2000;7:1336–7.

[15] Krenzelok EP, Guharoy SL, Johnson DR. Toxicology screening in the emergency department: ethanol, barbiturates, and salicylates. Am J Emerg Med 1984;2:331–2.

[16] Chan TY, Chan AY, Ho CS, Critchley JA. The clinical value of screening for salicylates in acute poisoning. Vet Hum Toxicol 1995;37:37–8.

[17] Chan TY, Chan AY. Use of a plasma salicylate assay service in a medical unit in Hong Kong: a follow-up study. Vet Hum Toxicol 1996;38:278–9.

[18] Sporer KA, Khayam-Bashi H. Acetaminophen and salicylate serum levels in patients with suicidal ingestion or altered mental status. Am J Emerg Med 1996;14:443–6.

[19] Leatherman JW, Schmitz PG. Fever, hyperdynamic shock, and multiple-system organ failure: a pseudo-sepsis syndrome associated with chronic salicylate intoxication. Chest 1991;100:1391–6.

[20] Chui PT. Anesthesia in a patient with undiagnosed salicylate poisoning presenting as intraabdominal sepsis. J Clin Anesth 1999;11:251–3.

[21] Paul BN. Salicylate poisoning in the elderly: diagnostic pitfalls. J Am Geriatr Soc 1972;20(8): 387–90.

[22] Anderson RJ, Potts DE, Gabow PA, et al. Unrecognized adult salicylate intoxication. Ann Intern Med 1976;85:745–8.

[23] McGuigan MA. A two-year review of salicylate deaths in Ontario. Arch Intern Med 1987; 147:510–2.

[24] Halla JT, Atchison SL, Hardin JG. Symptomatic salicylate ototoxicity: a useful indicator of serum salicylate concentration? Ann Rheum Dis 1991;50:682–4.

[25] Bailey RB, Jones SR. Chronic salicylate intoxication: a common cause of morbidity in the elderly. J Am Geriatr Soc 1989;37:556–61.

[26] Baer A, Holstege C, Eldridge D. Serum bicarbonate as a predictor of toxic salicylate levels. Presented at the European Association of Poison Centres and Clinical Toxicologists 25th International Congress. Berlin, Germany, 2005.

[27] Bizovi KE, Smilkstein MJ. Acetaminophen. In: Goldfrank LR, Flomenbaum NE, Lewin NA, et al, editors. Goldfrank's toxicologic emergencies. 7th ed. New York: McGraw-Hill; 2002. p. 480–501.

[28] Smilkstein MJ, Knapp GL, Kulig KW, Rumack BH. Efficacy of oral N-acetylcysteine in the treatment of acetaminophen overdose: analysis of the national multicenter study (1976 to 1985). N Engl J Med 1988;319:1557–62.

[29] Ashbourne JF, Olson KR, Khayam-Bashi H. Value of rapid screening for acetaminophen in all patients with intentional drug overdose. Ann Emerg Med 1989;18:1035–8.

[30] Chan TY, Chan AY, Ho CS, Critchley JA. The clinical value of screening for paracetamol in patients with acute poisoning. Hum Exp Toxicol 1995;14:187–9.

[31] Dargan PI, Ladhani S, Jones AL. Measuring plasma paracetamol concentrations in all patients with drug overdose or altered consciousness: does it change outcome? Emerg Med J 2001;18:178–82.

[32] Hartington K, Hartley J, Clancy M. Measuring plasma paracetamol concentrations in all patients with drug overdoses: development of a clinical decision rule and clinicians willingness to use it. Emerg Med J 2002;19:408–11.

[33] Suchard JR. Osmolal gap. In: Dart RC, editor. Medical toxicology. 3rd ed. Philadelphia: Lippincott Williams & Wilkins; 2004. p. 106–9.

[34] Kruse JA, Cadnapaphornchai P. The serum osmole gap. J Crit Care 1994;9:185–97.

[35] Erstad BL. Osmolality and osmolarity: narrowing the terminology gap. Pharmacotherapy 2003;23:1085–6.

[36] Glaser DS. Utility of the serum osmol gap in the diagnosis of methanol or ethylene glycol ingestion. Ann Emerg Med 1996;27:343–6.

[37] Worthley LI, Guerin M, Pain RW. For calculating osmolality, the simplest formula is the best. Anaesth Intensive Care 1987;15:199–202.

[38] Hoffman RS, Smilkstein MJ, Howland MA, Goldfrank LR. Osmol gaps revisited: normal values and limitations. J Toxicol Clin Toxicol 1993;31:81–93.

[39] Smithline N, Gardner KD Jr. Gaps—anionic and osmolal. JAMA 1976;236:1594–7.

[40] Glasser L, Sternglanz PD, Combie J, Robinson A. Serum osmolality and its applicability to drug overdose. Am J Clin Pathol 1973;60:695–9.

[41] McQuillen KK, Anderson AC. Osmol gaps in the pediatric population. Acad Emerg Med 1999;6:27–30.

[42] Aabakken L, Johansen KS, Rydningen EB, et al. Osmolal and anion gaps in patients admitted to an emergency medical department. Hum Exp Toxicol 1994;13:131–4.

[43] Darchy B, Abruzzese L, Pitiot O, et al. Delayed admission for ethylene glycol poisoning: lack of elevated serum osmol gap. Intensive Care Med 1999;25:859–61.

[44] Steinhart B. Case report: severe ethylene glycol intoxication with normal osmolal gap—"a chilling thought". J Emerg Med 1990;8:583–5.

[45] Chabali R. Diagnostic use of anion and osmolal gaps in pediatric emergency medicine. Pediatr Emerg Care 1997;13:204–10.

[46] Ishihara K, Szerlip HM. Anion gap acidosis. Semin Nephrol 1998;18:83–97.

[47] Gabow PA. Disorders associated with an altered anion gap. Kidney Int 1985;27:472–83.

[48] Hoffman RJ, Nelson LS, Hoffman RS. Use of ferric chloride to identify salicylate-containing poisons. J Toxicol Clin Toxicol 2002;40:547–9.

[49] King JA, Storrow AB, Finkelstein JA. Urine Trinder spot test: a rapid salicylate screen for the emergency department. Ann Emerg Med 1995;26:330–3.

[50] Ford M, Tomaszewski C, Kerns W, et al. Bedside ferric chloride urine test to rule out salicylate intoxication. Vet Hum Toxicol 1994;36:364.

[51] Weiner AL, Ko C, McKay CA Jr. A comparison of two bedside tests for the detection of salicylates in urine. Acad Emerg Med 2000;7:834–6.

[52] Wallace KL, Suchard JR, Curry SC, Reagan C. Diagnostic use of physicians' detection of urine fluorescence in a simulated ingestion of sodium fluorescein-containing antifreeze. Ann Emerg Med 2001;38:49–54.

[53] Winter ML, Ellis MD, Snodgrass WR. Urine fluorescence using a Wood's lamp to detect the antifreeze additive sodium fluorescein: a qualitative adjunctive test in suspected ethylene glycol ingestions. Ann Emerg Med 1990;19:663–7.

[54] Casavant MJ, Shah MN, Battels R. Does fluorescent urine indicate antifreeze ingestion by children? Pediatrics 2001;107:113–4.

[55] Kellermann AL, Fihn SD, LoGerfo JP, Copass MK. Impact of drug screening in suspected overdose. Ann Emerg Med 1987;16:1206–16.

[56] Mahoney JD, Gross PL, Stern TA, et al. Quantitative serum toxic screening in the management of suspected drug overdose. Am J Emerg Med 1990;8:16–22.

[57] Brett A. Toxicologic analysis in patients with drug overdose. Arch Intern Med 1988;148:2077.

[58] Bast RP, Helmer SD, Henson SR, et al. Limited utility of routine drug screening in trauma patients. South Med J 2000;93:397–9.

[59] Fabbri A, Marchesini G, Morselli-Labate AM, et al. Comprehensive drug screening in decision making of patients attending the emergency department for suspected drug overdose. Emerg Med J 2003;20:25–8.

[60] Milzman DP, Boulanger BR, Rodriguez A, et al. Pre-existing disease in trauma patients: a predictor of fate independent of age and injury severity score. J Trauma 1992;32:236–43.

[61] Perrone J, De Roos F, Jayaraman S, Hollander JE. Drug screening versus history in detection of substance use in ED psychiatric patients. Am J Emerg Med 2001;19:49–51.

[62] George S, Braithwaite RA. A preliminary evaluation of five rapid detection kits for on site drugs of abuse screening. Addiction 1995;90:227–32.

[63] Gennari FJ. Current concepts: serum osmolality: uses and limitations. N Engl J Med 1984; 310:102–5.

[64] Sklar AH, Linas SL. The osmolal gap in renal failure. Ann Intern Med 1983;98:481–2.

[65] Yaucher NE, Fish JT, Smith HW, Wells JA. Propylene glycol-associated renal toxicity from lorazepam infusion. Pharmacotherapy 2003;23:1094–9.

[66] Schelling JR, Howard RL, Winter SD, Linas SL. Increased osmolal gap in alcoholic ketoacidosis and lactic acidosis. Ann Intern Med 1990;113:580–2.

[67] Seifert SA. Unexplained acid-base and anion gap disorders. In: Dart RC, editor. Medical toxicology. 3rd edition. Philadelphia: Lippincott Williams & Wilkins; 2004. p. 43–51.

ELSEVIER
SAUNDERS

CLINICS IN
LABORATORY
MEDICINE

Clin Lab Med 26 (2006) 31–48

Differentiating the Causes of Metabolic Acidosis in the Poisoned Patient

Bryan S. Judge, MD[a,b],*

[a]DeVos Children's Hospital Regional Poison Center, Grand Rapids, MI, USA
[b]Grand Rapids MERC/Michigan State University Program in Emergency Medicine,
Grand Rapids, MI, USA

Metabolic acidosis may be a significant consequence of a vast array of toxins. Hence, determining which drugs or toxins might be responsible for metabolic acidosis in a patient with an unknown ingestion, accidental exposure, or exposure from therapeutic drug use can present daunting diagnostic and therapeutic challenges. More importantly, vital cellular functions and metabolic processes become impaired with increasing acidosis [1,2]. Therefore, it is paramount that clinicians recognize the substances that can result in metabolic acidosis so that timely and appropriate therapy may be instituted.

Metabolic acidosis is defined as a process that lowers serum bicarbonate (HCO_3^-) and occurs when H^+ ion production exceeds the body's ability to compensate adequately through buffering or increased minute ventilation. Acidemia should not be confused with acidosis. Acidemia refers to a blood pH less than 7.40. Comprehensive discussion of acid-base disturbances is beyond the scope of this article, and the reader is referred elsewhere for further information [1,3,4].

Approach to the poisoned patient who has metabolic acidosis

Evaluating a poisoned patient may pose numerous challenges to the treating physician. First, patients may present with altered mental status, substantially limiting the ability to take an adequate history. Second,

---

Portions of this article were previously published in Holstege CP, Rusyniak DE: Medical Toxicology. 89:6, Med Clin North Am, 2005; with permission.

* DeVos Children's Hospital Regional Poison Center, 1300 Michigan NE, Suite 203, Grand Rapids, MI 49503.

E-mail address: bryan.judge@spectrum-health.org

significant clues at the scene suggestive of the nature of the poisoning may be absent, may be overlooked by personnel at the scene, or may be inadequately conveyed to health care providers. Third, family members or friends, who are often able to provide critical information, may not immediately accompany the patient to the hospital. The exposure history can be enhanced by specific findings on the physical examination. The patient may have a characteristic toxidrome (eg, anticholinergic, cholinergic, opioid, or sympathomimetic), odor, track marks, or other physical examination clues.

Because many poisoned patients are unable or unwilling to provide an accurate history, laboratory evaluation is essential. Specific diagnostic tests, such as a comprehensive metabolic panel and 12-lead ECG, should be considered. They provide invaluable information regarding end-organ toxicity and may assist with diagnosis and treatment, gauge the gravity of the toxicologic process, and provide insight into potential deterioration in a patient's condition [5]. A quantitative test for acetaminophen, aspirin, carboxyhemoglobin, ethylene glycol, iron, methanol, or theophylline may delineate the cause of an elevated anion gap metabolic acidosis. An arterial blood gas serves as a useful adjunct in differentiating acid-base disturbances; however, serum HCO_3^- remains an important initial diagnostic test, because a depressed level is an early indicator of many metabolic toxins.

The routine use of serum and urine drug screens in the acutely poisoned patient is rarely beneficial. Standard urine drug screens test for a limited number of common drugs, and a negative screen does not exclude toxins as the cause of illness. A positive result on the urine drug screen may confirm exposure to a particular substance, but that substance may not be the cause of the patient's clinical condition. Few institutions have readily available comprehensive toxicology laboratory services, a situation which delays turnaround time for comprehensive drug testing [6]. Furthermore, the results of comprehensive drug screens rarely affect either treatment or outcomes, and often medical decision making is best accomplished through routine diagnostic testing and thoroughly assessing and reassessing the patient's clinical condition [7–9].

Once the comprehensive metabolic panel has been obtained, an anion gap (AG) should be determined using the following equation: $AG = [Na^+] - ([Cl^-] + [HCO_3^-])$. Historically, a normal AG has been defined as 12 ± 4 mEq/L. However, a study by Winter and colleagues [10] suggests that a normal AG should be 7 ± 4 mEq/L, because of an increase in measured chloride from improved instrumentation [11]. Therefore, it is important to recognize that the previously accepted range for the AG may not be suitable with newer laboratory technology. If the ingestion of a toxic alcohol (ie, ethylene glycol, isopropanol, methanol) is suspected, osmolarity should be estimated by the following equation: osmolarity $= 2 \times [Na^+] + [glucose]/18 + [blood urea nitrogen \{BUN\}]/2.8$ [12]. An osmol gap (OG) may then be determined by subtracting calculated osmolarity from measured osmolality (OG = measured osmolality − calculated osmolarity). Note that osmolarity refers to the number of particles in 1 L of solution (osmoles/L of solution), and osmolality refers to the number of particles per kilograms of solution (osmoles/kg of solution), but the terms are often used interchangeably because they are almost equivalent for body fluids [13].

Classification of toxicants associated with metabolic acidosis

Although there is no ideal way to classify poisons that cause metabolic acidosis, a clinically useful and systematic approach is to differentiate toxins based on whether they are associated with an elevated AG (Boxes 1 and 2) or a normal AG (Box 3). Many medical conditions are also associated with an increased or normal AG metabolic acidosis and should be included in the differential diagnosis. An elevated AG metabolic acidosis occurs when an acid is paired with an unmeasured anion (eg, lactate), whereas a normal AG metabolic acidosis results from a gain of both H^+ and Cl^- ions or a loss of HCO_3^- and retention of Cl^-, preserving electroneutrality. This classification method has several limitations. The AG may be affected by inherent errors in calculation, laboratory anomalies, and numerous non–acid-base disorders and disease states that may disguise an elevated AG or augment a normal AG (Box 4) [14]. Also, a normal AG acidosis may occur with several of the toxins that produce an AG; therefore, a normal AG should not be used to exclude a possible cause of metabolic acidosis [15].

Many common toxicologic and illness-related causes of an increased AG metabolic acidosis may be remembered with the mnemonic MUDPILES (see Box 1). There are however, several other causes (see Box 2) for an elevated AG metabolic acidosis that should not be overlooked. In this author's experience, acetaminophen, amphetamines, carbon monoxide, cocaine, toluene, and valproic acid are toxins commonly encountered in the clinical setting that might contribute to an increased AG metabolic

---

Box 1. Toxins and disease states associated with an elevated anion gap metabolic acidosis

Methanol
Uremia
Diabetic ketoacidosis, alcoholic ketoacidosis, starvation
  ketoacidosis
Paraldehyde, phenformin
Iron, isoniazid
Lactic acidosis
Ethylene glycol
Salicylates

Box 2. Drugs and medical conditions not listed in MUDPILES mnemonic associated with an elevated anion gap metabolic acidosis

Acetaminophen
Aminocaproic acid
Amphetamines
Benzene
Carbon monoxide
Catecholamines
Citric acid
Cocaine
Cyanide
Didanosine
Diethylene glycol
Ephedrine
Fluoride
Formaldehyde
Hydrogen sulfide
Ibuprofen
Inborn errors of metabolism
Nalidixic acid
Metformin
Niacin
Nitroprusside
Nonsteroidal anti-inflammatory drugs
Polyethylene glycol
Propofol
Propylene glycol
Pseudoephedrine
Streptozotocin
Sulfur
Theophylline
Thiamine deficiency
Toluene
Triethylene glycol
Valproate
Zidovudine

From Seifert SA. Unexplained acid base and anion gap disorders. In: Dart RC, editor. Medical toxicology. 3rd edition. Philadelphia: Lippincott Williams & Wilkins; 2004. p. 1914; with permission.

Box 3. Drugs and medical conditions associated with a normal anion gap metabolic acidosis

Acetazolamide
Acids (ammonium chloride, calcium chloride, hydrochloric acid)
Cholestyramine
Diarrhea
Hyperalimentation
Magnesium chloride
Pancreatic fistula
Posthypocapnia
Rapid intravenous fluid administration
Renal tubular acidosis
Sulfamylon
Topiramate
Ureteroenterostomy

---

acidosis but are not listed in the MUDPILES mnemonic. Recognizing the many toxins associated with an increased AG metabolic acidosis is imperative, because the presence of a profoundly elevated AG may help identify specific causes of the acidosis and have prognostic value [16–18].

The osmol gap may provide additional information in a patient with an elevated AG acidosis who has ingested a toxic alcohol. Although the OG may be increased in the presence of toxic alcohols, several other medical conditions, such as ketoacidosis, renal failure, and shock states, may also increase the measured serum osmolality [19–21]. Toxins that elevate the OG can be memorized with the mnemonic MADGAS (Box 5) [13]. For simplicity, a "normal" OG is considered to be less than 10 ± 6 mOsm/L [22]. However, the use of the "normal" range for the OG has inherent limitations, owing to wide variability of the OG in the population [19,20,23] and potential errors in calculation and laboratory methodology (eg, freezing point depression should be used to measure serum osmolality and not vapor pressure) [24]. Furthermore, the absence of an OG cannot be used to rule out the presence of a toxic alcohol, because patients with a "normal" OG may have toxic and potentially lethal levels of a toxic alcohol [25,26]. Conversely, a significantly elevated OG (> 25 mOsm/L) is a potential indicator of a toxic alcohol ingestion [20].

Other methods of analyzing metabolic acidosis exist, including base excess/deficit and strong ion difference. Base excess/deficit is the quantity of acid or base necessary to restore pH to 7.40 in blood equilibrated at standard conditions [27]; strong ion difference is the apparent difference between entirely dissociated cations and entirely dissociated anions [28]. In a study by Fencl and colleagues [29], the strong ion difference was able to detect acid-base disorders that were missed using the anion gap. However, neither of these

---

Box 4. Conditions affecting the anion gap

Increased anion gap
  Carbenicillin
  Dehydration/Diarrhea
  Hypocalcemia
  Hypokalemia
  Hypomagnesemia
  Metabolic acidosis
  Metabolic alkalosis
  Nonketotic hyperosmolar coma
  Respiratory alkalosis
  Sodium penicillin
  Uremia

Decreased anion gap
  Halides (bromine, iodine)
  Hypercalcemia
  Hyperkalemia
  Hyperlipidemia
  Hypermagnesemia
  Hyperparathyroidism
  Hypoalbuminemia
  Hyponatremia
  Lithium intoxication
  Multiple myeloma
  Polymyxin

Data from Salem M, Mujais SK. Gaps in the anion gap. Arch Intern Med 1992;152:1625.

---

methods is clinically feasible, because base excess/deficit is prone to missing serious acid-base disorders, whereas the strong ion difference is difficult to calculate and requires additional laboratory testing [29,30].

Mechanisms of toxin-induced metabolic acidosis

Toxin-induced metabolic acidosis arises from increased acid production or impaired acid elimination. Toxins accomplish either of these effects by means of several important and distinct mechanisms. Increased acid production may occur with toxins that (1) are acidic or have acidic metabolites, (2) produce an imbalance between ATP consumption and production, or (3) cause metabolic derangements resulting in the generation of ketone bodies. Underlying impairment of renal function or nephrotoxic compounds may lead to

---

Box 5. Toxins associated with an elevated osmol gap

Mannitol
Alcohols: ethanol, ethylene glycol, isopropanol, methanol,
    propylene glycol
Diatrizoate
Glycerol
Acetone
Sorbitol

From Chabali R. Diagnostic use of anion and osmolal gaps in pediatric emergency medicine. Pediatr Emerg Care 1997;13:204; with permission.

---

diminished acid elimination and the development of a metabolic acidosis. Some toxins, such as salicylates, may produce metabolic acidosis through a combination of these mechanisms.

Toxins resulting in increased acid production

Toxins that are acids or have acid metabolites
    Metabolic acidosis may result from the ingestion of a substance that is an acid or has an acidifying metabolite. Several alcohols (eg, benzyl alcohol, ethanol, ethylene glycol, methanol) are not acidifying until they are metabolized to acidic intermediates [31]. Ethylene glycol has several acidic metabolites (ie, glycolic acid, glyoxylic acid, oxalic acid); however, glycolic acid is primarily responsible for the metabolic acidosis, whereas formic acid is the metabolite that causes metabolic acidosis from methanol poisoning [32]. Large ingestions of ethanol may produce metabolic acidosis by means of its metabolism to acetic acid. Benzyl alcohol is commonly used as a preservative in intravenous medications. The use of such preparations in neonates has caused gasping respirations, hypotension, hepatic and renal failure, and fatal metabolic acidosis owing to formation of benzoic acid and hippuric acid, the products of benzyl alcohol metabolism [33].
    Salicylates are weak acids that may produce metabolic acidosis through numerous mechanisms. In toxic concentrations, salicylates interfere with energy production by uncoupling oxidative phosphorylation [34] and may produce renal insufficiency that causes accumulation of phosphoric and sulfuric acids [35]. The metabolism of fatty acids is likewise increased in patients with salicylate toxicity, generating ketone body formation. These processes all contribute to the development of an elevated AG metabolic acidosis in patients with salicylate poisoning.
    Caustic agents, both acid and alkali, may cause significant tissue damage after ingestion and produce metabolic acidosis. In some instances of acid

injury, a metabolic acidosis may occur from the absorption of nonionized acid from the gastric mucosa. The ingestion of hydrochloric acid may initially produce a normal AG metabolic acidosis, because both H^+ and Cl^- ions are systemically absorbed and accounted for in the measurement of the AG. Other acids, such as sulfuric acid, may produce an increased AG metabolic acidosis, because the sulfate anion is not accounted for in the measurement of the AG [36].

Toxins affecting ATP consumption and production

Many poisons may interfere with cellular energy production and consumption, resulting in metabolic acidosis. Toxins may disrupt mito-chondrial function and subsequent energy production either by uncoupling oxidative phosphorylation or by inhibiting cytochromes of the electron transport chain. Excessive energy consumption may result from toxins that produce a hyperadrenergic state.

Acetaminophen is a readily available over-the-counter analgesic that is commonly ingested or coingested during a suicide attempt and may cause an increased AG metabolic acidosis [37,38]. In fact, a pH of less than 7.30 is used as one of the indicators for a poor prognosis in acetaminophen-induced hepatotoxicity [39]. Although the exact mechanism of acetaminophen-induced metabolic acidosis remains unknown, several animal studies suggest that acetaminophen and its hepatotoxic metabolite N-acetyl-p-benzoquino-neimine inhibit oxidative phosphorylation, which subsequently leads to metabolic acidosis [40–42].

HIV-positive patients taking antiretroviral therapy are at risk for developing lactic acidosis syndrome. Stavudine, zidovudine, and other nucleoside analogue reverse transcriptase inhibitors impair oxidative phosphorylation by inhibiting mitochondrial DNA polymerase γ [43]; this process may result in hepatic dysfunction and steatosis, lactic acidosis, and death [44,45]. Mortality in patients who develop this condition ranges between 25% and 57% [43,46]. Patients who are on chronic antiretroviral therapy may also develop hyperlactatemia without acidosis [47]. Case reports suggest that mortality in patients with lactic acidosis syndrome may be decreased with the administration of carnitine and riboflavin; however, larger studies are required to assess the possible benefit of these therapies [46,48].

Metabolic acidosis is an important consequence of acute valproic acid toxicity, because profound acidosis after massive ingestions confers a poor prognosis [49–51]. Once ingested, valproic acid is extensively metabolized by the liver [52]. The net effect of valproic acid metabolites is depletion of intramitochondrial coenzyme A and carnitine, which inhibits the β-oxidation of fatty acids, impairing ATP production [53]. Carnitine supplementation may help restore β-oxidation to mitochondria, and, in 1996, the Pediatric Neurology Advisory Committee recommended that carnitine be administered to children with acute ingestions of valproic acid [54]. However, owing to lack of controlled studies, further research is required to evaluate the role of carnitine in valproic acid overdoses.

Historically, the biguanide phenformin is a well-known pharmacologic cause of acquired lactic acidosis (40 to 64 cases per 100,000 patient-years); it was withdrawn from the United States market because of its association with this life-threatening condition [55]. Metformin is another biguanide that became available in the United States in 1995. To date, no clear relationship exists between the therapeutic use of metformin and increased risk for lactic acidosis. Stang and colleagues [55] found the incidence of lactic acidosis in metformin users to be nine cases per 100,000 patient-years, which is similar to the background rate of lactic acidosis in patients with type 2 diabetes mellitus who are not on metformin therapy (~ 10 cases per 100,000 patient-years) [56]. Furthermore, most cases of lactic acidosis related to therapeutic metformin use have occurred in the presence of a severe underlying disease state [57], such as renal failure, that could have caused the lactic acidosis. A recent meta-analysis finds no evidence to support the association of metformin therapy with an increased risk for lactic acidosis compared with other hypoglycemic agents [58]. However, metformin does inhibit the electron transport chain by binding to complex I, and the intentional overdose of metformin has resulted in lactic acidosis and even death [59–61].

Several mitochondrial poisons are responsible for a profound metabolic acidosis that may require prompt antidotal intervention. Examples of such toxins include carbon monoxide, cyanide, hydrogen sulfide, iron, methanol, and salicylates. Carbon monoxide, cyanide, hydrogen sulfide, and the metabolite of methanol (formic acid) impair oxidative metabolism by inhibiting complex IV of the electron transport chain [62–64]. Iron and salicylates hinder energy production by disrupting oxidative phosphorylation [34,65]. Following toxicity with these agents, cellular energy stores are quickly diminished, resulting in disruption of critical electrolyte gradients, ATP-dependent processes, and the H^+ ion consumption in the aerobic synthesis of ATP [63]. Furthermore, many of these toxins (eg, carbon monoxide, cyanide, iron) impair tissue perfusion, disrupting aerobic cellular energy production and worsening metabolic acidosis.

Excessive adrenergic stimulation from agents such as amphetamines, caffeine, cocaine, β-2 agonists, ephedrine, phencyclidine, and theophylline may result in hyperglycemia, hypokalemia, leukocytosis, and metabolic acidosis [66–68]. In the presence of catecholamines, β-adrenoreceptor stimulation results in the hydrolysis of ATP and augments cyclic adenosine monophosphate activity within cells, which stimulates $Na^+K^+-ATPase$ and causes K^+ ions to shift intracellularly. Excess catecholamines also stimulate glycogenolysis and the breakdown of fatty acids, resulting in hyperglycemia and metabolic acidosis, respectively. Poisoning with an agent that causes hyperadrenergic stimulation should be strongly suspected in a patient who has the aforementioned laboratory abnormalities and a sympathomimetic toxidrome.

Special mention should be made of lactic acidosis, because this terminology is misleading and erroneous. When glucose is converted to lactate during anaerobic metabolism to generate two molecules of ATP, net H^+ ions are not produced [69,70]. Other pieces of evidence supporting the concept that lactate does not cause metabolic acidosis include (1) the parenteral administration of lactate causes a rise in pH, because it is hepatically metabolized to HCO_3^-; (2) as many as 25% of patients with an increased AG metabolic acidosis have normal lactic acid levels [17]; (3) lactate levels do not always correlate with the AG [17]; and (4) lactic acid levels may rise without acidosis (eg, with strenuous exercise [71] and the ingestion of ethanol [72]).

Net H^+ ions are produced when ATP is used as a cellular energy source [69]. The electron transport chain then uses the H^+ ions that are generated from the hydrolysis of ATP in the aerobic synthesis of ATP, thus maintaining a normal pH under typical physiologic conditions [73]. However, metabolic acidosis may ensue in the presence of a toxin or other physiologic derangement, resulting in an imbalance of ATP hydrolysis and synthesis. The imbalance of ATP hydrolysis and synthesis is acidifying, not the production of lactate. Lactate should only serve as an indicator of anaerobic metabolism [69,74].

Metabolic derangements causing increased acid production

Certain toxins may induce metabolic derangements, resulting in the increased production of ketone bodies (ie, acetoacetate, acetone, β-hydroxybutyrate). The generation of ketoacids may also occur secondary to uncontrolled diabetes and is a normal response to fasting and prolonged exercise [75]. Alcoholic ketoacidosis (AKA) is a prime example in which toxin-induced (ie, ethanol) metabolic derangements and an acute starvation state result in the production of ketoacids and an elevated AG metabolic acidosis. Patients who develop AKA are usually chronic ethanol abusers who have been binge drinking and develop a gastrointestinal illness (eg, gastritis, hepatitis, pancreatitis) that limits oral intake [76]. The diagnosis of AKA should be considered in a patient who (1) recently binged on ethanol and has had a decrease in ethanol consumption, (2) has a history of vomiting or decreased oral intake, (3) has a blood glucose level of less than 300 mg/dL, and (4) has an elevated AG metabolic acidosis for which other causes have been excluded [77].

Isoniazid (INH) poisoning is characterized by refractory seizures, elevated AG metabolic acidosis, and coma. Survival from acute INH toxicity has been reported in a patient with an arterial pH as low as 6.49 [78]. The mechanism underlying the development of metabolic acidosis in patients poisoned with INH remains unclear. Plausible explanations include muscular activity from seizures, acidifying INH metabolites, and enhanced fatty acid metabolism that produces ketoacids [79–81].

Toxins impairing the renal elimination of acids

Several substances may cause or exacerbate renal insufficiency. Renal dysfunction may lead to the accumulation of parent compounds or toxic intermediates and contribute to or produce a metabolic acidosis. Renal impairment, whether drug-induced or underlying, may result in uremia. Even in the absence of a toxin that produces metabolic acidosis, the build-up of nitrogenous compounds may cause an increased AG metabolic acidosis by means of impaired ammonia secretion and retention of unmeasured anions [18].

Toluene exposure may lead to a metabolic acidosis as a result of toluene's metabolism to an acidic metabolite, hippuric acid [82]. The chronic abuse of toluene may also result in the development of a distal renal tubular acidosis (RTA), with associated hypokalemia and metabolic acidosis [83]. The mechanism by which toluene induces this RTA has not been fully elucidated. Toluene and hippuric acid are most likely directly toxic to the distal renal tubule [84] and impair H^+ ion secretion. Impaired H^+ ion secretion results in the loss of Na^+ and K^+ ions, incapacity to acidify the urine, and a normal- or increased-AG metabolic acidosis [82,84,85].

Ethylene glycol is not by itself a nephrotoxin [86]. However, once hepatically metabolized, it forms nephrotoxic intermediates. Ethylene glycol–associated renal insufficiency has been attributed to the deposition of calcium oxalate crystals in the renal tubules [87]; however, urinary calcium oxalate crystals are only present in 50% to 65% of patients who have ethylene glycol poisoning [88,89]. Therefore, another mechanism may be responsible for or contribute to ethylene glycol–associated renal insufficiency, and the absence of calcium oxalate crystalluria cannot be used to rule out ethylene glycol poisoning. Ethylene glycol–associated renal dysfunction may exacerbate the metabolic acidosis produced by its metabolites (glycolic acid, glyoxylic acid, oxalic acid).

Propylene glycol is commonly employed as a diluent and preservative in numerous pharmaceutical preparations, including chlordiazepoxide, diazepam, digoxin, esmolol, etomidate, lorazepam, nitroglycerin, phenobarbital, phenytoin, and trimethoprim/sulfamethoxazole. Although it is considered to be generally safe, problems arise with the prolonged or rapid administration of agents containing propylene glycol, especially in patients with renal insufficiency. Cardiac dysrhythmias, hypotension, conduction abnormalities, and death have occurred with the rapid administration of phenytoin, because of the presence of propylene glycol in its intravenous product [90,91]. Patients receiving continuous infusions of propylene glycol–containing sedatives may develop an elevated AG metabolic acidosis and increased osmolality [1]. These metabolic abnormalities resolve quickly once the offending medication has been discontinued. Because propylene glycol is metabolized to lactate by alcohol dehydrogenase, some authors [92] have proposed this as a mechanism for propylene glycol–induced metabolic acidosis. A study by Morshed and colleagues [93] suggests that the prolonged administration of a propylene glycol–containing medication causes proximal renal tubule damage and subsequent renal dysfunction. However, the concentrations needed to produce renal tubule damage in the study would only occur if very high doses of propylene glycol were administered to a patient.

Treatment considerations for toxin-induced metabolic acidosis

The most important measures in treating toxin-induced metabolic acidosis are to recognize and treat the underlying cause and to provide excellent supportive care, including airway control and fluid resuscitation. Discontinuing the offending agent or agents in a patient who develops metabolic acidosis while taking therapeutic quantities of certain drugs (eg, topiramate, metformin) may be all that is necessary. Many patients who develop a mild metabolic acidosis after an intentional ingestion experience improvement with close observation and supportive care. However, when poisoned patients have progressive worsening of their metabolic acidosis despite supportive care (ie, fluid resuscitation, oxygen therapy), then alternative causes for their metabolic acidosis should be sought. Therapy for specific toxin-induced metabolic acidoses is variable, with some of the more common management strategies discussed in the following section.

Role of buffer therapy

Many clinicians may be inclined to treat toxin-induced metabolic acidosis with a buffer, such as sodium bicarbonate, to increase serum pH. However, this practice should be discouraged. The administration of sodium bicarbonate has not been definitively shown to improve outcomes in patients who have metabolic acidosis, and it can be detrimental in some [74]. Paradoxical intracellular acidosis may occur because of increased production of carbon dioxide [94]. Sodium bicarbonate administration may also impair oxygen delivery to tissues by shifting the oxyhemoglobin dissociation curve to the left [95]. Other methods of alkalinization, such as carbicarb [96] and tris-hydroxymethyl aminomethane (THAM), are not routinely used in the treatment of toxin-induced metabolic acidosis, owing to the scarcity of carbicarb and lack of improvement in patient outcomes with THAM [1].

Patients who may benefit from the use of sodium bicarbonate are those poisoned with agents whose elimination may be increased through alkalinization (eg, salicylates) and those poisoned with drugs that cause blockade of cardiac Na^+ channels (eg, cyclic antidepressants). Sodium bicarbonate is useful in decreasing tissue levels of salicylates and in facilitating the elimination of salicylates in the urine [97,98]. Hemodialysis should be instituted in those salicylate-poisoned patients who have altered mental status, pulmonary edema, renal failure, severe electrolyte and metabolic abnormalities, or a salicylate level greater than 100 mg/dL after an acute ingestion. Sodium bicarbonate is also effective in treating drug-induced cardiac sodium channel blockade [99]. For cyclic antidepressant–induced cardiotoxicity, 1 to 2 mEq/kg of sodium bicarbonate should be given as an intravenous bolus and repeated as needed until a blood pH of 7.55 is attained [100,101].

Antidotal therapy

Ingestion of a toxic alcohol requires antagonism of alcohol dehydrogenase with ethanol or fomepizole and consideration of hemodialysis in patients who are profoundly acidotic or have had a massive ingestion. Neither ethanol nor fomepizole affects the toxic metabolites of ethylene glycol or methanol. Complications associated with the administration of ethanol include central nervous system (CNS) depression, hypoglycemia, and fluctuating levels due to patient variability in its metabolism. Advantages of fomepizole include ease of dosing, no need for monitoring of serum levels, and lack of CNS-depressant activity. Specific vitamins may be used as adjuvant therapy in ethylene glycol and methanol poisoning. Folate enhances the metabolism of formic acid to carbon dioxide and water, whereas thiamine and pyridoxine help metabolize toxic ethylene glycol intermediates to less toxic compounds [89,102].

Treatment for acute INH toxicity should focus on termination of seizures, reversal of metabolic acidosis, and stabilization of vital signs through supportive measures. INH causes toxicity by diminishing the synthesis of γ-amino butyric acid in the CNS through antagonism of pyridoxine. The antidote for INH-induced neurotoxicity is pyridoxine [103,104]. Pyridoxine rapidly terminates INH-induced seizures, reverses coma, and corrects metabolic acidosis.

Management of patients with cyanide and hydrogen sulfide toxicity is complicated by the nature of these extremely rapidly acting and potent toxins; hence most victims succumb to a rapid death or are moribund with a severe metabolic acidosis on presentation. The cyanide antidote kit containing amyl nitrite, sodium nitrite, and sodium thiosulfate should be considered early in the management of toxicity. Hydrogen sulfide is detoxified when it binds to methemoglobinemia to form sulfmethemoglobin [105]. Several case reports demonstrated improvement in the condition of patients when nitrites were administered soon after exposure to hydrogen sulfide [106–108]. Therefore, sodium nitrite should be considered for patients with suspected severe hydrogen sulfide toxicity.

Summary

Metabolic acidosis may arise from several drugs and toxins through a variety of mechanisms. Differentiating the causes of metabolic acidosis in the poisoned patient is an indispensable skill in clinical practice. Comprehension of toxin-induced metabolic acidosis, combined with a thorough history, physical examination, appropriate use of laboratory tests, and a stepwise approach, should aid the clinician in determining the cause of metabolic acidosis in the poisoned patient. When confronted with such a patient, it is imperative that one administer appropriate antidotal therapy, when necessary, and provide the patient with exceptional supportive care.

References

[1] Gauthier PM, Szerlip HM. Metabolic acidosis in the intensive care unit. Crit Care Clin 2002;18:289.

[2] Swenson ER. Metabolic acidosis. Respir Care 2001;46:342.

[3] Hoffman RS. Fluid, electrolyte, and acid-base principles. In: Goldfrank LR, Howland MA, Hoffman RS, et al, editors. Goldfrank's toxicologic emergencies. 7th edition. New York: McGraw-Hill; 2002. p. 2170.

[4] Seifert SA. Unexplained acid-base and anion gap disorders. In: Dart RC, editor. Medical toxicology. 3rd edition. Philadelphia: Lippincott Williams & Wilkins; 2004. p. 1914.

[5] Kirk M, Pace S. Pearls, pitfalls, and updates in toxicology. Emerg Med Clin North Am 1997;15:427–49.

[6] College of American Pathologists Participant Summaries. Toxicology Survey T-B; Therapeutic Drug Monitoring (General) Survey Set Z-B; Urine Toxicology Survey Set UT-B; Serum Alcohol/Volatiles Survey Set AL2-B; Chemistry Survey Set C4-B. Northfield (IL): College of American Pathologists; 1999.

[7] Brett AS. Implications of discordance between clinical impression and toxicology analysis in drug overdose. Arch Intern Med 1988;148:437–41.

[8] Kellermann AL, Fihn SD, LoGerfo JP, et al. Impact of drug screening in suspected overdose. Ann Emerg Med 1987;16:1206–16.

[9] Sporer KA, Ernst AA. The effect of toxicologic screening on management of minimally symptomatic overdoses. Am J Emerg Med 1992;10:173–5.

[10] Winter SD, Pearson JR, Gabow PA, et al. The fall of the serum anion gap. Arch Intern Med 1990;150:311–3.

[11] Oh MS, Carroll HJ. The anion gap. N Engl J Med 1977;297:814–7.

[12] Epstein FB. Osmolality. Emerg Med Clin North Am 1986;4:253–61.

[13] Chabali R. Diagnostic use of anion and osmolal gaps in pediatric emergency medicine. Pediatr Emerg Care 1997;13:204–10.

[14] Salem MM, Mujais SK. Gaps in the anion gap. Arch Intern Med 1992;152:1625–9.

[15] Gabow PA, Anderson RJ, Potts DE, et al. Acid-base disturbances in the salicylate-intoxicated adult. Arch Intern Med 1978;138:1481–4.

[16] Brenner BE. Clinical significance of the elevated anion gap. Am J Med 1985;79:289–96.

[17] Gabow PA, Kaehny WD, Fennessey PV, et al. Diagnostic importance of an increased serum anion gap. N Engl J Med 1980;303:854–8.

[18] Ishihara K, Szerlip HM. Anion gap acidosis. Semin Nephrol 1998;18:83–97.

[19] Inaba H, Hirasawa H, Mizuguchi T. Serum osmolality gap in postoperative patients in intensive care. Lancet 1987;1:1331–5.

[20] Schelling JR, Howard RL, Winter SD, et al. Increased osmolal gap in alcoholic ketoacidosis and lactic acidosis. Ann Intern Med 1990;113:580–2.

[21] Sklar AH, Linas SL. The osmolal gap in renal failure. Ann Intern Med 1983;98:481–2.

[22] Dorwart WV, Chalmers L. Comparison of methods for calculating serum osmolality from chemical concentrations, and the prognostic value of such calculations. Clin Chem 1975;21: 190–4.

[23] Hoffman RS, Smilkstein MJ, Howland MA, et al. Osmol gaps revisited: normal values and limitations. J Toxicol Clin Toxicol 1993;31:81–93.

[24] Eisen TF, Lacouture PG, Woolf A. Serum osmolality in alcohol ingestions: differences in availability among laboratories of teaching hospital, nonteaching hospital, and commercial facilities. Am J Emerg Med 1989;7:256–9.

[25] Glaser DS. Utility of the serum osmol gap in the diagnosis of methanol or ethylene glycol ingestion. Ann Emerg Med 1996;27:343–6.

[26] Steinhart B. Case report: severe ethylene glycol intoxication with normal osmolal gap— "a chilling thought." J Emerg Med 1990;8:583–5.

[27] Mizock BA. Utility of standard base excess in acid-base analysis. Crit Care Med 1998;26: 1146–7.

[28] Stewart PA. Modern quantitative acid-base chemistry. Can J Physiol Pharmacol 1983;61: 1444–61.

[29] Fencl V, Jabor A, Kazda A, et al. Diagnosis of metabolic acid-base disturbances in critically ill patients. Am J Respir Crit Care Med 2000;162:2246–51.

[30] Kowalchuk JM, Scheuermann BW. Acid-base regulation: a comparison of quantitative methods. Can J Physiol Pharmacol 1994;72:818–26.

[31] Gabow PA, Clay K, Sullivan JB, et al. Organic acids in ethylene glycol intoxication. Ann Intern Med 1986;105:16–20.

[32] Moreau CL, Kerns W II, Tomaszewski CA, et al. Glycolate kinetics and hemodialysis clearance in ethylene glycol poisoning. META Study Group. J Toxicol Clin Toxicol 1998; 36:659–66.

[33] Gershanik JJ, Boecler G, Ensley H, et al. The gasping syndrome and benzyl alcohol poisoning. N Engl J Med 1982;307:1384–8.

[34] Alberti KG, Cohen RD, Woods HF. Lactic acidosis and hyperlactataemia. Lancet 1974;2: 1519–60.

[35] Insel PA. Analgesic-antipyretic and anti-inflammatory agents and drugs employed in the treatment of gout. In: Harmon JG, Limbird LE, editors. Goodman & Gilman's The pharmacologic basis of therapeutics. 9th edition. New York: McGraw-Hill; 1996. p. 1905.

[36] Rao RB, Hoffman RS. Caustics and batteries. In: Goldfrank LR, Howland MA, Hoffman RS, et al, editors. Goldfrank's toxicologic emergencies. 7th edition. New York: McGraw-Hill; 2002. p. 2170.

[37] Flanagan RJ, Mant TG. Coma and metabolic acidosis early in severe acute paracetamol poisoning. Hum Toxicol 1986;5:179–82.

[38] Zezulka A, Wright N. Severe metabolic acidosis early in paracetamol poisoning. Br Med J (Clin Res Ed) 1982;285:851–2.

[39] O'Grady JG, Alexander GJ, Hayllar KM, et al. Early indicators of prognosis in fulminant hepatic failure. Gastroenterology 1989;97:439–45.

[40] Esterline RL, Ji S. Metabolic alterations resulting from the inhibition of mitochondrial respiration by acetaminophen in vivo. Biochem Pharmacol 1989;38:2390–2.

[41] Esterline RL, Ray SD, Ji S. Reversible and irreversible inhibition of hepatic mitochondrial respiration by acetaminophen and its toxic metabolite, N-acetyl-p-benzoquinoneimine (NAPQI). Biochem Pharmacol 1989;38:2387–90.

[42] Porter KE, Dawson AG. Inhibition of respiration and gluconeogenesis by paracetamol in rat kidney preparations. Biochem Pharmacol 1979;28:3057–62.

[43] Tripuraneni NS, Smith PR, Weedon J, et al. Prognostic factors in lactic acidosis syndrome caused by nucleoside reverse transcriptase inhibitors: report of eight cases and review of the literature. AIDS Patient Care STDS 2004;18:379–84.

[44] Mokrzycki MH, Harris C, May H, et al. Lactic acidosis associated with stavudine administration: a report of five cases. Clin Infect Dis 2000;30:198–200.

[45] Sundar K, Suarez M, Banogon PE, et al. Zidovudine-induced fatal lactic acidosis and hepatic failure in patients with acquired immunodeficiency syndrome: report of two patients and review of the literature. Crit Care Med 1997;25:1425–30.

[46] Falco V, Rodriguez D, Ribera E, et al. Severe nucleoside-associated lactic acidosis in human immunodeficiency virus–infected patients: report of 12 cases and review of the literature. Clin Infect Dis 2002;34:838–46.

[47] John M, Moore CB, James IR, et al. Chronic hyperlactatemia in HIV-infected patients taking antiretroviral therapy. AIDS 2001;15:717–23.

[48] Dalton SD, Rahimi AR. Emerging role of riboflavin in the treatment of nucleoside analogue–induced type B lactic acidosis. AIDS Patient Care STDS 2001;15:611–4.

[49] Anderson GO, Ritland S. Life-threatening intoxication with sodium valproate. J Toxicol Clin Toxicol 1995;33:279–84.

[50] Ishikura H, Matsuo N, Matsubara M, et al. Valproic acid overdose and L-carnitine therapy. J Anal Toxicol 1996;20:55–8.

[51] Murakami K, Sugimoto T, Woo M, et al. Effect of L-carnitine supplementation on acute valproate intoxication. Epilepsia 1996;37:687–9.

[52] Dupuis RE, Lichtman SN, Pollack GM. Acute valproic acid overdose. Clinical course and pharmacokinetic disposition of valproic acid and metabolites. Drug Saf 1990;5:65–71.

[53] Raskind JY, El-Chaar GM. The role of carnitine supplementation during valproic acid therapy. Ann Pharmacother 2000;34:630–8.

[54] DeVivo DC, Bohan TP, Coulter DL, et al. L-carnitine supplementation in childhood epilepsy: current perspectives. Epilepsia 1998;39:1216–25.

[55] Stang M, Wysowski DK, Butler-Jones D. Incidence of lactic acidosis in metformin users. Diabetes Care 1999;22:925–7.

[56] Brown JB, Pedula K, Barzilay J, et al. Lactic acidosis rates in type 2 diabetes. Diabetes Care 1998;21:1659–63.

[57] Chan NN, Brain HP, Feher MD. Metformin-associated lactic acidosis: a rare or very rare clinical entity? Diabet Med 1999;16:273–81.

[58] Salpeter SR, Greyber E, Pasternak GA, et al. Risk of fatal and nonfatal lactic acidosis with metformin use in type 2 diabetes mellitus: systematic review and meta-analysis. Arch Intern Med 2003;163:2594–602.

[59] Owen MR, Doran E, Halestrap AP. Evidence that metformin exerts its anti-diabetic effects through inhibition of complex 1 of the mitochondrial respiratory chain. Biochem J 2000;3: 607–14.

[60] Palatnick W, Meatherall R, Tenenbein M. Severe lactic acidosis from acute metformin overdose [abstract]. J Toxicol Clin Toxicol 1999;37:638–9.

[61] Spiller HA, Weber J, Hofman M, et al. Multicenter case series of adult metformin ingestion [abstract]. J Toxicol Clin Toxicol 1999;37:639.

[62] Brown SD, Piantadosi CA. In vivo binding of carbon monoxide to cytochrome c oxidase in rat brain. J Appl Physiol 1990;68:604–10.

[63] Delaney KA. Biochemical principles. In: Goldfrank LR, Howland MA, Hoffman RS, et al, editors. Goldfrank's toxicologic emergencies. 7th edition. New York: McGraw-Hill; 2002. p. 2170.

[64] Way JL. Cyanide intoxication and its mechanism of antagonism. Annu Rev Pharmacol Toxicol 1984;24:451–81.

[65] Robotham JL, Lietman PS. Acute iron poisoning. A review. Am J Dis Child 1980;134: 875–9.

[66] Brown MJ. Hypokalemia from beta 2–receptor stimulation by circulating epinephrine. Am J Cardiol 1985;56:3D–9D.

[67] Liem EB, Mnookin SC, Mahla ME. Albuterol-induced lactic acidosis. Anesthesiology 2003;99:505–6.

[68] Wong KM, Chak WL, Cheung CY, et al. Hypokalemic metabolic acidosis attributed to cough mixture abuse. Am J Kidney Dis 2001;38:390–4.

[69] Mizock BA. Lactic acidosis. Dis Mon 1989;35:233–300.

[70] Stacpoole PW. Lactic acidosis. Endocrinol Metab Clin North Am 1993;22:221–45.

[71] Ahlborg G, Wahren J, Felig P. Splanchnic and peripheral glucose and lactate metabolism during and after prolonged arm exercise. J Clin Invest 1986;77:690–9.

[72] Fulop M, Bock J, Ben-Ezra J, et al. Plasma lactate and 3-hydroxybutyrate levels in patients with acute ethanol intoxication. Am J Med 1986;80:191–4.

[73] Mizock BA. Controversies in lactic acidosis. Implications in critically ill patients. JAMA 1987;258:497–501.

[74] Stacpoole PW, Wright EC, Baumgartner TG, et al. Natural history and course of acquired lactic acidosis in adults. DCA—Lactic Acidosis Study Group. Am J Med 1994; 97:47–54.

[75] Mitchell GA, Kassovska-Bratinova S, Boukaftane Y, et al. Medical aspects of ketone body metabolism. Clin Invest Med 1995;18:193–216.

[76] Fulop M. Alcoholism, ketoacidosis, and lactic acidosis. Diabetes Metab Rev 1989;5: 365.

[77] Soffer A, Hamburger S. Alcoholic ketoacidosis: a review of 30 cases. J Am Med Womens Assoc 1982;37:106–10.

[78] Hankins DG, Saxena K, Faville RJ Jr, et al. Profound acidosis caused by isoniazid ingestion. Am J Emerg Med 1987;5:165–6.

[79] Chin L, Sievers ML, Herrier RN, et al. Convulsions as the etiology of lactic acidosis in acute isoniazid toxicity in dogs. Toxicol Appl Pharmacol 1979;49:377–84.

[80] Pahl MV, Vaziri ND, Ness R, et al. Association of beta hydroxybutyric acidosis with isoniazid intoxication. J Toxicol Clin Toxicol 1984;22:167–76.

[81] Weber WW, Hein DW. Clinical pharmacokinetics of isoniazid. Clin Pharmacokinet 1979; 4:401–22.

[82] Carlisle EJ, Donnelly SM, Vasuvattakul S, et al. Glue-sniffing and distal renal tubular acidosis: sticking to the facts. J Am Soc Nephrol 1991;1:1019–27.

[83] Kao KC, Tsai YH, Lin MC, et al. Hypokalemic muscular paralysis causing acute respiratory failure due to rhabdomyolysis with renal tubular acidosis in a chronic glue sniffer. J Toxicol Clin Toxicol 2000;38:679–81.

[84] Kamijima M, Nakazawa Y, Yamakawa M, et al. Metabolic acidosis and renal tubular injury due to pure toluene inhalation. Arch Environ Health 1994;49:410–3.

[85] Batlle DC, Sabatini S, Kurtzman NA. On the mechanism of toluene-induced renal tubular acidosis. Nephron 1988;49:210–8.

[86] Cheng JT, Beysolow TD, Kaul B, et al. Clearance of ethylene glycol by kidneys and hemodialysis. J Toxicol Clin Toxicol 1987;25:95–108.

[87] Clay KL, Murphy RC. On the metabolic acidosis of ethylene glycol intoxication. Toxicol Appl Pharmacol 1977;39:39–49.

[88] Brent J, McMartin K, Phillips S, et al. Fomepizole for the treatment of ethylene glycol poisoning. N Engl J Med 1999;344:424–9.

[89] Jacobsen D, Hewlett TP, Webb R, et al. Ethylene glycol intoxication: evaluation of kinetics and crystalluria. Am J Med 1988;84:145–52.

[90] Gellerman GL, Martinez C. Fatal ventricular fibrillation following intravenous sodium diphenylhydantoin therapy. JAMA 1967;200:337–8.

[91] Unger AH, Sklaroff HJ. Fatalities following intravenous use of sodium diphenylhydantoin for cardiac arrhythmias. Report of two cases. JAMA 1967;200:335–6.

[92] Cate JC, Hedrick R. Propylene glycol intoxication and lactic acidosis. N Engl J Med 1980; 303:1237.

[93] Morshed KM, Jain SK, McMartin KE. Acute toxicity of propylene glycol: an assessment using cultured proximal tubule cells of human origin. Fundam Appl Toxicol 1994;23:38–43.

[94] Nakashima K, Yamashita T, Kashiwagi S, et al. The effect of sodium bicarbonate on CBF and intracellular pH in man: stable Xe-CT and 31P-MRS. Acta Neurol Scand Suppl 1996; 166:96–8.

[95] Sing RF, Branas CA. Bicarbonate therapy in the treatment of lactic acidosis: medicine or toxin? J Am Osteopath Assoc 1995;95:52–7.

[96] Bersin RM, Arieff AI. Improved hemodynamic function during hypoxia with Carbicarb, a new agent for the management of acidosis. Circulation 1988;77:227–33.

[97] Hill JB. Experimental salicylate poisoning: observations on the effects of altering blood pH on tissue and plasma salicylate concentrations. Pediatrics 1971;47:658–65.

[98] Reimold EW, Worthen HG, Reilly TP Jr. Salicylate poisoning. Comparison of acetazolamide administration and alkaline diuresis in the treatment of experimental salicylate intoxication in puppies. Am J Dis Child 1973;125:668–74.

[99] Hoffman JR, Votey SR, Bayer M, et al. Effect of hypertonic sodium bicarbonate in the treatment of moderate-to-severe cyclic antidepressant overdose. Am J Emerg Med 1993;11: 336–41.

[100] Pentel PR, Benowitz NL. Tricyclic antidepressant poisoning. Management of arrhythmias. Med Toxicol 1986;1:101–21.

[101] Smilkstein MJ. Reviewing cyclic antidepressant cardiotoxicity: wheat and chaff. J Emerg Med 1990;8:645–8.

[102] Smith EN, Taylor RT. Acute toxicity of methanol in the folate-deficient acatalasemic mouse. Toxicology 1982;25:271–87.

[103] Wason S, Lacouture PG, Lovejoy FH Jr. Single high-dose pyridoxine treatment for isoniazid overdose. JAMA 1981;246:1102–4.

[104] Howland MA. Pyridoxine. In: Goldfrank LR, Howland MA, Hoffman RS, et al, editors. Goldfrank's toxicologic emergencies. 7th edition. New York: McGraw-Hill; 2002. p. 2170.

[105] Beck JF, Bradbury CM, Connors AJ, et al. Nitrite as antidote for acute hydrogen sulfide intoxication? Am Ind Hyg Assoc J 1981;42:805–9.

[106] Hoidal CR, Hall AH, Robinson MD, et al. Hydrogen sulfide poisoning from toxic inhalations of roofing asphalt fumes. Ann Emerg Med 1986;15:826–30.

[107] Peters JW. Hydrogen sulfide poisoning in a hospital setting. JAMA 1981;246:1588–9.

[108] Stine RJ, Slosberg B, Beacham BE. Hydrogen sulfide intoxication. A case report and discussion of treatment. Ann Intern Med 1976;85:756–8.

ELSEVIER
SAUNDERS

Clin Lab Med 26 (2006) 49–65

CLINICS IN
LABORATORY
MEDICINE

Acetaminophen Poisoning

Adam K. Rowden, DO[a,*], Jeffrey Norvell, MD[b],
David L. Eldridge, MD, MA[c], Mark A. Kirk, MD[a]

[a]Division of Medical Toxicology, Department of Emergency Medicine,
University of Virginia, Charlottesville, VA, USA
[b]University of Missouri–Kansas City Truman Medical Center, Kansas City, MO, USA
[c]Department of Pediatrics, Brody School of Medicine, East Carolina University,
Greenville, NC, USA

In 2003, the American Association of Poison Control Centers reported more than 127,000 exposures involving acetaminophen (acetyl-para-aminophenol or APAP). Of these exposures, 65,000 patients received treatment in a medical facility, and 16,500 received N-acetylcysteine (NAC). There were 214 deaths involving overdose where an analgesic agent was thought to be primarily responsible. In 62 of these cases, APAP was the single agent involved [1]. APAP toxicity is also a major cause of fulminant hepatic failure (FHF) and is implicated in as many as 39% of cases presenting to tertiary care hospitals [2].

The objective of this current literature review is to enable the clinician to recognize which patients need to be treated for APAP toxicity. In addition, this article discusses NAC treatment protocols and provides clinicians with guidance in the selection of patients who would benefit from transfer to a tertiary care facility capable of liver transplantation.

Diagnosis

Prompt recognition of APAP toxicity is essential to preventing morbidity and mortality. This recognition is made difficult by the nonspecific clinical findings early in the course of APAP toxicity. The first 24 hours are considered the first phase of APAP poisoning and are characterized by

Portions of this article were previously published in Holstege CP, Rusyniak DE: Medical Toxicology. 89:6, Med Clin North Am, 2005; with permission.

* Corresponding author. Division of Medical Toxicology, Department of Emergency Medicine, 1222 Jefferson Park Avenue, 4th Floor, Room 4601, PO Box 800774, Charlottesville, VA 22908.

E-mail address: ar6r@virginia.edu (A.K. Rowden).

nonspecific findings, such as nausea, vomiting, anorexia, pallor, and lethargy. In this phase, however, the patient may appear normal. In the second phase of APAP poisoning, the patient begins to develop clinical and laboratory evidence of hepatotoxicity. Classically, it is taught that APAP-induced liver dysfunction occurs only after a latent period of 24 to 48 hours. However, Singer and colleagues [3] demonstrated that liver enzymes often become elevated in the initial 24 hours. In the third phase, the patient progresses to FHF with all its associated complications. Phase four, usually occurring 72 to 96 hours after ingestion, is the resolution of liver function and complete recovery if the patient survives the initial insult.

APAP toxicity should be suspected in all intentional overdoses because of the ubiquitous nature of APAP. The early symptoms of APAP ingestion are often vague or absent, leading to concern that potentially toxic ingestions could be missed owing to the poor histories often encountered in the overdose patient. To address this concern, several studies have attempted to evaluate the role of screening all intentional ingestions with serum APAP levels. Ashbourne and colleagues [4] found that, in patients without history of APAP ingestion, approximately 1 in 70 had detectable APAP levels and approximately 1 in 500 had potentially hepatotoxic APAP levels. A large retrospective study by Sporer and colleagues [5] found similar results: the rate of potentially hepatotoxic APAP levels in patients without history of ingestion was 0.3%.

Based on the wide availability of APAP, the low cost of quantitative APAP levels, and the potentially disastrous consequences of unrecognized APAP ingestion, all intentional overdoses should be screened for APAP toxicity. Since all overdose patients should be screened for APAP, it is equally important that all acute care facilities have the ability to rapidly run an APAP assay.

It should be noted the false positive APAP levels have been seen in patients with hyperbilirubinemia. The actual threshold for bilirubin's interference with the APAP assay is unclear. Because of the treatment and prognostic decisions that could follow a misdiagnosis of APAP induced hepatitis, caution is warranted and the clinician should be aware of this lab phenomenon [6,7].

APAP and histopathology

Predicatable histopathologic changes occur following acetaminophen poisoning. From autopsy and liver biopsy specimens, a characteristic pattern is observed in the liver [8–10]. Microscopic examination shows necrosis of the centrilobular hepatocytes. Associated findings include passive congestion, scattered mononucleated and polynucleated leukocytes and no fatty infiltration. Reticulin stain reveals maintenace of the hepatic architecture in areas of hepatocyte necrosis. In one case, a liver biopsy during the acute phase of an acetaminophen poisoning demonstrated the above changes. A wedge biopsy was obtained 4 years after that showed normal liver architecture and no fibrosis or cirrhosis [8]. However, additional fibrotic changes have been observed months after acute poisoning in association with chronic alcoholism [11]. The kidneys show diffuse acute tubular necrosis with tubular epithelial swelling and fatty vacuolization [9,10]. Autopsies have also demonstrated diffuse acute pancreatitis and diffuse cerebral edema with brainstem herniation [9,10].

Risk factors

Several populations of patients are at increased risk for hepatotoxicity from APAP. An understanding of the pathophysiology is necessary to evaluate the need for treatment in those who may be at increased risk.

With therapeutic dosing, 90% of APAP is conjugated with glucuronide or sulfate to form nontoxic metabolites. Approximately 5% of APAP is metabolized by the hepatic cytochrome p450 mixed-function oxidase enzyme to a toxic metabolite, N-acetyl-p-benzoquinoneimine (NAPQI). In normal dosing, NAPQI is rapidly detoxified by glutathione (GSH) to nontoxic metabolites. Acetaminophen overdoses overwhelm conjugation pathways, resulting in increased use of the cytochrome p450 pathway and increased formation of NAPQI, increased depletion of GSH, and, ultimately, hepatic injury. Because APAP is metabolized to its toxic metabolite, NAPQI, by the p450 system, any agent that induces this system theoretically increases the risk for APAP hepatotoxicity. However, few interactions have been reported or formally studied [12–16]. Ethanol is the best-studied inducer, with chronic alcohol ingestion inducing the p450 enzyme system and in turn making the liver capable of metabolizing more APAP to the toxic metabolite NAPQI. This interaction has been demonstrated in animal models, but its clinical relevance is unknown. Currently, chronic alcoholics who acutely ingest APAP should be treated in the same manner as other patients, by obtaining a 4-hour APAP level and plotting it on the nomogram [16–20].

Chronic alcoholics have been shown to have significantly lower levels of plasma GSH than controls: this may be a risk factor for APAP toxicity [20]. To investigate the influence of acute and chronic alcohol intake on the clinical course and outcome, one study looked at 209 patients who had an acute APAP overdose. This study showed that, after one has corrected for all other factors, chronic alcohol intake is associated with a fivefold increase in the relative risk of developing hepatic encephalopathy. The study was unable, however, to demonstrate a significant change in mortality [21].

Because alcohol and APAP are metabolized by the same enzymes system, some have speculated that they may competitively inhibit each other's metabolism. Acute alcohol intake does not independently influence the clinical course of APAP overdose in humans [21]. By contrast, some animal studies have shown a marginal benefit from acute alcohol ingestion in APAP overdoses [12,22,23]. The clinical significance of acute alcohol ingestion is probably minimal and should not affect treatment decisions.

Specific drugs metabolized by the p450 system may theoretically play a role in the formation of NAPQI. For example, isoniazid is often implicated as an inducer of the p450 system and thereby may play a role in APAP toxicity [24–28]. APAP is metabolized through a specific subset of enzymes (CYP2E) in the p450 system, and only drugs actually inducing this subset of enzymes affect the formation of NAPQI [16].

GSH is essential for the detoxification of NAPQI. Patients who are at increased risk for APAP hepatotoxicity also include those with decreased GSH stores. The most common reason for decreased GSH stores is malnutrition—for example, anorexia nervosa [29] and chronic alcoholism [19]. Reports also exist of APAP-induced hepatotoxicity associated with fasting from febrile illnesses and chronic disease [30,31]. These risk factors do not appear to play a major role in acute ingestions but may play an important one in nonacute ingestions.

Treatment

The Rumack-Mathew treatment nomogram is the primary tool used to guide treatment after acute ingestion of APAP. A firm understanding of the nomogram's use and its limitations is essential in the management of APAP exposure. The nomogram was first studied retrospectively in 64 cases of acute ingestion of APAP in an attempt to correlate APAP serum levels with hepatotoxicity. Hepatotoxicity was arbitrarily defined as an aspartate aminotransferase (AST) level of 1000 IU/L. Serum APAP levels at or above a line connecting 200 µg/mL at 4 hours postingestion and 6.25 µg/mL at 24 hours postingestion consistently predicted hepatotoxicity [32]. This line is referred to as the probable toxicity line. In Europe, a level above this line is an indication for NAC therapy. When the nomogram was introduced in the United States, the US Food and Drug Administration (FDA) insisted on a 25% reduction of this treatment threshold. A line connecting 150 µg/mL at 4 hours and 4.7 µg/mL at 24 hours, which is considered the possible toxicity line, is used for a treatment threshold [16]. The nomogram was later validated in a large trial using the 72-hour NAC protocol [33].

Acute poisoning, which has not been well defined in the literature, is generally regarded as a single ingestion of APAP over less than a 4-hour time period. The Rumack-Mathew nomogram can only be used to determine the need for NAC treatment after an acute ingestion [16]. All other ingestions are not applicable to the nomogram. Typically, the potentially toxic dose is 150 mg/kg, or 15 g in the healthy adult [34]. These doses would correspond to a potentially toxic level on the nomogram.

After an acute ingestion, the serum APAP levels should be drawn 4 hours after ingestion or at any time thereafter and plotted on the nomogram. Patients with APAP levels falling above the possible toxicity line should be treated with NAC. The period of 4 hours after ingestion was arbitrarily chosen to assume full absorption and a peak serum APAP level [16].

The time of ingestion is an essential piece of history when plotting levels on the nomogram. However, the exact time of ingestion is not always clear. Patients' histories are frequently unreliable or intentionally misleading. When possible, it is helpful to corroborate a patient's history with a third party. The earliest possible time of ingestion should be used when no reliable history is available. When in doubt, treatment with NAC is always the safest option when the time of ingestion remains uncertain.

Patients who present late after acute APAP ingestion may present some difficulties in determining the need for NAC therapy, because, as the time after ingestion approaches 24 hours, the treatment line on the nomogram approaches the lower limits of detection of some laboratories. In these cases, the need for NAC treatment is determined using a serum APAP, AST, and ALT levels, along with the patient's reported amount of ingestion (usually > 7.5 g in an adult or 140 mg/kg in a child [33]) and the patient's risk factors for APAP toxicity. If APAP is detectable, it should be plotted on the nomogram, and treatment should follow if indicated. When APAP is undetectable and AST and ALT are elevated, it should be assumed that the patient is in the second clinical phase of APAP toxicity, and NAC therapy should be initiated. In patients who have undetectable APAP and normal AST and ALT, NAC may probably be safely withheld. Concern exists that impending APAP-induced hepatotoxicity may be preceded by a brief window of time, 24 hours after ingestion but before AST and ALT begin to rise, in which APAP is undetectable and AST and ALT are normal. Such cases are not reported in the literature. However, because of this theoretic concern, some physicians institute NAC therapy in patients who are at increased risk for APAP-induced hepatotoxicity despite normal laboratory values.

Originally, it was believed that NAC therapy was ineffective when started after 15 hours; therefore, it was frequently withheld from late presenters [34–37]. It has since been shown that NAC provides significant benefit to patients presenting with APAP-induced FHF regardless of the time after ingestion [38,39], and it is recommended in any patient with APAP-induced elevations in liver enzymes.

Tylenol Extended Relief

Acute ingestion of Tylenol Extended Relief (TER) is another challenging problem. TER is available in 650-mg caplets intended to provide 325 mg of immediate release and 325 mg more slowly. Because of delayed absorption and possible delayed time to peak serum concentration, the standard 4-hour APAP level plotted on the nomogram may not be a reliable predictor of toxicity.

If an initial 4-hour level falls above the treatment line, NAC therapy should be initiated and further APAP levels are not necessary. If an initial

4-hour APAP serum level falls below the treatment line, obtaining a repeat level at 6 hours should be considered; if a second level falls above the treatment line, NAC therapy should be started [40,41]. Cases have been reported where APAP levels crossed the treatment line as late as 14 hours after ingestion, but their clinical significance is not fully understood [40,42–44]. These case reports suggest the need to check multiple APAP levels in patients who have ingested extended-release formulations; however, other authors have suggested that their pharmacokinetics are so similar to those of regular-release formulations that no change in standard protocol is needed [45].

Nonacute overdoses

Nonacute ingestions of APAP, frequently referred to as subacute or chronic, are ingestions that take place over a period longer than 4 hours. In these cases, the nomogram offers no guidance in treatment, because it is intended only for use with acute ingestions. Furthermore, few studies exist to guide management or determine who warrants screening, making management of nonacute ingestions problematic.

Most cases of nonacute ingestion of APAP that result in hepatotoxicity involve persons taking supratherapeutic doses who are at increased risk for APAP-induced hepatotoxicity [31,46–48]. Based on these observations, a reasonable approach to screening would take into account the overall APAP dosage per day (usually > the manufacturer-recommended 4 g and typically >10 g per day [19,49]) and the existence of risk factors for hepatotoxicity (see previous discussion). In patients where there is concern about possible toxicity from nonacute ingestion of APAP, a serum level along with AST and ALT should be drawn. Patients with detectable APAP or abnormal AST and ALT should be treated with a course of NAC. In patients who have excessive dosing or who have increased risk factors for APAP-induced hepatotoxicity, treatment may be warranted despite normal laboratory testing.

Two small studies provide data to support this approach. In a prospective, observational study of nonacute APAP ingestion, Daly and colleagues [48] found that no patient with chronic APAP ingestion and an AST below 50 IU at presentation went on to develop hepatotoxicity, whereas 15% of those with an AST between 50 and 1000 IU at presentation went on to develop hepatotoxicity. This study has limitations: it reported on a small number of patients, 50% of the normal AST group received NAC therapy, it had no standard treatment protocol, and risk factors were not addressed. A smaller study by Kozer and colleagues [47] found similar results in children but had the same limitations. Despite the studies' limitations, these data support the approach outlined by these authors for chronic APAP ingestions until further prospective studies can be done.

Mechanism of action of N-acetylcysteine

NAC has two roles in the treatment of APAP toxicity. In patients who present <8 hours after ingestion, NAC has preventive mechanisms that rapidly detoxify toxic metabolites or prevent their formation. In patients who already manifest laboratory and clinical evidence of APAP-induced hepatic injury, NAC appears to have secondary mechanisms that improve overall patient outcomes; these are far less effective than its primary effects and are poorly understood.

NAC is an extremely effective antidote when administered within 8 hours after ingestion of a potentially toxic dose of APAP [32–34,37,50,51]. NAC is a precursor of GSH and increases GSH synthesis [52]. Animal models show that significant hepatotoxicity does not occur until total body stores of GSH fall to 30% of baseline [53]. Because it takes a significant time to deplete body stores of GSH, NAC is equally effective whether started immediately after ingestion or within 8 hours.

Ample supplies of GSH, which may be secured by NAC administration, ensure that NAPQI will bind to the thiol groups of GSH instead of binding to hepatocytes. Once the thiol group is bound to NAPQI, it produces cysteine and mercapturic acid conjugates, which are no longer reactive and pose less danger to the liver cells [52,54]. NAC also appears to increase the sulfation of APAP to nontoxic metabolites [55] and may reverse the formation of NAPQI [14].

Clear evidence now exists that NAC is effective no matter how late the therapy is initiated or how profoundly the patient appears to have suffered clinical toxic effects [38]. Improved oxygen delivery by means of increased hepato-splanchnic circulation and increased oxygen extraction have been proposed as mechanisms to explain improved outcomes of late presenters treated with NAC [56–58], but these mechanisms have also been disputed [59]. Improved cerebral blood flow has been demonstrated with NAC therapy [60]. Reversal of the covalent bond between NAPQI and hepatocytes and decreased protein arylation of specific hepatocyte proteins have been reported with NAC administration [61]. A protective antioxidant effect of NAC against oxidative stress has also been reported [62,63], but some evidence suggests that the effect is minimal [64,65], and no human data exist to support a clinical benefit. Another mechanism of NAC's effectiveness may be its limitation of lipid peroxidation, which has been established in mice as another hepatotoxic effect of APAP ingestion [66].

Duration of N-acetylcysteine therapy

Once the decision to treat with NAC is made, the clinician must decide how long to continue therapy. This decision is complicated by the existence of several published protocols, varying in length from 20 to 72 hours.

For more than 20 years in Europe, Australia, and Canada, the standard treatment for potentially toxic APAP ingestions has been 20 hours of intravenous (IV) NAC. In this 20-hour protocol, NAC is administered as a loading dose of 150 mg/kg over 15 minutes, followed by 50 mg/kg of NAC infused over 4 hours. Over the remaining 16 hours, an additional 100 mg/kg are administered as a constant infusion [34]. Several studies and a long clinical experience validate this protocol as both safe and effective [50]. In 2004, the US FDA approved this same 20-hour protocol for use in the United States [67].

In the United States, before 2004, the standard treatment for APAP toxicity was a 72-hour protocol of oral NAC. Under the FDA approval, the oral dosing protocol of NAC is a 140 mg/kg loading dose followed by a maintenance dose of 70 mg/kg every 4 hours for 17 more doses. Given that nausea and vomiting are reported in 33% of APAP overdoses before NAC and in an estimated 51% during oral NAC therapy [68], vomiting within 1 hour of dosing requires a repeat dose. This protocol has been well studied and found to be both safe and effective, and, until recently, it was the only FDA-approved treatment for APAP toxicity in the United States [16,33,37]. A 48-hour IV protocol [69] and a 36-hour oral protocol [70] have also been described. Both have been found to be safe and effective but are not widely used. Given the recent approval of the 20-hour IV protocol in the United States and the body of evidence to support both 20-hour and 72-hour protocols, it is unlikely that these intermediate protocols will receive much more attention.

The 72-hour oral, 48-hour IV, and 20-hour IV protocols have been compared by retrospective study and through meta-analysis [71]. When started within 8 hours of ingestion, no protocol shows advantage over another. Although there is general consensus that IV administration is preferable in the face of intractable vomiting, no study shows clear evidence that IV therapy is more or less effective than oral NAC therapy [71,72].

In cases of presentation after 8 hours, the 72- and 48-hour protocols appear to have an advantage over the 20-hour IV protocol [71]. Some evidence suggests that longer courses of NAC are more effective in late presenters, especially in the face of FHF [33,39]. In cases with documented elevation in AST and ALT, NAC therapy should be continued indefinitely until significant improvement, liver transplantation, or death [38].

Oral versus intravenous N-acetylcysteine

Until recently, the decision to use IV NAC was complicated by the lack of an FDA-approved preparation for IV administration. Traditionally, the oral NAC solution was diluted in 5% dextrose (D5W) and administered by the IV route through a filter. In 2004, Acetadote became the first NAC solution approved by the FDA for IV use, allowing the United States to join the rest of the industrialized world, which has been using IV NAC since its introduction in 1977. It should be noted that dosing miscalculations occur more frequently with IV dosing and appear to be associated with more serious adverse reactions [73].

Although serious adverse drug reactions (ADR) have been reported with the use of IV NAC, they appear to be rare. Oral NAC has been reported to cause ADR at a lower rate than IV therapy. Most ADR appear to be anaphylactoid in nature and are dose- and rate-related [74,75]. ADR tend to occur during the initial loading dose. The overall rate of ADR from IV NAC ranges from 3% to 25% in most studies; however, one recent small prospective study found the rate of ADR to approach 50% [76]. Children, although less thoroughly studied, appear to have a similar incidence of ADR [77].

Nausea and vomiting are frequently reported ADR with IV NAC therapy [71,72,74–76,78,79]. Antiemetics and IV maintenance fluids are the only treatment required, and the infusion should be continued if no other reactions are observed. Because these symptoms are expected in the natural course of APAP toxicity, it is difficult to separate typical APAP poisoning from ADR associated with antidote therapy. Because most studies include nausea and vomiting as ADR, the true rate of ADR may actually be lower than reported.

The most common reported ADR are cutaneous skin reactions, but more serious ADR, such as bronchospasm, angioedema, and hypotension, have been reported. Treatment of cutaneous reactions by stopping the NAC infusion and administering antihistamines is usually adequate. The NAC infusion may usually be restarted at a slower rate after the reaction has subsided without further incident [79]. More serious, systemic reactions have been reported, including bronchospasm, angioedema, hypotension, and even death, but these are unusual [73,74,80]. A past medical history of asthma does not appear to predict the risk of bronchospasm [78]. Reactive airway disease should be treated in the usual manner with nebulized bronchodilators and systemic corticosteroids after discontinuation of the NAC infusion. The more serious ADR of angioedema and hypotension require the clinician to pay special attention to the patient's airway, breathing, and circulation.

After any adverse reaction, a critical reassessment of the need for NAC therapy is warranted. If treatment is still indicated, evidence shows that restarting the infusion is safe [79]. The infusion is customarily restarted at a slower rate, based on the belief that the ADR are anaphylactoid and rate- and dose-related. Recurrence of ADR is rare but has been reported [79].

Although an FDA-approved NAC preparation now exists, it may not be available in some centers. Because oral NAC is effective and widely available, it will likely continue to be used to treat APAP toxicity. The clinician may be faced with the challenge of treating a patient who cannot tolerate oral NAC and for whom there is no IV NAC immediately available. In this situation, oral NAC may generally be considered safe to administer by way of IV. Dribben and colleagues [81] prospectively evaluated oral NAC suspensions and found them to be safe, sterile, and stable. Moreover, a considerable body of evidence shows that IV use of oral NAC is both safe and effective in clinical practice [78]. However, it is important to note that in all these studies the oral NAC was filtered before use.

Prognosis

Patients who are APAP poisoned have a wide spectrum of clinical presentations. Most present in the first 8 hours and before any signs of hepatotoxicity develop. ICU resources are limited and are not necessary for many APAP-poisoned patients. Close observation for progression of serious toxicity is the most common reason for critical care use. Most patients do not require critical care resources for invasive procedures. Patients who exhibit signs of serious hepatotoxicity, such as coagulopathy, encephalopathy, and metabolic derangements, will likely benefit from the ICU and may need invasive procedures. Patients who have renal failure or other end-organ effects are also candidates for the ICU. Patients who have coingestants with a potential for serious toxic effects may also need close monitoring.

NAC therapy is not an indication for critical care admission. Asymptomatic patients presenting early after ingestion may be cared for on a general ward unless concerns about suicide or self-harm warrant otherwise.

It is important for the clinician to identify patients at increased risk for FHF so as to begin the process of transfer to a specialized center should hepatic transplant become necessary. Although the AST and ALT levels are frequently the first laboratory sign of liver injury in APAP toxicity, the rate of rise and peak level give no indication of prognosis. A collection of clinical parameters and laboratory findings known as the King's College Criteria have been established and well validated to predict poor outcome from APAP toxicity. Patients who have isolated APAP overdoses and develop significant metabolic acidosis (pH < 7.3 after adequate fluid resuscitation), a serum creatinine > 3.3 mg/dL, a prothrombin time > 1.8 times control (> 100 seconds or an international normalized ratio [INR] > 6.5), or grade III or higher encephalopathy have a poorer prognosis [82]. Any patient meeting any one of these criteria should be transferred to a tertiary care center in anticipation of FHF and possible transplantation [82]. These criteria have also been validated by subsequent studies [83–85].

The King's College Criteria (KCC) are well established, but they are not without their limitations. With the exception of fluid resuscitation, therapeutic interventions affecting these criteria may negate their predictive value. However, once criteria are met, further intervention is no longer problematic. For instance, creatinine levels of 3.3 mg/dL or greater already put the patient at higher risk; hence subsequent measurements with or without dialysis are irrelevant.

Monitoring of coagulopathy is also problematic. To establish a rise in prothrombin time, serial levels must be drawn, a process that again may delay identification of patients at risk for FHF. In one series, a prothrombin time > 180 at 4 days was highly suggestive of death [86]. Although this may provide useful information to the liver transplant service, waiting 4 days before transfer to a tertiary center is clearly not beneficial to the patient. The original KCC were developed before the widespread use of the INR, which makes comparison among prothrombin times difficult.

Reported cases also exist of prolongation of prothrombin time without clinical or laboratory signs of hepatotoxicity [87]. In fact, in both retrospective and small prospective studies, prothrombin time prolongation appeared to correlate with IV NAC use rather than hepatic failure [88–90]. This rise in INR without overt FHF may be due, in part, to decreased factor VII levels [88].

Coagulopathy in the face of FHF, and the associated increase in INR, is due to the reduction of clotting factors. The admission ratio of factor VIII to factor V, and the overall concentration of factor V have both been found to be helpful in predictors of outcome. Factor V levels less than 10 percent were a poor prognostic findings. A factor VIII/V ratio of greater than 30 is also a poor prognostic sign [91]. Because of these observations, some recommend factor monitoring [87]. While this may be useful for the transplant team, it should not be relied upon as a screening tool.

Treatment of coagulopathy can be accomplished with administration of FFP. While many clinicians treat this coagulopathy without signs of bleeding, there is evidence that it is safe to withhold treatment in APAP induced coagulopathy. Gazzard et al compared two groups with APAP induced coagulopathy. The control group was treated with FFP while the experimental group was not unless the INR was over 7. There was no difference in outcome or complications. In the face of bleeding FFP and factor administration is necessary, but with bleeding, it may be possible to with hold blood products [92].

The limitations of the KCC have led to a search for other screening tools. Although many parameters have been suggested and evaluated in small numbers, none are currently as well established or widely used as the KCC.

The acute physiology and chronic health evaluation II (APACHE II) score has shown promise as an early and accurate indicator of impending hepatic failure and the need for transplantation [93]. In a small study, this evaluation was found to be more sensitive and specific than KCC. It was based on patient assessment on the first day of hospital admission, making it possible to determine the need for transplant referral at an earlier time. The disadvantage of the APACHE is that it is cumbersome and difficult to remember. Although this evaluation is intriguing, further study is required.

Changes in serum phosphate levels have been suggested as a prognostic indicator in APAP-induced hepatotoxicity. One prospective study looking at 125 patients who had suspicion of severe APAP-induced hepatotoxicity evaluated the prognostic value of serial serum phosphate measurements [94]. The study revealed that a serum phosphate level >1.2 mmol/L 48 to 96 hours after an APAP overdose specifically and sensitively identifies patients with little chance of survival. The authors hypothesize that the liver consumes phosphate during hepatic regeneration. Thus, phosphate levels represent a balance of renal failure and liver regeneration. Similar findings in patients who have FHF have been reported [95]; however, other studies show mixed results [96]. Further study is needed to clarify the role of phosphate as a prognostic indicator.

Elevated arterial lactate has been proposed as a prognostic marker for poor outcomes in APAP overdose. A retrospective cohort study revealed that lactate levels >3.5 mmol/L before fluid resuscitation or >3.0 mmol/L after fluid resuscitation were sensitive and specific indicators of survival [97]. A subsequent prospective cohort study was performed for validation [97]. Comparison with the KCC revealed that early lactate levels >3.5 mmol/L identified at-risk patients earlier but had a lower sensitivity and accuracy than the KCC criteria. Postresuscitation lactate concentrations >3.0 mmol/L had equivalent sensitivity and higher specificity and accuracy than the KCC criteria. However, there was no significant difference in time to identification of patients between KCC criteria and postresuscitation lactate [97].

Recently, investigators have shown interest in hyperamylasemia as a possible prognostic indicator in APAP toxicity. A large retrospective study at a Danish referral center found amylase levels >1.5 times normal to correlate with poor outcome and the need for transplantation. Hyperamylasemia did not appear to be due to clinical pancreatitis; however, speciation of the amylase was not performed [98]. Prospective validation of amylase with speciation is needed.

Although it does not directly predict the need for transplantation, a novel approach using easily measurable criteria has been prospectively used to predict encephalopathy in APAP toxicity. Time to NAC therapy, platelet count, and INR are used to determine a prognostic index [99]. Because hepatic encephalopathy requires specialized care, referral based on these criteria may prove useful.

Level of alfa-fetoprotein (AFP) be used to predict favorable outcome in APAP induced FHF. A small increase in AFP one day after peak of ALT was found in survivors compared to non-survivors. Because this increase was small, a highly sensitive assay is required to make reliable predictions [100].

Summary

APAP is likely to remain a common toxic exposure and continue to cause significant morbidity and mortality. To minimize the harm to patients, it is necessary for the clinician to be aware of the current diagnostic and therapeutic management of APAP poisoning. Despite the bulk of literature on APAP, management strategies are likely to continue to change as more studies are conducted to improve our understanding of nonacute ingestions and the role of prognostic markers in defining those most at risk for life-threatening hepatotoxicity.

References

[1] Watson WA, Litovitz TL, Klein-Schwartz W, et al. 2003 annual report of the American Association of Poison Control Centers Toxic Exposure Surveillance System. Am J Emerg Med 2004;22(5):335–404.

[2] Ostapowicz G, Fontana RJ, Schiodt FV, et al. Results of a prospective study of acute liver failure at 17 tertiary care centers in the United States. Ann Intern Med 2002; 137(12):947–54.

[3] Singer AJ, Carracio TR, Mofenson HC. The temporal profile of increased transaminase levels in patients with acetaminophen-induced liver dysfunction. Ann Emerg Med 1995; 26(1):49–53.

[4] Ashbourne JF, Olson KR, Khayam-Bashi H. Value of rapid screening for acetaminophen in all patients with intentional drug overdose. Ann Emerg Med 1989;18(10): 1035–8.

[5] Sporer KA, Khayam-Bashi H. Acetaminophen and salicylate serum levels in patients with suicidal ingestion or altered mental status. Am J Emerg Med 1996;14(5):443–6.

[6] Bertholf RL, Johannsen LM, Bazooband A, et al. False-positive acetaminophen results in a hyperbilirubinemic patient. Clin Chem 2003;49(4):695–8.

[7] Beuhler MC, Curry SC. False Positive acetaminophen levels associated with hyperbilirubinemia. Clin Toxicol (Phila) 2005;43(3):167–70.

[8] Baeg NJ, Bodenheimer HC Jr, et al. Long-term sequellae of acetaminophen-associated fulfminant hepatic failure: relevance of early histology. Am J Gastroenterol 1988;83(5): 569–71.

[9] Blake KV, Beiley D, Zientek GM, et al. Death of a child associated with multiple overdoses of acetaminophen. Clin Pharm 1988;7(5):391–7.

[10] McJunkin B, Barwick KW, Little WC, et al. Fatal Massive hepatic necrosis following acetaminophen overdose. Jama 1976;236(16):1874–5.

[11] O'Dell JR, Zetterman RK, Burnett DA. Centilobular hepatic fibrosis following acetaminophen-induced hepatic necrosis in an alcoholic. Jama 1986;255(19):2636–7.

[12] Thummel KE, Slattery JT, Ro H, et al. Ethanol and production of the hepatotoxic metabolite of acetaminophen in healthy adults. Clin Pharmacol Ther 2000;67(6):591–9.

[13] Rumack BH. Acetaminophen misconceptions. Hepatology 2004;40(1):10–5.

[14] Corcoran GB, Mitchell JR, Vaishnav YN, et al. Evidence that acetaminophen and N-hydroxyacetaminophen form a common arylating intermediate, N-acetyl-p-benzoquinoneimine. Mol Pharmacol 1980;18(3):536–42.

[15] Mitchell JR, Corcoran GB, Smith CV, et al. Alkylation and peroxidation injury from chemically reactive metabolites. Adv Exp Med Biol 1981;136(Pt A):199–223.

[16] Rumack BH. Acetaminophen hepatotoxicity: the first 35 years. J Toxicol Clin Toxicol 2002;40(1):3–20.

[17] Tredger JM, Smith HM, Read RB, et al. Effects of ethanol ingestion on the metabolism of a hepatotoxic dose of paracetamol in mice. Xenobiotica 1986;16(7):661–70.

[18] Seeff LB, Cuccherini BA, Zimmerman HJ, et al. Acetaminophen hepatotoxicity in alcoholics. A therapeutic misadventure. Ann Intern Med 1986;104(3):399–404.

[19] Whitcomb DC, Block GD. Association of acetaminophen hepatotoxicity with fasting and ethanol use. JAMA 1994;272(23):1845–50.

[20] Lauterburg BH, Velez ME. Glutathione deficiency in alcoholics: risk factor for paracetamol hepatotoxicity. Gut 1988;29(9):1153–7.

[21] Schiodt FV, Lee WM, Bondesen S, et al. Influence of acute and chronic alcohol intake on the clinical course and outcome in acetaminophen overdose. Aliment Pharmacol Ther 2002; 16(4):707–15.

[22] Wong LT, Whitehouse LW, Solomonraj G, et al. Effect of a concomitant single dose of ethanol on the hepatotoxicity and metabolism of acetaminophen in mice. Toxicology 1980; 17(3):297–309.

[23] Sato C, Nakano M, Lieber CS. Prevention of acetaminophen-induced hepatotoxicity by acute ethanol administration in the rat: comparison with carbon tetrachloride–induced hepatoxicity. J Pharmacol Exp Ther 1981;218(3):805–10.

[24] Bray GP, Harrison PM, O'Grady JG, et al. Long-term anticonvulsant therapy worsens outcome in paracetamol-induced fulminant hepatic failure. Hum Exp Toxicol 1992;11(4): 265–70.

[25] Zand R, Nelson SD, Slattery JT, et al. Inhibition and induction of cytochrome P4502E1–catalyzed oxidation by isoniazid in humans. Clin Pharmacol Ther 1993;54(2):142–9.

[26] Murphy R, Swartz R, Watkins PB. Severe acetaminophen toxicity in a patient receiving isoniazid. Ann Intern Med 1990;113(10):799–800.

[27] Epstein MM, Nelson SD, Slattery JT, et al. Inhibition of the metabolism of paracetamol by isoniazid. Br J Clin Pharmacol 1991;31(2):139–42.

[28] Brackett CC, Bloch JD. Phenytoin as a possible cause of acetaminophen hepatotoxicity: case report and review of the literature. Pharmacotherapy 2000;20(2):229–33.

[29] Zenger F, Russmann S, Junker E, et al. Decreased glutathione in patients with anorexia nervosa. Risk factor for toxic liver injury? Eur J Clin Nutr 2004;58(2):238–43.

[30] Henretig FM, Selbst SM, Forrest C, et al. Repeated acetaminophen overdosing. Causing hepatotoxicity in children. Clinical reports and literature review. Clin Pediatr (Phila) 1989; 28(11):525–8.

[31] Kurtovic J, Riordan SM. Paracetamol-induced hepatotoxicity at recommended dosage. J Intern Med 2003;253(2):240–3.

[32] Rumack BH, Matthew H. Acetaminophen poisoning and toxicity. Pediatrics 1975;55(6): 871–6.

[33] Smilkstein MJ, Knapp GL, Kulig KW, et al. Efficacy of oral N-acetylcysteine in the treatment of acetaminophen overdose. Analysis of the national multicenter study (1976 to 1985). N Engl J Med 1988;319(24):1557–62.

[34] Prescott LF, Illingworth RN, Critchley JA, et al. Intravenous N-acetylcysteine: the treatment of choice for paracetamol poisoning. BMJ 1979;2(6198):1097–100.

[35] Peterson RG, Rumack BH. Toxicity of acetaminophen overdose. JACEP 1978;7(5):202–5.

[36] Prescott LF. Treatment of severe acetaminophen poisoning with intravenous acetylcysteine. Arch Intern Med 1981;141(3 Spec No):386–9.

[37] Rumack BH, Peterson RC, Koch GG, et al. Acetaminophen overdose. 662 cases with evaluation of oral acetylcysteine treatment. Arch Intern Med 1981;141(3 Spec No):380–5.

[38] Keays R, Harrison PM, Wendon JA, et al. Intravenous acetylcysteine in paracetamol induced fulminant hepatic failure: a prospective controlled trial. BMJ 1991;303(6809): 1026–9.

[39] Harrison PM, Keays R, Bray GP, et al. Improved outcome of paracetamol-induced fulminant hepatic failure by late administration of acetylcysteine. Lancet 1990;335(8705): 1572–3.

[40] Cetaruk EW, Dart RC, Horowitz RS, et al. Extended-release acetaminophen overdose. JAMA 1996;275(9):686.

[41] Temple AR. Dear Doctor, Tylenol ER letter [product insert]. Fort Washington (PA): McNeil Consumer Products Company; 1995.

[42] Vassallo S, Khan ANGA, Howland MA. Use of the Rumack-Matthew nomogram in cases of extended-release acetaminophen toxicity. Ann Intern Med 1996;125(11):940.

[43] Cetaruk EW, Dart RC, Hurlbut KM, et al. Tylenol Extended Relief overdose. Ann Emerg Med 1997;30(1):104–8.

[44] Bizovi KE, Aks SE, Paloucek F, et al. Late increase in acetaminophen concentration after overdose of Tylenol Extended Relief. Ann Emerg Med 1996;28(5):549–51.

[45] Douglas DR, Sholar JB, Smilkstein MJ. A pharmacokinetic comparison of acetaminophen products (Tylenol Extended Relief vs regular Tylenol). Acad Emerg Med 1996;3(8):740–4.

[46] Mathis RD, Walker JS, Kuhns DW. Subacute acetaminophen overdose after incremental dosing. J Emerg Med 1988;6(1):37–40.

[47] Kozer E, Barr J, Bulkowstein M, et al. A prospective study of multiple supratherapeutic acetaminophen doses in febrile children. Vet Hum Toxicol 2002;44(2):106–9.

[48] Daly FF, O'Malley GF, Heard K, et al. Prospective evaluation of repeated supratherapeutic acetaminophen (paracetamol) ingestion. Ann Emerg Med 2004;44(4):393–8.

[49] Kuffner EK, Dart RC, Bogdan GM, et al. Effect of maximal daily doses of acetaminophen on the liver of alcoholic patients: a randomized, double-blind, placebo-controlled trial. Arch Intern Med 2001;161(18):2247–52.

[50] Prescott LF, Illingworth RN, Critchley JA, et al. Intravenous N-acetylcysteine: still the treatment of choice for paracetamol poisoning. BMJ 1980;280(6206):46–7.

[51] Peterson RG, Rumack BH. N-acetylcysteine for acetaminophen overdosage (cont.). N Engl J Med 1977;296(9):515.

[52] Lauterburg BH, Corcoran GB, Mitchell JR. Mechanism of action of N-acetylcysteine in the protection against the hepatotoxicity of acetaminophen in rats in vivo. J Clin Invest 1983; 71(4):980–91.

[53] Mitchell JR, Thorgeirsson SS, Potter WZ, et al. Acetaminophen-induced hepatic injury: protective role of glutathione in man and rationale for therapy. Clin Pharmacol Ther 1974; 16(4):676–84.

[54] Buckpitt AR, Rollins DE, Mitchell JR. Varying effects of sulfhydryl nucleophiles on acetaminophen oxidation and sulfhydryl adduct formation. Biochem Pharmacol 1979; 28(19):2941–6.

[55] Slattery JT, Wilson JM, Kalhorn TF, et al. Dose-dependent pharmacokinetics of acetaminophen: evidence of glutathione depletion in humans. Clin Pharmacol Ther 1987; 41(4):413–8.

[56] Spies CD, Reinhart K, Witt I, et al. Influence of N-acetylcysteine on indirect indicators of tissue oxygenation in septic shock patients: results from a prospective, randomized, double-blind study. Crit Care Med 1994;22(11):1738–46.

[57] Harrison PM, Wendon JA, Gimson AE, et al. Improvement by acetylcysteine of hemodynamics and oxygen transport in fulminant hepatic failure. N Engl J Med 1991; 324(26):1852–7.

[58] Devlin J, Ellis AE, McPeake J, et al. N-acetylcysteine improves indocyanine green extraction and oxygen transport during hepatic dysfunction. Crit Care Med 1997;25(2): 236–42.

[59] Walsh TS, Hopton P, Philips BJ, et al. The effect of N-acetylcysteine on oxygen transport and uptake in patients with fulminant hepatic failure. Hepatology 1998;27(5):1332–40.

[60] Wendon JA, Harrison PM, Keays R, et al. Cerebral blood flow and metabolism in fulminant liver failure. Hepatology 1994;19(6):1407–13.

[61] Bruno MK, Cohen SD, Khairallah EA. Antidotal effectiveness of N-acetylcysteine in reversing acetaminophen-induced hepatotoxicity. Enhancement of the proteolysis of arylated proteins. Biochem Pharmacol 1988;37(22):4319–25.

[62] Cuzzocrea S, Costantino G, Mazzon E, et al. Protective effect of N-acetylcysteine on multiple organ failure induced by zymosan in the rat. Crit Care Med 1999;27(8): 1524–32.

[63] Bajt ML, Knight TR, Lemasters JJ, et al. Acetaminophen-induced oxidant stress and cell injury in cultured mouse hepatocytes: protection by N-acetyl cysteine. Toxicol Sci 2004; 80(2):343–9.

[64] Lewerenz V, Hanelt S, Nastevska C, et al. Antioxidants protect primary rat hepatocyte cultures against acetaminophen-induced DNA strand breaks but not against acetaminophen-induced cytotoxicity. Toxicology 2003;191(2–3):179–87.

[65] Brent JA, Rumack BH. Role of free radicals in toxic hepatic injury. II. Are free radicals the cause of toxin-induced liver injury? J Toxicol Clin Toxicol 1993;31(1):173–96.

[66] Knight TR, Fariss MW, Farhood A, et al. Role of lipid peroxidation as a mechanism of liver injury after acetaminophen overdose in mice. Toxicol Sci 2003;76(1):229–36.

[67] Acetadote package insert. Nashville (TN): Cumberland Pharmaceuticals; 2004.

[68] Miller LF, Rumack BH. Clinical safety of high oral doses of acetylcysteine. Semin Oncol 1983;10(1 Suppl 1):76–85.

[69] Smilkstein MJ, Bronstein AC, Linden C, et al. Acetaminophen overdose: a 48-hour intravenous N-acetylcysteine treatment protocol. Ann Emerg Med 1991;20(10):1058–63.

[70] Woo OF, Mueller PD, Olson KR, et al. Shorter duration of oral N-acetylcysteine therapy for acute acetaminophen overdose. Ann Emerg Med 2000;35(4):363–8.

[71] Buckley NA, Whyte IM, O'Connell DL, et al. Oral or intravenous N-acetylcysteine: which is the treatment of choice for acetaminophen (paracetamol) poisoning? J Toxicol Clin Toxicol 1999;37(6):759–67.

[72] Taylor SE. Acetaminophen intoxication and length of treatment: how long is long enough?—A comment. Pharmacotherapy 2004;24(5):694–6 [discussion: 696].

[73] Mant TG, Tempowski JH, Volans GN, et al. Adverse reactions to acetylcysteine and effects of overdose. Br Med J (Clin Res Ed) 1984;289(6439):217–9.

[74] Yip L, Dart RC, Hurlbut KM. Intravenous administration of oral N-acetylcysteine. Crit Care Med 1998;26(1):40–3.

[75] Bailey B, Amre DK, Gaudreault P. Fulminant hepatic failure secondary to acetaminophen poisoning: a systematic review and meta-analysis of prognostic criteria determining the need for liver transplantation. Crit Care Med 2003;31(1):299–305.

[76] Lynch RM, Robertson R. Anaphylactoid reactions to intravenous N-acetylcysteine: a prospective case controlled study. Accid Emerg Nurs 2004;12(1):10–5.

[77] Mullins ME, Schmidt RU Jr, Jang TB. What is the rate of adverse events with intravenous versus oral N-acetylcysteine in pediatric patients? Ann Emerg Med 2004; 44(5):547–9.

[78] Kao LW, Kirk MA, Furbee RB, et al. What is the rate of adverse events after oral N-acetylcysteine administered by the intravenous route to patients with suspected acetaminophen poisoning? Ann Emerg Med 2003;42(6):741–50.

[79] Bailey B, McGuigan MA. Management of anaphylactoid reactions to intravenous N-acetylcysteine. Ann Emerg Med 1998;31(6):710–5.

[80] Appelboam AV, Dargan PI, Knighton J. Fatal anaphylactoid reaction to N-acetylcysteine: caution in patients with asthma. Emerg Med J 2002;19(6):594–5.

[81] Dribben WH, Porto SM, Jeffords BK. Stability and microbiology of inhalant N-acetylcysteine used as an intravenous solution for the treatment of acetaminophen poisoning. Ann Emerg Med 2003;42(1):9–13.

[82] O'Grady JG, Alexander GJ, Hayllar KM, et al. Early indicators of prognosis in fulminant hepatic failure. Gastroenterology 1989;97(2):439–45.

[83] Mutimer DJ, Ayres RC, Neuberger JM, et al. Serious paracetamol poisoning and the results of liver transplantation. Gut 1994;35(6):809–14.

[84] Makin AJ, Wendon J, Williams R. A 7-year experience of severe acetaminophen-induced hepatotoxicity (1987–1993). Gastroenterology 1995;109(6):1907–16.

[85] Anand AC, Nightingale P, Neuberger JM. Early indicators of prognosis in fulminant hepatic failure: an assessment of the King's criteria. J Hepatol 1997;26(1):62–8.

[86] Harrison PM, O'Grady JG, Keays RT, et al. Serial prothrombin time as prognostic indicator in paracetamol induced fulminant hepatic failure. BMJ 1990;301(6758):964–6.

[87] Payen C, Dachraoui A, Pulce C, et al. Prothrombin time prolongation in paracetamol poisoning: a relevant marker of hepatic failure? Hum Exp Toxicol 2003;22(11):617–21.

[88] Whyte IM, Buckley NA, Reith DM, et al. Acetaminophen causes an increased International Normalized Ratio by reducing functional factor VII. Ther Drug Monit 2000;22(6):742–8.

[89] Schmidt LE, Knudsen TT, Dalhoff KP, et al. [Effect of N-acetylcysteine on prothrombin index in patients with uncomplicated paracetamol poisoning.] Ugeskr Laeger 2004;166(40): 3502–4.

[90] Schmidt LE, Knudsen TT, Dalhoff K, et al. Effect of acetylcysteine on prothrombin index in paracetamol poisoning without hepatocellular injury. Lancet 2002;360(9340):1151–2.

[91] Pereira LM, Langley PG, Hayllar KM, et al. Coagulation factor V and VIII/V ratio as predictors of outcome in paracetamol induced fulminant hepatic failure: relation to other prognostic indicators. Gut 1992;33(1):98–102.

[92] Gazzard BG, Henderson JM, Williams R. Early changes in coagulation following a paracetamol overdose and a controlled trial of fresh frozen plasma therapy. Gut 1975; 16(8):617–20.

[93] Mitchell I, Bihari D, Chang R, et al. Earlier identification of patients at risk from acetaminophen-induced acute liver failure. Crit Care Med 1998;26(2):279–84.

[94] Schmidt LE, Dalhoff K. Serum phosphate is an early predictor of outcome in severe acetaminophen-induced hepatotoxicity. Hepatology 2002;36(3):659–65.

[95] Chung PY, Sitrin MD, Te HS. Serum phosphorus levels predict clinical outcome in fulminant hepatic failure. Liver Transpl 2003;9(3):248–53.

[96] Ng KL, Davidson JS, Bathgate AJ. Serum phosphate is not a reliable early predictor of outcome in paracetamol induced hepatotoxicity. Liver Transpl 2004;10(1):158–9.

[97] Bernal W, Donaldson N, Wyncoll D, et al. Blood lactate as an early predictor of outcome in paracetamol-induced acute liver failure: a cohort study. Lancet 2002;359(9306):558–63.

[98] Schmidt LE, Dalhoff K. Hyperamylasaemia and acute pancreatitis in paracetamol poisoning. Aliment Pharmacol Ther 2004;20(2):173–9.

[99] Schiodt FV, Bondesen S, Tygstrup N, et al. Prediction of hepatic encephalopathy in paracetamol overdose: a prospective and validated study. Scand J Gastroenterol 1999; 34(7):723–8.

[100] Schmidt LE, Dalhoff K. Alpha-fetoprotein is a predictor of outcome in acetaminophen-induced liver injury. Hepatology 2004;41(1):26–31.

ELSEVIER
SAUNDERS

CLINICS IN
LABORATORY
MEDICINE

Clin Lab Med 26 (2006) 67–97

Heavy Metal Poisoning: Clinical Presentations and Pathophysiology

Danyal Ibrahim, MD[a], Blake Froberg, MD[a],
Andrea Wolf, MD[b], Daniel E. Rusyniak, MD[a],*

[a]*Department of Emergency Medicine, Division of Medical Toxicology,
Indiana University School of Medicine, 1050 Wishard Boulevard, Room 2200,
Indianapolis, IN 46202, USA*
[b]*Department of Emergency Medicine, Indiana University School of Medicine,
1050 Wishard Boulevard, Room 2200, Indianapolis, IN 46202, USA*

Heavy metals are natural components of the earth's crust and as such are the oldest toxins known to humans, having been used for thousands of years. Potential exposures to heavy metals include natural sources (eg, groundwater, metal ores), industrial processes, commercial products, folk remedies, and contaminated food and herbal products. Virtually all heavy metals are toxic in sufficient quantities. Several, however, are of particular interest because of their concentrations in the environment (lead, mercury, and arsenic) or their use in criminal poisonings (arsenic and thallium). Entering our bodies by way of food, drinking water, and air, metals produce toxicity by forming complexes with cellular compounds containing sulfur, oxygen, or nitrogen. The complexes inactivate enzyme systems or modify critical protein structures leading to cellular dysfunction and death. The most commonly involved organ systems include central nervous, gastrointestinal (GI), cardiovascular, hematopoietic, renal, and peripheral nervous systems. The nature and severity of toxicity vary with the heavy metal involved, its exposure level, chemical and valance states (inorganic versus organic), mode of exposure (acute versus chronic), and the age of the individual. Children, with their developing nervous systems, are particularly vulnerable to heavy metal intoxication (especially lead) and deserve special consideration. This article presents an overview of the aforementioned heavy metals with emphasis on clinical presentation and pathophysiology.

* Corresponding author.
E-mail address: drusynia@iupui.edu (D.E. Rusyniak).

0272-2712/06/$ - see front matter © 2006 Elsevier Inc. All rights reserved.
doi:10.1016/j.cll.2006.02.003
labmed.theclinics.com

Arsenic

Clinical scenario

A 46-year-old chemical engineer presented to the emergency department with symptoms of nausea, vomiting, fatigue, extremity paresthesias, and dark-brown urine. Symptoms began within a few hours after troubleshooting newly installed equipment for wastewater treatment. The facility at which he worked manufactures silicone wafers, a process that generates wastewater containing arsenic. Over the next 24 hours, he developed hemolytic anemia, jaundice, and oliguric renal failure. His initial urine arsenic level was 1470 μg/L. The patient was treated with red blood cell (RBC) exchange transfusions, plasmapheresis, and hemodialysis, with eventual full recovery of his renal function. It was determined later that arsine gas was produced when arsenic inadvertently reacted with an acid in the electrocoagulation chamber of the equipment on which he was working.

Background

Over the centuries, arsenic has been used for various purposes. Hippocrates prescribed a paste of arsenic sulfide to treat skin conditions [1]. Arsenic is derived from the Greek word *arsenikon*, meaning potent. Fowler's solution, a 1% arsenic trioxide preparation, was used widely during the nineteenth century in various medical conditions [1,2]. In fact, before penicillin was discovered arsenic was one of the primary treatments for syphilis [1]. Along with its use in medicine, arsenic was common in makeup and pigments. Paints with copper acetoarsenite pigment were known commonly as Paris green. Frank Capra's film *Arsenic and Old Lace* presented arsenic as the perfect poison. In the film, two ladies use arsenic powder as part of a concoction added to elderberry wine to poison lonely old men and transients. Commonly known as aqua toffana after the famous 18th century poisoner Madame Guilina Toffana, mixtures of arsenic have provided a ready means of criminal poisoning throughout history and have been suspected in many famous deaths, including Mozart [3] and Napoleon [4]. Although its physical properties place arsenic in the category of metalloids, its similar pathophysiology and toxicity often result in its being categorized as a heavy metal in clinical papers. In industry, arsenic has been used to manufacture paints, fungicides, insecticides, pesticides, herbicides, wood preservatives, and cotton desiccants. Arsenide crystals, such as aluminium gallium arsenide, are common components of semiconductors and electronic devices [5]. Medicinally, arsenic trioxide is used to induce remission in patients who have acute promyelocytic leukemia [6] and is a common constituent or contaminant of many nonwestern traditional medicine remedies. Most cases of acute arsenic poisoning occur from accidental ingestion of arsenic-containing pesticides and less commonly from attempted suicide or homicide [5,7]. The major cause of chronic human arsenic toxicity is from geological contamination of drinking water, with tragic examples recently demonstrated in Bangladesh and West Bengal, India [8,9].

Toxicity

Arsenic compounds occur in three oxidation states: trivalent arsenite, pentavalent arsenate, and elemental. Arsenite is ten times more toxic than arsenate; elemental is nontoxic. Arsenic also exists in three chemical forms: organic, inorganic, and arsine gas, with organic arsenic having little acute toxicity whereas inorganic arsenic and arsine gas are toxic [10]. Exposure to arsenic primarily occurs by ingestion, but inhalation and absorption through the skin are possible. Arsenic occurs naturally in seafood as nontoxic organic compounds, such as arsenobetaine, which can cause elevated urine arsenic levels [11,12].

The lethal dose of inorganic arsenic has been estimated to be 0.6 mg/kg [5,13]. After absorption, inorganic arsenic rapidly binds to hemoglobin in erythrocytes [14]. Blood arsenic is redistributed quickly (within 24 hours) to the liver, kidneys, heart, lungs, and to a lesser degree the nervous system, GI tract, and spleen. Arsenic undergoes hepatic biomethylation to form monomethylarsonic and dimethylarsinic acids that have less acute toxicity. A small amount of inorganic arsenic also is excreted unchanged [15–17]. About 50% of ingested arsenic can be eliminated in the urine in three to five days with residual amounts remaining in the keratin-rich tissues, such as nails, hair, and skin [5].

Depending on its oxidative state arsenic poisons cells by one of two key mechanisms [18]. By binding the sulfhydryl groups on critical enzymes, trivalent arsenite depletes lipoate, which is involved in the synthesis of key intermediates in the Krebs cycle. Lipoate depletion results in inhibition of the Krebs cycle and oxidative phosphorylation leading to ATP depletion [19]. Pentavalent arsenate, on the other hand, can replace the stable phosphate ester bond in ATP with the arsenate ester bond rapidly hydrolyzing (arsenolysis) uncoupling oxidative phosphorylation and depleting ATP stores [14]. The combination of inhibiting cellular respiration and uncoupling oxidative phosphorylation results in cellular energy depletion, resulting in cell death in high energy dependent tissues [18].

In acute arsenic poisoning, the clinical features initially are GI, including nausea, vomiting, abdominal pain, and bloody rice water diarrhea [10,20,21]. Hypovolemic shock may follow in severe cases as a result of endothelial damage and third spacing of fluid [22]. Hematologic abnormalities, including bone marrow depression, pancytopenia, anemia, and basophilic stippling, usually appear within 4 days of large ingestions [23]. QT interval prolongation and ventricular arrhythmias, such as torsade de pointes, can occur several days after initial improvement in GI symptoms [24,25]. Neurologic manifestations include a distal symmetric peripheral neuropathy commonly presenting with burning and numbness in the hands and feet

[26,27]. In cases of severe poisoning, however, a syndrome of rapidly developing ascending weakness similar to Guillain-Barré may be seen [28,29]. Along with the peripheral nervous system, the central nervous system may be affected, with the development of encephalopathy [29].

In chronic arsenic exposure, a wide range of clinical features are seen [30]. Dermatologic changes include hyperpigmentation and keratosis on the palms and soles [31,32]. The nails may exhibit transverse white bands known as Mees lines (Fig. 1) [33]. Mees lines are the result of interruption of the nail matrix, can be seen in acute and chronic poisoning, and are not specific to arsenic. They may not be evident until weeks after the exposure and may not be present in all patients. Cardiovascular effects include an increased incidence of hypertension and peripheral vascular disease. Sporadic outbreaks of peripheral vascular gangrene known as black foot disease have occurred in Taiwan and have been linked to high levels of arsenic in the drinking water [34]. A stocking-glove distribution sensory greater than motor peripheral neuropathy is the most frequent neurologic manifestation of chronic arsenic toxicity [27]. Chronic arsenic exposure has been associated with various malignancies including skin, lung, liver, bladder, and kidney [35]. Inorganic arsenic crosses the placenta and may be teratogenic in animals [36].

Diagnosis

Diagnosis of arsenic poisoning is based on incorporating clinical presentation (history and physical findings) with history of exposure in the presence of elevated body burden of arsenic. Laboratory tests should survey multiorgan functions, including a complete blood count with smear and a comprehensive metabolic panel. Some arsenic compounds are radiopaque and visible on abdominal radiograph [37]. An electrocardiogram is indicated to assess the QT interval, which may be prolonged [24]. Nerve conduction testing typically shows evidence of distal symmetric sensorimotor axonopathy [27]. In massive ingestions, however, conduction slowing may be evident, resulting in the false diagnosis of Guillain-Barré [29].

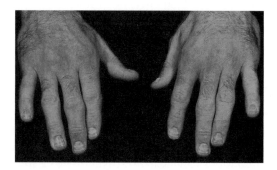

Fig. 1. Arsenic poisoning and Mees lines. (Courtesy of R. Pascuzzi, MD, Indianapolis, IN.)

The most important and reliable diagnostic test is a quantitative 24-hour urinary arsenic excretion [5,10]. Normal values are less than 50 μg/L. Recent seafood ingestion, however, may cause significantly elevated urinary arsenic values, and speciation of the urinary arsenic can be performed to differentiate inorganic from organic forms [12]. Although blood arsenic may be elevated initially in the acute poisoning, levels rapidly decline in the next 24 to 48 hours despite continued symptoms and increased urinary arsenic excretion. Whole blood arsenic level is usually less than 1 μg/dL. Residual arsenic in hair and nails may persist for prolonged periods, but external contamination may render interpretation difficult and unreliable [38].

Management

Treatment of arsenic poisoning begins with the removal from the exposure source. Supportive measures and chelation therapy are the mainstays of management. Volume resuscitation is of paramount importance in the severely poisoned patient, and chelation with dimercaprol or succimer (2,3-dimercaptosuccinic acid, DMSA) should be considered in patients who have symptoms or increased body burden of arsenic [39–42]. Hemodialysis maybe considered for patients who have renal failure [43].

Arsine gas

Arsine gas is considered the most toxic of all arsenic compounds. It is a dense, colorless, nonirritating gas with a garlic-like odor. It has poor warning characteristics allowing for significant exposure and toxicity to occur before detection [44]. Exposure to arsine gas occurs whenever inorganic arsenic-containing solutions or compounds are exposed to acids or nascent hydrogen. At-risk occupations include the smelting of metals and ores, galvanizing, and microelectronics semiconductor manufacturing [45].

Toxicity

Inhaled arsine gas rapidly diffuses into the bloodstream binding with RBCs and causing a rapid and severe Coombs negative intravascular hemolysis [46]. The mechanism of hemolysis is not elucidated fully, but is believed to involve oxidative stress and depletion of glutathione stores in the RBCs [47–54]. Along with hemolysis, arsine gas exposure causes acute renal failure [55]. The pathophysiology of oliguric renal failure from arsine is multifactorial, including direct toxic effects by arsine and arsenite on renal tubular cells, hemoglobin pigment deposition on the renal tubular cells, and tissue hypoxia secondary to severe hemolysis [56,57].

Between 2 and 24 hours following a significant exposure to arsine gas, patients present with general nonspecific symptoms, including malaise, fatigue, headache, dizziness, fever and chills, nausea, vomiting, and abdominal pain [13,46,58–60]. Within 4 to 12 hours, patients report dark red urine followed by oliguria or anuria, and by 24 to 48 hours of exposure a bronze discoloration of the skin may appear. The triad of abdominal pain, hemolysis, and hematuria are characteristic diagnostic features of arsine toxicity. Symptoms of sensorimotor peripheral neuropathy also may appear within weeks of exposure.

Diagnosis

Diagnosis of arsine gas poisoning is based on incorporating the clinical presentation (history and physical findings) with the history of exposure. The clinical triad of abdominal pain, hematuria, and hemolysis together with a history of recent potential occupational exposure is highly suggestive of arsine toxicity [13,46,58,59]. Laboratory tests, such as CBC with peripheral smear, serum chemistry, a negative Coombs test, decreased serum haptoglobin levels, and urinalysis, should help reveal and quantify the intravascular hemolysis. Even though blood and urine arsenic concentrations would be elevated following significant exposure to arsine gas, the diagnosis usually can be established by clinical presentation. Prompt treatment should not be delayed pending arsenic laboratory analysis.

Management

The first component of intervention following arsine gas poisoning is the removal from the source of exposure. In a severely poisoned patient who has evidence of hemolysis prompt whole blood exchange transfusion is of paramount importance based on case reports in the literature [13,46,50,55,58–63]. The benefits of exchange transfusion include restoring functional RBCs, clearance of hemoglobin pigment released by hemolysis (Fig. 2), and removal

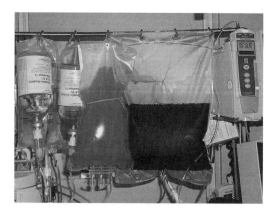

Fig. 2. Arsine hemolysis. The bag on the right represents the plasma removed from an arsine-poisoned patient compared with normal fresh frozen plasma on the left. (Courtesy of D. Rusyniak, MD, Indianapolis, IN.)

of toxic products formed as a result of arsine–hemoglobin reaction. Hemodialysis and exchange transfusion may be required if there is evidence of renal insufficiency [63]. Chelation with British anti lewisite does not appear to alter the natural history of arsine-induced hemolysis [7]. Because arsine poisoning produces significant arsenite concentrations chelation therapy might be of benefit [64]. It is not clear whether chelation therapy affects the evolution of peripheral neuropathy associated with arsine poisoning.

Thallium

Clinical scenario

After a weekend of work at a local automotive plant five middle-aged men simultaneously began to complain of pain and paresthesias in their feet. Over the next 10 days their symptoms progressed to include pain and numbness in the lower extremities and hands. In several of the men the pain was severe enough to make the weight of a bed sheet intolerable. Although the diagnosis eluded various physicians, the development of alopecia in these five men ultimately lead to testing for and diagnosis of acute thallium poisoning. A workplace investigation by Occupational Health and Safety Administration (OSHA) and criminal authorities ultimately revealed nine poisoned patients and the source of thallium to be the malicious contamination of two workroom coffee pots [65].

Background

Thallium is a heavy metal, the toxicity of which has been known since shortly after its initial discovery in the late 1800s. Before 1930, thallium's depilatory properties were used in treatment of scalp ringworm until reports of pediatric deaths resulted in its clinical abandonment [66]. Thallium salts are tasteless, odorless, water soluble, and rapidly and completely absorbed by the GI tract. These properties made them excellent rodenticides until outbreaks of accidental and criminal poisonings led to their removal from the United States market in 1975 [67,68]. Thallium continues to be used today in the manufacturing of optic lenses and semiconductors. Because of its rapid uptake and distribution in the myocardium, small nontoxic doses of radioactive thallium are likewise still used today in the detection of cardiac dysfunction. Despite its limited access to the general public, thallium persists as a significant source of accidental and intentional poisonings in humans and animals [65,69–75].

Toxicity

Thallium is absorbed rapidly from the GI tract with measurable urinary and fecal levels as early as one hour after oral administration [76]. Thallium has wide distribution throughout the organism with the highest concentrations found in the kidney and the lowest in the serum, fat, and central nervous system. Secondary to its entero-entero circulation, the fecal removal of thallium serves as the primary means of elimination [76]. Several theories exist as to the mechanisms of thallium's toxicity in biologic systems. Because potassium and thallium are univalent cations with similar atomic radii, Tl+ (1.50 Å) and K+ (1.38 Å), thallium may interfere with K^+-dependent processes, including pyruvate kinase and Na+/K+ ATPase [77–79]. This interference results in a decrease in catabolism of carbohydrates and impaired ATP generation through oxidative phosphorylation [79,80]. Thallium's affinity for sulfhydryl groups also results in the inhibition of several sulfhydryl-containing enzymes, including pyruvate dehydrogenase complex, succinate dehydrogenase, hydrolases, oxidoreductases, and transferases [79]. The clinical manifestations of thallium poisoning vary depending on the dose, age of victim, and whether the exposure is acute or chronic. In general, however, the presentation of a rapidly progressive peripheral neuropathy with the development of alopecia accurately describes acute thallium toxicity. Dysesthesias and paraesthesias of the feet, and less commonly the hands, classically occur within 1 week of exposure. Hyperesthesias predominate in the feet and occur with weight bearing [65,81]. Moderate exposures may progress to significant sensorimotor peripheral neuropathies with sensory symptoms predominating [65]. Alopecia is the best-known complication of thallium poisoning (Fig. 3). The onset of alopecia generally begins about 2 weeks after exposure with complete alopecia occurring by 3 to 4 weeks. This latent period corresponds to the maturation period of the new epithelial cells of the hair matrix [82]. If patients survive, hair typically starts to regrow by the fourth month after poisoning and may be fine and occasionally unpigmented [65,83]. Alopecia typically involves

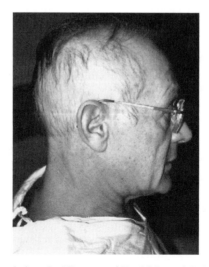

Fig. 3. Thallium-induced alopecia. (Courtesy of Daniel Rusyniak, MD, Indianapolis, IN.)

not only the scalp but also the lateral half of the eyebrows and the entire body, including pubic hair and axillary hair [82–85]. The cause of alopecia is not known but is believed to be either secondary to thallium interruption of cysteine in the synthesis of keratin or its ability to disturb energy metabolism in the growing cells of the hair matrix. Not all thallium-poisoned patients develop alopecia, and peripheral neuropathies can occur without its development [65].

Along with the neurologic and dermatologic manifestations of thallium poisoning, GI symptoms, including pain, diarrhea, and more commonly constipation, have been reported. Unlike arsenic, however, they do not dominate the early clinical picture. Other clinical manifestations of thallium poisoning include diffuse myalgias, pleuritic chest pain [65,67,72], insomnia, optic neuritis, hypertension, nonspecific ST-T wave changes, nail dystrophy (Mees lines), hepatitis, chronic neuropsychiatric manifestations [86], and cranial nerve deficits [87].

Diagnosis

Early diagnosis in thallium poisoning may be problematic because it is an uncommon poison with its initial symptoms often attributed to other causes [65]. Further complicating the early recognition of thallium poisoning is that alopecia, the most recognizable feature of thallium poisoning [73], may not be evident for up to 14 days [82]. Hair analysis may offer the potential for early diagnosis. In cases in which the hair of thallium-poisoned patients has been examined it has been found to be in anagen effluvium [82,88]. Other microscopic findings include dysplastic hair roots, changes in the diameter of the fiber, and a disorganized cortex, which appears dark under a light microscope [82]. The most interesting and perhaps diagnostic feature in acute thallium-poisoned patients is the finding of darkened hair roots when examined under a light-powered microscope (Fig. 4) [65,83]. This finding is reported to occur as early as 3 hours in rats and 4 days in humans after thallium poisoning [83]. The pigment is reported to be present in up to 95% of scalp hair and in 50% to 60% of chest and leg hair, but only 30% of tactile hair (eyebrows and eyelids) [83]. If poisoning occurs in repeated doses several bands can be seen, analogous to multiple Mees lines [83]. Although some investigators have suggested that the dark roots actually represent an accumulation of pigment [83], the cause of the blackened roots is not a pigment or the metal itself but rather an optical phenomenon. It is believed that in the hair root the disorganized matrix results in the accumulation of gaseous inclusions, which results in diffracting light and the appearance of a black stain [82,84]. When these hairs are treated with thioglycolic acid or mechanical pressure the gas bubbles have been noted to escape, with subsequent disappearance of the darkened strip [89].

Nerve conduction studies also may be a useful modality in diagnosing and monitoring patients who have thallium poisoning because the severity of abnormalities of nerve conduction studies seems to correlate with the

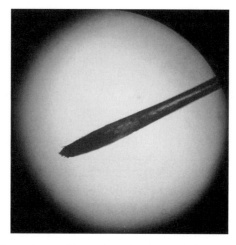

Fig. 4. Blackened hair root in a thallium-poisoned patient under light microscopy. (Courtesy of D. Rusyniak, MD, Indianapolis, IN.)

severity of other symptoms and findings [65]. In severe poisoning nerve biopsy may reveal Wallerian degeneration with axonal destruction and secondary myelin loss [87,90,91].

A definitive diagnosis of thallium poisoning, however, requires the identification of elevated thallium concentrations in urine or hair. As in other metals a 24-hour urine is considered the gold standard in thallium poisoning, with normal levels generally less than 20 µg per specimen. Hair also can be tested, with normal levels being less than 15 ng thallium per gram of hair [79].

Management

The primary objective in treating thallium poisoning is to increase its elimination and prevent further toxicity. Currently the best-studied and most effective antidote for thallium poisoning is Prussian blue. Prussian blue is a poorly absorbed complex of potassium hexacyanoferrate and is available in soluble (colloidal) and insoluble formulations [92]. Recently the insoluble formulation received approval from the US Food and Drug Administration as an antidote for cesium and thallium poisoning, although the soluble formulation may be more efficacious [79,92]. The current manufacturer-recommended dose of Prussian blue is 3 g orally three times a day with others recommending 250 mg/kg given two times a day [93]. Prussian blue's mechanism of action is through the exchange of potassium for thallium in the molecular lattice of the hexacyanoferrate complex resulting in the fecal excretion of a thallium–Prussian blue complex. Numerous animal studies show Prussian blue to decreased mortality, increase elimination, and decrease CNS thallium concentrations [94–101]. Good outcomes in a few human case reports have supported the safety and efficacy of Prussian blue in thallium poisoning [71,72]. Prussian blue is an exceedingly safe compound with few if any reported cases of toxicity in either animal or human studies [102]. Based on thallium's affinity for sulfhydryl groups, several commonly used sulfur chelators have been used in models of poisoning but without significant improvement [101,103,104]. Because some hospitals may not carry Prussian blue some authors have recommended activated charcoal until Prussian blue is available. In vitro studies demonstrate excellent adsorbent properties of thallium with activated charcoal [105,106]. Although thallium's entero-entero circulation makes charcoal an excellent choice for treatment, animal studies are contradictory [95,103] and human data is largely anecdotal.

Mercury

Clinical scenario

A 14-year-old male presented to an outpatient clinic with the chief complaint of bilateral thigh pain. Over the preceding 8 weeks his mother had noticed his becoming withdrawn and currently described him "like a hermit". His physical examination revealed profuse sweating, tachycardia, hypertension, tremor, ataxia, and a desquamating erythematous rash on the palms, soles, toes, and fingertips. Although initially believed to have pheochromocytoma, a 24-hour urine mercury concentration was found to be 264 μg/L. Environmental testing of his house, a former TV repair shop, showed high levels of elemental mercury vapor. He was removed from the exposure and treated with oral DMSA chelation therapy with resolution of his rash and symptoms.

Background

Mercury is a naturally occurring metal, the name of which comes from the Greek word Ύδραργυρος (hydrargyros), meaning water and silver. It exists in three forms, each with characteristic and distinct toxicities: elemental mercury, inorganic mercury salts, and organic mercury. Given its liquid, silvery appearance, the elemental form of mercury has also been called quicksilver or liquid silver [107]. Elemental mercury use was documented as early as 1500 BC in Egypt, where it was used to decorate the tombs of wealthy citizens [108]. Evidence of its use for cosmetic purposes was found in ancient Greece and Rome [109] and it has been used for medicinal purposes in Eastern Asia for centuries. In the 1400s mercury was used in Western Europe as a syphilitic, and is the origin of the phrase "two minutes with Venus, two years with mercury" [110]. Until the late 1800s, a tablespoon of quicksilver was a commonly used laxative in children [107], but the medicinal use of mercury largely fell out of favor by the nineteenth century when it was first suspected of causing toxic effects [108–110]. Reliance on mercury during the industrial revolution, however, resulted in increased workplace exposure. The most striking example of this occurred among hat makers, who combed elemental mercury through animal fur to prepare the fibers for use in felt production, a process called carroting. The term carroting came from to the orange hue the fur took on during this process. A large number of hatters developed mercury toxicity, resulting in the common phrase "mad as a hatter" [107].

Elemental mercury

Elemental mercury is one of only two metals that are known to be liquid at room temperature [111]. It is a heavy, nonwetting liquid that is able to volatilize to an odorless gas in quantities sufficient to cause clinical toxicity at room temperature [112]. Its uniform expansion over a wide range of temperatures and its ability to alloy easily with other metals led to mercury's use in several commercial applications [109], including thermometers, barometers, thermostats, electronics, batteries, dental amalgams, home folk remedies, and a host of other uses [109,113]. Because of recent concerns regarding exposure and toxicity, the use of mercury in the manufacture of most of these products has been abandoned in favor of less toxic substances [109]. Many older mercury-containing products are still in use, however, and continue to be a source for potential toxicity.

Toxicity

Exposure to elemental mercury occurs by way of inhalation of the vapor, ingestion of the liquid, or cutaneous exposure. Intravenous mercury injection is a rare route of exposure in cases of attempted self-harm [114]. Ingestion of elemental mercury rarely is of clinical consequence. The metal is poorly absorbed in the gut and is eliminated in the feces [108,109,113]. Although in patients who have normal GI mucosa toxicity rarely develops after ingestion, patients who have abnormal GI mucosa may absorb enough mercury for toxicity to occur [115]. Occasionally mercury becomes trapped within the appendix, but without signs of mercury toxicity or appendicitis it can be safely monitored and allowed to pass on its own [116,117]. If vomiting with subsequent aspiration of elemental mercury occurs the risk for toxicity is increased because mercury is well absorbed within the lungs [113]. In most cases cutaneous exposure also is of little clinical consequence [112] with the main risk to individuals who handle elemental mercury being inhalation of the vapor rather than direct contact with the metal. Toxicity from elemental mercury occurs from inhalation of the vapor because mercury is well absorbed into the pulmonary circulation allowing distribution to the brain, kidneys, gut, and lungs [108,112,113]. Elemental mercury readily crosses the blood–brain barrier where it concentrates in neuronal lysosomal dense bodies [108]. Mercury combines with sulfhydryl groups on cell membranes and interferes with numerous cellular processes, including protein and nucleic acid synthesis, oxidative stress, calcium homeostasis, and protein phosphorylation [118].

The manifestations of elemental mercury toxicity have great variability depending on the chronicity of the exposure. Acute toxicity may manifest within hours of a large exposure with GI upset, chills, weakness, cough, and dyspnea, with severe cases developing adult respiratory distress syndrome [119] and renal failure [120]. Chronic mercury toxicity may develop over a period of weeks to months, depending on the level of exposure. Initial symptoms commonly include GI upset, constipation, abdominal pain, and poor appetite, and may mimic a viral illness [108,121]. Other symptoms include dry mouth, headache, and muscle pains [108,113,121]. Chronic exposure results in two distinct clinical syndromes, acrodynia and erethism [108,113,121]. Known as pink disease, Feer syndrome, Feer-Swift disease, erythroderma, and raw-beef hands and feet [113,122,123], acrodynia is a complex of symptoms occurring in chronic toxicity from elemental and inorganic mercury. It occurs more commonly in infants and children, but has been reported in adults [113,124]. Characteristic findings include sweating, hypertension, tachycardia, pruritus, weakness, poor muscle tone, insomnia, anorexia, and an erythematous, desquamating rash to the palms and soles (Fig. 5) [108,112,113,121]. Oral findings including reddened, swollen gums, subsequent mucosal ulcerations, and possible tooth loss [108,113,123]. By an unknown mechanism, mercury may result in proximal weakness primarily involving the pelvic and pectoral girdle [113,121]. Patients who have mercury poisoning often develop characteristic personality changes collectively termed erethism. These patients may exhibit memory loss, drowsiness, withdrawal, lethargy, depression, and irritability [113]. Another common finding in mercury poisoning is incoordination and a fine motor intention tremor primarily involving the hands [125,126]. It has been suggested that erethism may be a Parkinsonian-like syndrome involving the basal ganglia and cerebellum, though dose relationships have not been shown clearly [113].

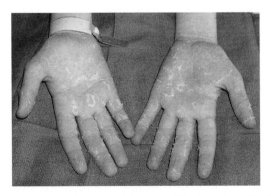

Fig. 5. Acrodynia from elemental mercury. (Courtesy of D. Rusyniak, MD, Indianapolis, IN.)

Whether these changes are reversible with the removal of the offending agent remains unclear also. The sweating, tremor, hypertension, and tachycardia associated with acrodynia may mimic the presentation of pheochromocytoma [127–129]. These patients often are misdiagnosed early in their clinical course, and while the patient is worked up for neuroendocrine disease the diagnosis of mercury toxicity may be delayed [127]. Mercury inhibits the enzyme catechol-o-methyltransferase by inactivation of the coenzyme S-adenosylmethionine, producing elevated levels of catecholamines in the body [127–129]. The increase in catecholamines results in hypertension, sweating, and tachycardia that may be clinically indistinguishable from pheochromocytoma. A 24-hour urine collection on these patients reveals elevated levels of urinary catecholamines, although typically to a lesser degree than that seen in true neuroendocrine disease [129]. This finding suggests that mercury toxicity should be considered in the differential for any patient presenting with symptoms of pheochromocytoma.

Diagnosis

The diagnosis of elemental mercury poisoning involves incorporating clinical presentation (history and physical findings), history of exposure, and an elevated body burden of mercury. Blood mercury levels have limited usefulness because of mercury's short half-life in the blood [108,112]. Whole blood mercury concentrations typically are less than 10 μg/L. Urine levels are obtained more commonly in chronically exposed patients, with 24-hour collections more reliable than spot urine levels. Normal levels typically are less than 50 μg of mercury in a 24-hour period [108,113]. Patients undergoing chelation therapy at the time of collection have elevated levels of mercury in a 24-hour sample making interpretation difficult if not impossible [130].

Management

Removal of the patient from the source of the toxic exposure is the most important intervention [63,108,112,113,121]. Because elemental mercury typically has minimal toxicity when ingested, there is little role for GI decontamination.

Although chelation therapy is considered the mainstay of treatment several controversies remain regarding its use. Chelators are charged molecules capable of binding the metal ion forming a neutral complex excreted by the kidney [112]. The goal of chelation therapy is to reduce the total body burden of heavy metal. Several agents are available, the most commonly cited including succimer, dimercaprol, and D-penicillamine [63]. Patients may require chelation for several months depending on the total body burden of mercury. The usefulness of chelation therapy remains unclear, because there is a lack of studies showing a clear long-term benefit in patients treated with this therapy [112,131]. In patients who have developed renal failure, hemodialysis may be required, with or without the inclusion of a chelation agent.

Inorganic mercury

Inorganic mercury occurs naturally as mercuric and mercurous salts, the most common being mercury(II) sulfide (HgS), also known commonly as cinnabar and vermillion. This red, earthy-appearing ore also is found in a crystal form prized for its rich red color, and was equally prized as a source of mercury throughout its history [132]. Other common mercurial salts include mercuric chloride, mercuric oxide, mercuric sulfide, mercurous chloride, mercuric iodide, ammoniated mercury, and phenylmercuric salts [108,113]. Historically, these compounds have been used in cosmetics and skin treatments, particularly as skin-lightening agents [113,133]. Mercurial teething powders containing calomel (mercuric chloride) were in common use until the mid-twentieth century and were prescribed to infants to soothe the discomfort of teething [122]. Although these treatments no longer are prescribed, some dermatologic preparations still are available over the counter in the United States [113]. Patients also may develop local or systemic toxicity after using mercurial compounds found in old topical antiseptics, skin creams, and folk remedies. Currently, most exposures in the United States occur from exposure to germicides, pesticides, and mercury-containing antiseptics [113].

Toxicity

Inorganic mercury is absorbed readily by multiple routes, including GI, inhalational, and dermal. Ingestion typically results in the greatest degree of absorption, followed by inhalational and dermal, but the absolute amount of mercury absorbed depends on the degree of exposure. In contrast to elemental mercury, inorganic mercury is severely corrosive to the GI mucosa [63,113,134]. Patients may present acutely after ingestion of mercurial salts complaining of oral pain or burning, nausea, vomiting, diarrhea, hematemesis, bloody stools, or abdominal discomfort [113,134]. Frank colitis with necrosis or sloughing of the GI mucosa may develop with severe toxicity [108,134]. In some cases, volume loss from GI losses or hemorrhage may require large volume fluid resuscitation. Because mercury salts are absorbed through the GI mucosa [135] significant blood levels can be achieved after ingestion, with resultant systemic toxicity.

Prolonged use of topical preparations containing mercury can result in several cutaneous changes, including worsening of hyperpigmentation, swelling, and a vesicular or scaling rash [113]. Hyperpigmentation manifests as a gray-brown discoloration in the skin and is most pronounced in the skin folds of the face and neck [113]. Topical use of calomel (mercuric chloride) on the oral mucosa was common in the nineteenth and early twentieth centuries and was associated with development of loose teeth, bluish discoloration of the gums, and systemic toxicity [113,122]. Contact stomatitis or irritation of the oral mucosa from dental amalgams has been reported also and may represent an allergic reaction [136–138]. Inorganic mercury is absorbed readily through the

skin, so patients may develop systemic mercury toxicity even if using only topical preparations [113]. Inorganic mercury has a half-life in the blood of 24 to
40 days with mercurial ions being excreted by the kidneys and resultant concentration of mercuric and mercurous ions in the renal tissues [108]. Acute renal failure may develop because of the toxic effect of mercury on the renal
tubular cells with the proximal tubular cells being particularly susceptible to
injury, although the mechanism remains unclear [139]. Acute tubular necrosis
may develop up to two weeks after exposure. Cases of nearly complete recovery have been reported, however, even after prolonged renal failure [140].

Chronic inorganic mercury exposure can cause membranous glomerulo-
nephritis and nephrotic syndrome [141]. The mechanism for this injury
is unclear, although animal studies suggest that it may be related to an
immune-modulated process with production of autoantibodies against components of the glomerular basement membrane [141]. In some cases the nephrotic syndrome has resolved spontaneously with removal of the offending
agent [141]. Like elemental mercury, inorganic mercury can cause acrodynia
and erethism [108,113].

Diagnosis

Diagnosis of inorganic mercury poisoning is the same as that of elemental
mercury poisoning, with 24-hour urine testing being the gold standard.

Management

The target organs of acute inorganic mercury poisoning are the GI tract
and the kidneys. The corrosive injury to the GI tract in serious inorganic
mercury ingestion may necessitate aggressive volume resuscitation. Also,
prompt and expedient chelation is critical in preventing or reducing renal injury. Dimercaprol has been reported to be most effective if administered
within 4 hours of inorganic mercury ingestion, but succimer may be
substituted for dimercaprol once patients are able to tolerate oral intake.
Hemodialysis is indicated in oliguric or anuric renal failure because it may
contribute to the elimination of dimercaprol–Hg complex.

Organic mercury

Although the toxicity of elemental and inorganic mercury has been known
for centuries, toxicity from organic mercury was not appreciated fully until
several large outbreaks brought it to the forefront of environmental toxicology. Of the organic mercurial compounds, methylmercury has resulted in
the largest number of poisonings. Used primarily as preservatives, antiseptics,
and in seed dressings, organic mercurial compounds were used commonly for
industrial and medicinal purposes in the early twentieth century. Merbromin
(mercurochrome) still is used today as a topical antiseptic and ethyl mercury

(thimerosal) was only recently removed from multidose vaccine vials. Today the most common source of organic mercury exposure, however, is dietary consumption of predatory fish. Through a process known as bioamplification, soil and marine microorganisms methylate inorganic and elemental mercury from industrial waste ultimately resulting in methylmercury concentrating in the tissues of large predatory fish, such as tuna and swordfish. In 1956 people in the Japanese finishing village of Minamata were stricken with a mysterious illness primarily affecting the central nervous system [142,143]. Secondary to the rising costs of recycling, a local industrial company had begun dumping mercury-laden waste directly into the bay [144], ultimately resulting in greater than 100 tons contaminating the waters and marine life for decades [145]. In total, methylmercury contamination in Japan resulted in 2263 cases of adult and 63 cases of congenital organic mercury poisoning [146]. A similar outbreak occurred in Iraq in 1972, at which time more than 6000 people were poisoned and 459 died after eating grain treated with a methylmercury fungicide that had been made into bread instead of planted [147].

Toxicity

Unlike the elemental and inorganic forms, organic mercury is well absorbed by the GI tract with greater than 90% of an ingested dose absorbed [148]. Likewise, organic mercury readily crosses the blood–brain barrier and the placenta. Once absorbed, organic mercury is distributed from the blood into the brain reaching levels three to six times those of the blood [149]. Organic mercury poisoning most commonly presents with clinical findings of marked concentric constriction of the bilateral visual fields, paresthesias of the extremities and mouth, ataxia, incoordination, tremor, dysarthria, and auditory impairments [142,147]. Autopsy findings commonly consist of neuronal damage in the gray matter of the cerebral and cerebellar cortex with the most-affected areas being the calcarine region of the occipital lobe and the pre- and postcentral and temporal cortex. In the cerebellum there is loss of granule cells typically with preservation of the neighboring Purkinje cells [142,146]. Along with the damage to the central nervous system peripheral nerve damage, largely in the sensory fibers, can occur [146,150].

One of the most devastating effects of methylmercury exposure in Japan was on children born to exposed mothers, who developed a syndrome similar to cerebral palsy [151] termed congenital Minamata disease. Symptoms seen in cases of congenital Minamata disease included mental retardation (100%), primitive reflexes (100%), cerebellar ataxia (100%), limb deformities (100%), dysarthria (100%), chorea (95%), hypersalivation (95%), and microcephaly (60%) [142,144,151]. The incidence of congenital Minamata disease between 1955 and 1958 in the Minamata area was estimated to involve as many as 29% of children born to exposed mothers [151]. Pathologic changes in congenital Minamata disease are similar to the adult form, with general atrophy of the cortex, hypoplasia of the corpus callosum, demyelination of the pyramidal tracts, and hypoplasia of the granula cell layer of the cerebellum [151]. Likewise in the Iraqi grain outbreak severe neurologic deficits were noted in children born to exposed mothers, including mental retardation and blindness [152]. To date, Minamata represents the best example of the sensitivity and risk for the developing central nervous system to methylmercury. More recently, ethyl mercury used as a preservative in vaccines has been a subject of intense debate as a possible cause of autism and other developmental disorders. Epidemiologic studies, however, have not established a link between mercury and autism [153].

Diagnosis

As with elemental and inorganic mercury poisoning, making the diagnosis of organic mercury poisoning requires recognition of the clinical effects with corroborating mercury levels in the person or the environment. Unlike inorganic and elemental poisoning, organic mercury is identified best in victims by analysis of whole blood or hair [147,152]. In the blood more than 90% of methylmercury is bound to hemoglobin within the RBCs [148]. Because methylmercury is eliminated primarily in the bile, urinary mercury levels are unreliable. Normal values for whole blood mercury typically are less than 0.006 mg/L, but diets rich in fish can increase blood mercury levels to as high as 0.200 mg/L or higher [154]. In the Iraq grain disaster, whereas the amount of mercury consumed was correlated strongly with blood levels and symptoms, there was wide individual variability with respect to blood levels and symptoms [147].

Management

The treatment of organic mercury poisoning requires early recognition and removal of the source. For those patients who have significant symptoms or exposures various chelating agents have been tried including D-Penicillamine, N-acetyl-D-L-penicillamine, 2,3-dimercaptopropane sulphonate, and succimer [147,152,155]. Although all treatments are believed to decrease whole blood mercury concentrations [156] no clinical studies have demonstrated appreciable clinical improvement. Because most cases are not identified until appreciable symptoms have developed it is unclear what role early chelation might play on outcomes. Animal studies have suggested that chelation reduces brain mercury concentrations but has to be administered early in the poisoning to see improved outcomes [157,158].

Lead

Clinical scenario

A 2-year-old white male presented to the emergency room with lethargy. He had not been to his pediatrician in the last year, but had reached all of his developmental milestones. Along with the lethargy the parents described him as being irritable and less interested in playing with his toys over the last two months. His father worked at a factory and the family lived in an urban area in a house that was built in the 1950s. On examination the patient had a depressed level of consciousness without focal neurologic findings. During the patient's workup for altered mental status a blood lead level was measured at 145 µg/dL. CT of the brain showed mild cerebral edema and blood work showed a microcytic anemia. A flat-plate radiograph did not show any foreign bodies. On admission the patient was started on oral succimer and intravenous CaEDTA. Two days later the patient's blood lead level was down to 60 µg/dL and his mental status had improved greatly. He was discharged from the hospital and continued on a 3-week course of oral succimer. The Department of Public Health evaluated the child's house and noticed teeth marks along many of the windowsills throughout the house. After removal of the lead paint from the house, the patient continued to have fluctuating lead levels for the next 3 years ranging from 10 to 45 µg/dL and received several more courses of oral succimer. His pediatrician reports his developmental progress is slightly delayed.

Background

A gray-silver heavy metal comprising approximately 0.002% of the earth's crust, lead has various industrial uses but no physiologic use. Any evidence of lead within the human body, therefore, can be viewed as contamination. The earliest evidence of lead use by humans dates back to 40,000 BC, found in paints at Neanderthal burial sites. Many prominent ancient cultures have mined lead, including the ancient Egyptians, Hebrews, Phoenicians, Greeks, and Romans [159]. The Industrial Revolution resulted in an increase in lead machinery used in the workplace and lead products distributed to consumers. Leaded gasoline and lead-based paints were two common forms of lead that achieved widespread use starting in the early twentieth century [159]. Today the only metal with more commercial use than lead is iron. The first written records of lead toxicity were by the ancient Egyptians. Historians speculate that the personality changes of the leaders of Rome, along with sterility and stillbirths, could have been a direct effect of lead toxicity [160]. Lead continued to cause medical problems throughout the ages. In 1763, Benjamin Franklin recognized abdominal colic and peripheral neuropathy as two consequences of chronic lead exposure. It was not until 1972, however, that the United States passed a law banning residential use of lead paint. Leaded gasoline, first used in the 1920s for its antiknock effects, has led to the contamination of air, soil, and crops. In the early 1990s leaded gasoline was no longer used in the United States, but continues to be a source of lead pollution in nondeveloped countries [159].

Modern occupational exposure is the main source for plumbism in adults. The main route of occupational toxicity is through respiratory exposure. The occupations that are associated with the highest risk for lead poisoning are battery plant workers, metal welders, painters, construction workers, crystal glass makers, firing-range operators, shipbuilders, and lead miners [161,162]. Our present-day environment also is a source of lead. Houses built before 1978 commonly were painted with lead-based paint and are a major source of lead exposure, especially in the urban pediatric population. Leaded paints deteriorate and cause contamination of surrounding dust and soil. Older plumbing also may contain lead and can cause lead exposure through tap water [161].

Toxic lead levels also can result from the lead contained in many modern products, such as retained lead bullets, curtain weights, lead-glazed ceramics, and lead fishing weights [1,163]. Most lead toxicity from lead-containing products is a result of misuse, such as ingestion. Some folk remedies used in some Hispanic populations, such as azarcon and greta, still contain lead [161].

Pediatric toxicity

Young children use hand-to-mouth activity to explore their environment. Children who live in an environment that is contaminated with lead (ie, those who live in and around houses with lead-based paints) are more likely to suffer the effects of lead poisoning [161]. Children are at the greatest risk for accidental ingestions, including lead-based objects, around the age of 2 years. Children are more at risk for lead exposure during the summer months, which may be a result of increased amounts of lead-containing dust and increased child activity during these months [164].

The most common childhood presentation of lead poisoning is central neurotoxicity. Although blood lead levels cannot be correlated strictly with symptoms, there tend to be some cutoff values that are predictive of certain features. At lower levels (1–50 μg/dL) lead may cause subtle cognitive and behavioral changes difficult to differentiate from normal developmental variance [165]. At moderate levels (50–70 μg/dL) children may display a global decrease in activity, presenting as a children who do not enjoy playing or who developmentally fall behind their peers. These symptoms have been classified as pre-encephalopathic symptoms and are most prominent between 1 and 5 years of age. With severe lead toxicity (>70 μg/dL) children may be encephalopathic with coma, seizures, altered mental status, and symptoms consistent with increased intracranial pressure [1,166]. Encephalopathy from lead occurs most commonly between the ages of 15 and 30 months.

Although there is no debate as to the harmful effects of high lead levels, there is continued controversy over the effects of low lead levels on childhood cognitive development. Although studies have shown a relationship between increased lead levels and decreased IQ [165], critics of these studies have pointed out that the design and number of confounders in these studies prohibit the proof of direct causality. Other symptoms of childhood lead toxicity include anemia; peripheral motor neuropathy; GI complaints, such as anorexia, vomiting, and abdominal pain; and growth delay. Lead readily crosses the placenta and has been reported to cause fetal toxicity [161].

The primary route of lead exposure in children is through the GI tract [161]. Lead probably is taken up at calcium absorption sites, which have increased activity at times of rapid growth [167].

The central neurotoxicity caused by lead is caused by disruption of the intercellular junction that seals the capillary endothelium. The mechanism of this disruption is interference with cellular calcium metabolism and second messenger signaling systems. With the loss of its tight seal, the blood–brain barrier is less effective and the capillaries leak, resulting in an increase in intracranial fluid and a resultant increase in intracranial pressure. This effect of lead is more prominent in young children because of their immature blood–brain barrier before the exposure [167,168].

Chronic exposure to lead affects numerous neurotransmitter systems, increasing the spontaneous release of dopamine, acetylcholine, and gamma-amino butyric acid; blocking N-methyl-D-aspartate glutamate receptors; and increasing levels of the intracellular messenger protein kinase C [161]. These effects result in an increase in random synaptic signals, termed synaptic noise, and a decrease in the ability of the neuron to produce a synaptic signal in response to a true stimulus. A human has the most neurologic synapses at the age of 2, after which the body, through apoptosis, rapidly starts to prune faulty and unnecessary synapses. The determination of whether a synapse is kept or destroyed is related to feedback from neurotransmitters and neurotransmitter receptors. Because lead interferes with neurotransmitters and their receptors it results in a disruption of synapse formation and synapse destruction [168].

Lead has two main toxic effects on the hematologic system: reduction of erythrocyte lifespan and decreased hemoglobin biosynthesis [169]. Lead causes inhibition of pyrimidine-5′-nucleotidase and inhibition of $Na+$ $-K+$-ATPase leading to decreased energy use by the erythrocyte and a decrease in cell membrane stability. Pyrimidine-5′−nucleotidase is necessary for the removal of degraded RNA, and its inhibition by lead causes erythrocytes to form clumps, giving the cells the classic basophilic stippling appearance. Lead interferes with several enzymes in the heme synthesis pathway, including aminolevulinic acid synthetase, δ-aminolevulinic dehydratase (ALA-D), ferrochelatase, and coproporphyrinogen decarboxylase. ALA-D in particular can be inhibited by minimal lead exposure [161].

Diagnosis

Blood lead levels are the best indicator of lead exposure. Venous blood samples are necessary because capillary samples can give false positives because of skin contamination [1]. All children who fit into a high-risk category (mainly based on socioeconomic factors) should be screened with a blood lead level at 1 and 2 years of age [1]. A complete blood count may show a hypochromic microcytic anemia and stippling of the RBCs [1].

Management

The most effective treatment for lead toxicity is removal of the patient from the lead-containing environment and cessation of exposure. Pediatric patients who present with symptoms of lead encephalopathy or with blood levels greater than 70 µg/dL should be considered candidates for parenteral chelation therapy with either dimercaprol or succimer and CaNa2EDTA [170]. Chelation with oral succimer should be considered in children who are asymptomatic with blood lead levels between 45 and 69 µg/dL [1,171]. Two recent studies have shown no neurologic benefit from chelation for children with blood lead levels between 20 and 44 µg/dL, and based on these studies chelation is not recommended for levels less than 44 µg/dL [172,173]. Children who present with lead foreign body ingestion may also benefit from cathartics, whole-bowel irrigation, or endoscopic removal [163].

Adult toxicity

Most adult lead poisonings occur from occupational respiratory exposures. Lead-induced hypertension is the most common symptom attributed to lead exposure in adults, but patients can also develop anemia, gastric colic, muscle and joint pain, decreased fertility, renal failure, and peripheral motor neuropathy [174]. Rarely, adults with blood lead levels greater than 100 µg/dL present with encephalopathy [175]. Adults more commonly suffer from subtle neurologic deficits, such as fatigue and emotional lability, after lead exposure. The main mechanism of lead-induced hypertension seems to be related to changes in vascular smooth muscle because of increased activity of the Na+–Ca+ exchange pump and interference of Na+–K+ ATPase activity. Lead-induced gastric colic may have a similar mechanism to that of vascular hypertension, with increased contractility of vascular smooth muscle. The progressive development of renal failure may result after long-term environmental exposures or the chronic release of deposited bone lead. Lead disrupts mitochondrial phosphorylation and oxidation within the kidney, leading to a decrease in energy-dependent transport. The end result of this disrupted transport is phosphaturia, glycosuria, and aminoaciduria [161]. With chronic lead exposure the kidneys are found to have lead–protein complex inclusion bodies [161]. There is some evidence that these inclusion bodies are the main pathway for lead excretion. As chronic lead exposure progresses fewer of these inclusion bodies are seen, and the renal tubules begin to show signs of intersitial fibrosis [161]. Peripheral neuropathy from lead exposure is caused by Schwann cell destruction followed by demyelination and axonal atrophy. Upper extremity motor neurons are more susceptible to damage from lead than sensory or lower extremity neurons, resulting in the classic, albeit rare, presentation of bilateral wrist drop [176].

Lead's total body burden is stored mainly in bone, with 70% of a child's and 95% of an adult's total body burden stored in bone [174]. Within bone there are two main storage areas: the cortical bone, which is a stagnant store, and the trabecular bone, which is a more bioavailable store. Blood lead levels may increase during times of increased bone metabolism during pregnancy, osteoporosis, and fractures. The half-life of lead in human bone is estimated to be up to 30 years [177]. Lead objects retained within the body can serve as an artificial store of lead. The exposure of the object to an acidic environment in synovial or gastric fluid and mechanical stresses to the object within a joint space can cause increased systemic absorption of lead (Fig. 6) [178].

Diagnosis

Lead toxicity should be considered in the differential in anyone who displays unexplained hypertension, encephalopathy, peripheral motor neuropathy, gastric colic, and renal failure. Adults with histories of large exposures as children may also warrant screening because of the long half-life of lead in bone. OSHA guidelines mandate periodic screening for workers exposed to air lead levels of 30 μg/m^3 for 30 days or more. Workers with blood lead levels greater than 60 μg/dL or three consecutive levels greater than 50 μg/dL should have a repeat level every month, those with a level between 40 and

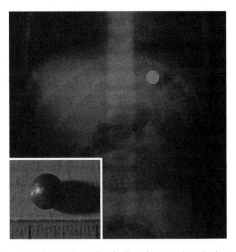

Fig. 6. A 3-year-old swallowed a lead musket ball at daycare (*inset*). A radiograph revealed the ball retained in the stomach. The lead ball was removed by endoscopy without complication. A venous blood lead level approximately 48 hours postingestion was 89 μg/dL. The child was treated with a course of succimer, and a repeat lead level 1 week after chelation was 5 μg/dL. The child never developed symptoms. (Courtesy of C. Holstege, MD, Charlottesville, VA.)

60 µg/dL should have a repeat level every 2 months, and those with elevated levels less than 40 µg/dL should have repeat levels every 6 months [162]. Currently the best screening test is a venous blood lead level. A complete blood count may show a hypochromic microcytic anemia and red blood cell stippling. A urinalysis and basic metabolic panel may be used to screen for renal toxicity. X-ray fluorescence technology may be a useful screening test in the future to determine bone lead burden; however, at this time it primarily serves as a research tool [179].

Management

The most effective therapy is limitation of exposure. In the workplace this may include using personal protective gear, improving industrial engineering, and adhering to safe work practices [162]. Chelation usually is reserved for adults who are symptomatic or who have a blood lead level greater than 70 µg/dL. Mildly symptomatic patients who have levels between 70 and 100 µg/dL may require a course of oral succimer, whereas those patients who have encephalopathy or levels greater than 100 µg/dL require intramuscular dimercaprol or oral succimer and intravenous CaNa2EDTA. A pregnant patient who has elevated lead levels should be treated using the same standards as a nonpregnant adult.

Summary

Acute and chronic toxicities from exposure to heavy metals are uncommon but pose significant morbidity and mortality if unrecognized. Diagnosis of heavy metal poisoning is based on incorporating clinical presentation (history and physical findings) with history of exposure in the presence of elevated body burden of the particular heavy metal. The key to managing heavy metal intoxication is the removal from offending exposure and the reduction of total body burden.

References

[1] Jolliffe DM. A history of the use of arsenicals in man. J R Soc Med 1993;86:287–9.
[2] Waxman S, Anderson KC. History of the development of arsenic derivatives in cancer therapy. Oncologist 2001;6(Suppl 2):3–10.
[3] Hirschmann JV. What killed Mozart? Arch Intern Med 2001;161:1381–9.
[4] Lin X, Alber D, Henkelmann R. Elemental contents in Napoleon's hair cut before and after his death: did Napoleon die of arsenic poisoning? Anal Bioanal Chem 2004;379:218–20.
[5] Yip L, Dart R. Arsenic. In: Sullivan JB, Krieger GR, editors. Clinical environmental health and toxic exposures. 2nd edition. Philadelphia: Lippincott, William and Williams; 2001. p. 858–66.
[6] Soignet SL, Maslak P, Wang ZG, et al. Complete remission after treatment of acute promyelocytic leukemia with arsenic trioxide. N Engl J Med 1998;339:1341–8.
[7] Kosnett M. Arsenic. In: Brent J, Wallace KL, Burkhart KK, et al, editors. Critical care toxicology. Philadelphia: Mosby; 2005. p. 799–815.

[8] Rahman MM, Chowdhury UK, Mukherjee SC, et al. Chronic arsenic toxicity in Bangladesh and West Bengal, India: a review and commentary. Clin Toxicol 2001;39: 683–700.

[9] Subramanian KS, Kosnett MJ. Human exposures to arsenic from consumption of well water in West Bengal, India. Int J Occup Environ Health 1998;4:217–30.

[10] Gorby MS. Arsenic poisoning. West J Med 1988;149:308–15.

[11] Lai VW, Sun Y, Ting E, et al. Arsenic speciation in human urine: are we all the same? Toxicol Appl Pharmacol 2004;198:297–306.

[12] Le XC, Lu X, Ma M, et al. Speciation of key arsenic metabolic intermediates in human urine. Anal Chem 2000;72:5172–7.

[13] Pinto SS, Nelson KW. Arsenic toxicology and industrial exposure. Annu Rev Pharmacol Toxicol 1976;16:95–100.

[14] Winski SL, Carter DE. Arsenate toxicity in human erythrocytes: characterization of morphologic changes and determination of the mechanism of damage. J Toxicol Environ Health A 1998;53:345–55.

[15] Carter DE, Aposhian HV, Gandolfi AJ. The metabolism of inorganic arsenic oxides, gallium arsenide, and arsine: a toxicochemical review. Toxicol Appl Pharmacol 2003;193: 309–34.

[16] Mahieu P, Buchet JP, Roels HA, et al. The metabolism of arsenic in humans acutely intoxicated by As2O3. Its significance for the duration of BAL therapy. Clin Toxicol 1981;18:1067–75.

[17] Radabaugh TR, Aposhian HV. Enzymatic reduction of arsenic compounds in mammalian systems: reduction of arsenate to arsenite by human liver arsenate reductase. Chem Res Toxicol 2000;13:26–30.

[18] Abernathy CO, Liu YP, Longfellow D, et al. Arsenic: health effects, mechanisms of actions, and research issues. Environ Health Perspect 1999;107:593–7.

[19] Webb J. Arsenicals. Volume 3. New York: Academic Press; 1966.

[20] Gillies AJ, Taylor AJ. Acute arsenical poisoning in Dunedin. N Z Med J 1979;89:379–81.

[21] Levin-Scherz JK, Patrick JD, Weber FH, et al. Acute arsenic ingestion. Ann Emerg Med 1987;16:702–4.

[22] Mathieu D, Mathieu-Nolf M, Germain-Alonso M, et al. Massive arsenic poisoning effect of hemodialysis and dimercaprol on arsenic kinetics. Intensive Care Med 1992;18:47–50.

[23] Kyle RA, Pease GL. Hematologic aspects of arsenic intoxication. N Engl J Med 1965;273: 18–23.

[24] Fennell JS, Stacy WK. Electrocardiographic changes in acute arsenic poisoning. Ir J Med Sci 1981;150:338–9.

[25] Glazener FS, Ellis JG, Johnson PK. Electrocardiographic findings with arsenic poisoning. Calif Med 1968;109:158–62.

[26] Murphy MJ, Lyon LW, Taylor JW. Subacute arsenic neuropathy: clinical and electrophysiological observations. J Neurol Neurosurg Psychiatry 1981;44:896–900.

[27] Oh SJ. Electrophysiological profile in arsenic neuropathy. J Neurol Neurosurg Psychiatry 1991;54:1103–5.

[28] Donofrio PD, Wilbourn AJ, Albers JW, et al. Acute arsenic intoxication presenting as Guillain-Barre-like syndrome. Muscle Nerve 1987;10:114–20.

[29] Jenkins RB. Inorganic arsenic and the nervous system. Brain 1966;89:479–98.

[30] Hall AH. Chronic arsenic poisoning. Toxicol Lett 2002;128:69–72.

[31] Shannon RL, Strayer DS. Arsenic-induced skin toxicity. Hum Toxicol 1989;8:99–104.

[32] Tay CH. Cutaneous manifestations of arsenic poisoning due to certain Chinese herbal medicine. Australas J Dermatol 1974;15:121–31.

[33] Mees RA. Een verschijnsel bij polyneuritis arsenicosa. Ned Tijdschr Verloskd Gynaecol 1919;1:391–6.

[34] Tseng CH. Blackfoot disease and arsenic: a never-ending story. J Environ Sci Health C Environ Carcinog Ecotoxicol Rev 2005;23:55–74.

[35] Jackson R, Grainge JW. Arsenic and cancer. Can Med Assoc J 1975;113:396–401.

[36] Lugo G, Cassady G, Palmisano P. Acute maternal arsenic intoxication with neonatal death. Am J Dis Child 1969;117:328–30.

[37] Vantroyen B, Heilier JF, Meulemans A, et al. Survival after a lethal dose of arsenic trioxide. Clin Toxicol 2004;42:889–95.

[38] Shamberger RJ. Validity of hair mineral testing. Biol Trace Elem Res 2002;87:1–28.

[39] Aposhian HV. DMSA and DMPS—water soluble antidotes for heavy metal poisoning. Annu Rev Pharmacol Toxicol 1983;23:193–215.

[40] Aposhian HV, Carter DE, Hoover TD, et al. DMSA, DMPS, and DMPA—as arsenic antidotes. Fundam Appl Toxicol 1984;4:S58–70.

[41] Aposhian HV, Maiorino RM, Gonzalez-Ramirez D, et al. Mobilization of heavy metals by newer, therapeutically useful chelating agents. Toxicology 1995;97:23–38.

[42] Stocken L, Thompson R. British Anti-Lewisite: 2, Dithiol compounds as antidotes for arsenic. Biochem J 1946;40:535–48.

[43] Vaziri ND, Upham T, Barton CH. Hemodialysis clearance of arsenic. Clin Toxicol 1980; 17:451–6.

[44] Klimecki WT, Carter DE. Arsine toxicity: chemical and mechanistic implications. J Toxicol Environ Health 1995;46:399–409.

[45] Romeo L, Apostoli P, Kovacic M, et al. Acute arsine intoxication as a consequence of metal burnishing operations. Am J Ind Med 1997;32:211–6.

[46] Fowler BA, Weissberg JB. Arsine poisoning. N Engl J Med 1974;291:1171–4.

[47] Amante L, Magistretti M, Pernis B. The action of arsine on reduced glutathione. Med Lav 1961;52:11–3.

[48] Ayala-Fierro F, Barber DS, Rael LT, et al. In vitro tissue specificity for arsine and arsenite toxicity in the rat. Toxicol Sci 1999;52:122–9.

[49] Blair PC, Thompson MB, Bechtold M, et al. Evidence for oxidative damage to red blood cells in mice induced by arsine gas. Toxicology 1990;63:25–34.

[50] Kensler C, Abels J, Rhoads C. Arsine poisoning, mode of action and treatment. J Pharmacol Exp Ther 1946;5:99–108.

[51] Pernis B, Magistretti M. A study of the mechanism of acute hemolytic anemia from arsine. Med Lav 1960;51:37–41.

[52] Peterson DP, Bhattacharyya MH. Hematological responses to arsine exposure: quantitation of exposure response in mice. Fundam Appl Toxicol 1985;5:499–505.

[53] Rael LT, Ayala-Fierro F, Carter DE. The effects of sulfur, thiol, and thiol inhibitor compounds on arsine-induced toxicity in the human erythrocyte membrane. Toxicol Sci 2000;55:468–77.

[54] Winski SL, Barber DS, Rael LT, et al. Sequence of toxic events in arsine-induced hemolysis in vitro: implications for the mechanism of toxicity in human erythrocytes. Fundam Appl Toxicol 1997;38:123–8.

[55] Coles GA, Davies HJ, Daley D, et al. Acute intravascular haemolysis and renal failure due to arsine poisoning. Postgrad Med J 1969;45:170–2.

[56] Ayala-Fierro F, Carter DE. LLC-PK1 cells as a model for renal toxicity caused by arsine exposure. J Toxicol Environ Health A 2000;60:67–79.

[57] Uldall PR, Khan HA, Ennis JE, et al. Renal damage from industrial arisine poisoning. Br J Ind Med 1970;27:372–7.

[58] Macaulay DB, Stanley DA. Arsine poisoning. Br J Ind Med 1956;13:217–21.

[59] McKinstry WJ, Hickes JM. Emergency; arsine poisoning. AMA Arch Ind Health 1957; 16:32–41.

[60] Pino P, Walter T, Oyarzun MJ, et al. Rapid drop in infant blood lead levels during the transition to unleaded gasoline use in Santiago, Chile. Arch Environ Health 2004;59: 182–7.

[61] Hesdorffer CS, Milne FJ, Terblanche J, et al. Arsine gas poisoning: the importance of exchange transfusions in severe cases. Br J Ind Med 1986;43:353–5.

[62] Hocken AG, Bradshaw G. Arsine poisoning. Br J Ind Med 1970;27:56–60.
[63] Teitelbaum DT, Kier LC. Arsine poisoning. Report of five cases in the petroleum industry and a discussion of the indications for exchange transfusion and hemodialysis. Arch Environ Health 1969;19:133–43.
[64] Apostoli P, Alessio L, Romeo L, et al. Metabolism of arsenic after acute occupational arsine intoxication. J Toxicol Environ Health 1997;52:331–42.
[65] Rusyniak DE, Furbee RB, Kirk MS. Thallium and arsenic poisoning in a small midwest town. Ann Emerg Med 2002;39:307–11.
[66] Lynch GR, Lond MB. The toxicology of thallium. Lancet Dec 1930;20:1340–4.
[67] Bank WJ, Pleasure DE, Suzuki K, et al. Thallium Poisoning. Arch Neurol 1972;26:456–64.
[68] Reed D, Crawley J, Faro SN, et al. Thallotoxicosis. JAMA 1963;183:516–22.
[69] Desenclos JC, Wilder MH, Coppenger GW, et al. Thallium poisoning: an outbreak in Florida 1988. South Med J 1992;85:1203–6.
[70] Insley BM, Grufferman S, Ayliffe HE. Thallium poisoning in cocaine abusers. Am J Emerg Med 1986;4:545–8.
[71] Malbrain ML, Lambrecht GL, Zandijk E, et al. Treatment of severe thallium intoxication. Clin Toxicol 1997;35:97–100.
[72] Meggs WJ, Hoffman RS, Shih RD, et al. Thallium poisoning from maliciously contaminated food. Clin Toxicol 1994;32:723–30.
[73] Moore D, House I, Dixon A. Thallium poisoning: diagnosis may be elusive but alopecia is the clue. BMJ 1993;306:1527–9.
[74] Questel F, Dugarin J, Dally S. Thallium-contaminated heroin. Ann Intern Med 1996;124:616.
[75] Waters CB, Hawkins EC, Knapp DW. Acute thallium toxicosis in a dog. J Am Vet Med Assoc 1992;201:883–5.
[76] Lund A. Distribution of thallium in the organism and its elimination. Acta Pharmacol Toxicol (Copenh) 1956;12:251–9.
[77] Douglas KT, Bunni MA, Baindur SR. Thallium in biochemistry. Int J Biochem 1990;22:429–38.
[78] Gehring PJ, Hammond PB. The interrelationship between thallium and potassium in animals. J Pharmacol Exp Ther 1967;155:187–201.
[79] Mulkey JP, Oehme FW. A review of thallium toxicity. Vet Hum Toxicol 1993;35:445–53.
[80] Melnick RL, Monti LG, Motzkin SM. Uncoupling of mitochondrial oxidative phosphorylation by thallium. Biochem Biophys Res Commun 1976;69:68–73.
[81] Cavanagh JB, Fuller NH, Johnson HRM. The effects of thallium salts, with particular reference to the nervous system changes: a report of three cases. Q J Med 1974;170:293–319.
[82] Tromme I, Van Neste D, Dobbelaere F, et al. Skin signs in the diagnosis of thallium poisoning. Br J Dermatol 1998;138:321–5.
[83] Moeschlin S. Thallium poisoning. Clin Toxicol 1980;17:133–46.
[84] Feldman J, Levisohn DR. Acute alopecia: clue to thallium toxicity. Pediatr Dermatol 1993;10:29–31.
[85] Heyl T, Barlow RJ. Thallium poisoning: a dermatological perspective. Br J Dermatol 1989;121:787–91.
[86] McMillan TM, Jacobson RR, Gross M. Neuropsychology of thallium poisoning. J Neurol Neurosurg Psychiatry 1997;63:247–50.
[87] Davis LE, Standefer JC, Kornfeld M, et al. Acute thallium poisoning: toxicological and morphological studies of the nervous system. Ann Neurol 1980;10:38–44.
[88] Koblenzer PJ, Weiner LB. Alopecia secondary to thallium intoxication. Arch Dermatol 1969;99:777.
[89] Metter D, Vock R. [Structure of the hair in thallium poisoning]. Z Rechtsmed 1984;91:201–14.
[90] Cavanagh JB. The 'dying back' process. A common denominator in many naturally occurring and toxic neuropathies. Arch Pathol Lab Med 1979;103:659–64.

[91] Cavanagh JB. What have we learnt from Graham Frederick Young? Reflections on the mechanism of thallium neurotoxicity. Neuropathol Appl Neurobiol 1991;17:3–9.

[92] Thompson DF, Callen ED. Soluble or insoluble Prussian blue for radiocesium and thallium poisoning? Ann Pharmacother 2004;38:1509–14.

[93] Hoffman RS. Thallium toxicity and the role of Prussian blue in therapy. Toxicol Rev 2003; 22:29–40.

[94] Barroso-Moguel R, Villeda-Hernandez J, Mendez-Armenta M, et al. Combined D-penicillamine and Prussian blue as antidotal treatment against thallotoxicosis in rats: evaluation of cerebellar lesions. Toxicology 1994;89:15–24.

[95] Heydlauf H. Ferric-cyanoferrate (II):An effective antidote in thallium poisoning. Eur J Pharmacol 1969;6:340–4.

[96] Kamerbeek HH, Rauws AG, Ham MT, et al. Prussian blue in therapy of thallotoxicosis: an experimental and clinical investigation. Acta Med Scand 1971;189:321–4.

[97] Manninen V, Malkonen M, Skulskii IA. Elimination of thallium in rats as influenced by Prussian blue and sodium chloride. Acta Pharmacol Toxicol (Copenh) 1976;39: 256–61.

[98] Meggs WJ, Cahill-Morasco R, Shih RD, et al. Effects of Prussian blue and N-acetylcysteine on thallium toxicity in mice. Clin Toxicol 1997;35:163–6.

[99] Rauws AG. Thallium pharmacokinetics and its modification by Prussian blue. Naunyn Schmiedebergs Arch Pharmacol 1974;284:295–306.

[100] Rios C, Monroy-Noyola A. D-penicillamine and Prussian blue as antidotes against thallium intoxication in rats. Toxicology 1992;74:69–76.

[101] Rusyniak DE, Kao LW, Nanagas KA, et al. Dimercaptosuccinic acid and Prussian blue in the treatment of acute thallium poisoning in rats. Clin Toxicol 2003;41:137–42.

[102] Pearce J. Studies of any toxicological effects of Prussian blue compounds in mammals–a review. Food Chem Toxicol 1994;32:577–82.

[103] Lund A. The effect various substances on the excretion and the toxicity of thallium in the rat. Acta Pharmacol Toxicol (Copenh) 1956;12:260–8.

[104] Van der Stock J, Schepper J. The effect of Prussian blue and sodium-ethylenediaminetetraacetic acid on the faecal and urinary elimination of thallium by the dog. Res Vet Sci 1978;25: 337–42.

[105] Hoffman RS, Stringer JA, Feinberg RS, et al. Comparative efficacy of thallium adsorption by activated charcoal, Prussian blue, and sodium polystyrene sulfonate. Clin Toxicol 1999; 37:833–7.

[106] Lehmann PA, Favari L. Parameters for the adsorption of thallium ions by activated charcoal and Prussian blue. Clin Toxicol 1984;22:331–9.

[107] Goldwater LJ. Hat industry. In: Goldwater LJ, editor. Mercury: a history of quicksilver. Baltimore (MD): York Press; 1955.

[108] Graeme KA, Pollack CV. Heavy metal toxicity, Part I: arsenic and mercury. J Emerg Med 1998;16:45–56.

[109] Richer J, DeWoskin R. ATSDR. Toxicological profile for MERCURY. In: US Department of Health and Human Services. Atlanta (GA): Agency for Toxic Substances and Disease Registry; 1999. p. 3–676.

[110] O'Shea JG. "Two minutes with Venus, two years with mercury": mercury as an antisyphilitic chemotherapeutic agent. J R Soc Med 1990;83:392–5.

[111] Lide Dr., editor. CRC handbook of chemistry and physics. 86th edition. Boca Raton (FL): CRC Press; 2005.

[112] Rishler JF, Amler SN. Mercury exposure: evaluation and intervention in the inappropriate use of chelation agents in the diagnosis and treatment of putative mercury poisoning. Neurotoxicology 2005;26:691–9.

[113] Boyd AS, Seger D, Vannucci S, et al. Mercury exposure and cutaneous disease. J Am Acad Dermatol 2000;43:81–90.

[114] Gutierrez F, Lucio L. Elemental mercury embolism to the lung. N Engl J Med 2000;342:1791.

[115] Bredfeldt JE, Moeller DD. Systemic mercury intoxication following rupture of a Miller-Abbott tube. Am J Gastroenterol 1978;69:478–80.

[116] McKinney PE. Elemental mercury in the appendix: an unusual complication of a Mexican-American folk remedy. Clin Toxicol 1999;37:103–7.

[117] Nanagas KA, O'Connor AD, Potts ME, et al. Conservative management of elemental mercury sequestration in the appendix. Clin Toxicol 2003;41:A52.

[118] Chang LW, Verity MA. Mercury neurotoxicity: effects and mechanisms. In: Chang LW, Dyer RS, editors. Handbook of neurotoxicology. New York: Marcel Dekker; 1995. p. 31–59.

[119] Rowens B, Guerrero-Betancourt D, Gottlieb CA, et al. Respiratory failure and death following acute inhalation of mercury vapor: a clinical and histologic perspective. Chest 1991;99:185–90.

[120] Aguado S, de Quiros IF, Marin R, et al. Acute mercury vapour intoxication: report of six cases. Nephrol Dial Transplant 1989;4:133–6.

[121] Clarkson TW, Magos L, Myers GJ. The toxicology of mercury: current exposures and clinical manifestations. N Engl J Med 2003;349:1731–7.

[122] Dally A. The rise and fall of pink disease. Soc Hist Med 1997;10:291–304.

[123] Sedano HO. Mercury poisoning and acrodynia. Oral Surg Oral Med Oral Pathol Oral Radiol Endod 1998;85:349.

[124] Harrop-Griffiths H. Adult pink disease. BMJ 1970;1:298.

[125] Beuter A, de Geoffroy A. Can tremor be used to measure the effect of chronic mercury exposure in human subjects? Neurotoxicology 1996;17:213–27.

[126] Netterstrom B, Guldager B, Heeboll J. Acute mercury intoxication examined with coordination ability and tremor. Neurotoxicol Teratol 1996;18:505–9.

[127] Henningsson C, Hoffmann S, McGonigle L. Acute mercury poisoning (acrodynia) mimicking pheochromocytoma in an adolescent. J Pediatr 1993;122:252–3.

[128] Torres AD, Ashok NR, Hardiek ML. Mercury intoxication and arterial hypertension: report of two patients and review of the literature. Pediatrics 2000;105:E34.

[129] Wossmann W, Kohl M, Gruning G, et al. Mercury intoxication presenting with hypertension and tachycardia. Arch Dis Child 1999;80:556–7.

[130] Archbold GP, McGuckin RM, Campbell NA. Dimercaptosuccinic acid loading test for assessing mercury burden in healthy individuals. Ann Clin Biochem 2004;41: 233–6.

[131] Kosnett MJ. Unanswered questions in metal chelation. Clin Toxicol 1992;30:529–47.

[132] Martin-Gil J, Martin-Gil FJ, Delibes-de-Castro G, et al. The first known use of vermillion. Experientia 1995;51:759–61.

[133] DeBont B, Lauwerys R, Govaerts H, et al. Yellow mercuric oxide ointment and mercury intoxication. Eur J Pediatr 1986;145:217–8.

[134] Dargan P, Giles L, Wallace C, et al. Case report: severe mercuric sulphate poisoning treated with 2,3-dimercaptopropane-1-sulphonate and haemodiafiltration. Crit Care 2003;7:R1–6.

[135] Endo T, Nakaya S, Kimura R, et al. Gastrointestinal absorption of inorganic mercuric compounds in vivo and in situ. Toxicol Appl Pharmacol 1984;74:223–9.

[136] Fardal O, Johannessen AC, Morken T. Gingivo-mucosal and cutaneous reactions to amalgam fillings. J Clin Periodontol 2005;32:430–3.

[137] Laeijendecker R, Dekker SK, Burger PM, et al. Oral lichen planus and allergy to dental amalgam restorations. Arch Dermatol 2004;140:1434–8.

[138] Schrallhammer-Benkler K, Ring J, Przybilla B, et al. Acute mercury intoxication with lichenoid drug eruption followed by mercury contact allergy and development of antinuclear antibodies. Acta Derm Venereol 1992;72(4):294–6.

[139] Zalups RK, Ahmad S. Homocysteine and the renal epithelial transport and toxicity of inorganic mercury: role of basolateral transporter organic anion transporter 1. J Am Soc Nephrol 2004;15:2023–31.

[140] Newton JA, House IM, Volans GN, et al. Plasma mercury during prolonged acute renal failure after mercuric chloride ingestion. Hum Toxicol 1983;2:535–7.
[141] Aymaz S, Gross O, Krakamp B, et al. Membranous nephropathy from exposure to mercury in the fluorescent-tube-recycling industry. Nephrol Dial Transplant 2001;16:2253–5.
[142] Harada M. Minamata disease: methylmercury poisoning in Japan caused by environmental pollution. Crit Rev Toxicol 1995;25:1–24.
[143] Tsuchiya K. The discovery of the causal agent of Minamata disease. Am J Ind Med 1992; 21:275–80.
[144] Kondo K. Congenital Minamata disease: warnings from Japan's experience. J Child Neurol 2000;15:458–64.
[145] Tedeschi LG. The Minamata disease. Am J Forensic Med Pathol 1982;3:335–8.
[146] Eto K. Minamata disease. Neuropathology 2000;20(Suppl):S14–9.
[147] Bakir F, Damluji SF, Amin-Zaki L, et al. Methylmercury poisoning in Iraq. Science 1973; 181:230–41.
[148] Aberg B, Ekman L, Falk R, et al. Metabolism of methyl mercury (203Hg) compounds in man. Arch Environ Health 1969;19:478–84.
[149] Berlin M, Carlson J, Norseth T. Dose-dependence of methylmercury metabolism. A study of distribution: biotransformation and excretion in the squirrel monkey. Arch Environ Health 1975;30:307–13.
[150] Eto K, Tokunaga H, Nagashima K, et al. An autopsy case of Minamata disease (methyl-mercury poisoning): pathological viewpoints of peripheral nerves. Toxicol Pathol 2002; 30:714–22.
[151] Harada M. Congenital Minamata disease: intrauterine methylmercury poisoning. Teratology 1978;18:285–8.
[152] Bakir F, Rustam H, Tikriti S, et al. Clinical and epidemiological aspects of methylmercury poisoning. Postgrad Med J 1980;56:1–10.
[153] Hviid A, Stellfeld M, Wohlfahrt J, et al. Association between thimerosal-containing vaccine and autism. JAMA 2003;290:1763–6.
[154] Baselt RC. Disposition of toxic drugs and chemicals in man. 6th edition. Foster City (CA): Biomedical Publications; 2002.
[155] Nierenberg DW, Nordgren RE, Chang MB, et al. Delayed cerebellar disease and death after accidental exposure to dimethylmercury. N Engl J Med 1998;338:1672–6.
[156] Clarkson TW, Magos L, Cox C, et al. Tests of efficacy of antidotes for removal of methyl-mercury in human poisoning during the Iraq outbreak. J Pharmacol Exp Ther 1981;218: 74–83.
[157] Aaseth J, Frieheim EA. Treatment of methyl mercury poisoning in mice with 2,3-dimercaptosuccinic acid and other complexing thiols. Acta Pharmacol Toxicol (Copenh) 1978;42:248–52.
[158] Zimmer LJ, Carter DE. The efficacy of 2,3-dimercaptopropanol and D-penicillamine on methyl mercury induced neurological signs and weight loss. Life Sci 1978;23:1025–34.
[159] Hernberg S. Lead poisoning in a historical perspective. Am J Ind Med 2000;38:244–54.
[160] Gilfillan SC. Lead Poisoning and the fall of Rome. J Gnathol 1965;85:53–60.
[161] Lockitch G. Perspectives on lead toxicity. Clin Biochem 1993;26:371–81.
[162] Staudinger KC, Roth VS. Occupational lead poisoning. Am Fam Physician 1998;57: 719–26, 731–2.
[163] Mowad E, Haddad I, Gemmel DJ. Management of lead poisoning from ingested fishing sinkers. Arch Pediatr Adolesc Med 1998;152:485–8.
[164] Haley VB, Talbot TO. Seasonality and trend in blood lead levels of New York state children. BMC Pediatr 2004;4:8.
[165] Canfield RL, Henderson CR Jr, Cory-Slechta DA, et al. Intellectual impairment in children with blood lead concentrations below 10 microg per deciliter. N Engl J Med 2003;348: 1517–26.

[166] Lidsky TI, Schneider JS. Lead neurotoxicity in children: basic mechanisms and clinical correlates. Brain 2003;126:5–19.

[167] Goldstein GW. Neurologic concepts of lead poisoning in children. Pediatr Ann 1992; 21:384–8.

[168] Johnston MV, Goldstein GW. Selective vulnerability of the developing brain to lead. Curr Opin Neurol 1998;11:689–93.

[169] Slobozhanina EI, Kozlova NM, Lukyanenko LM, et al. Lead-induced changes in human erythrocytes and lymphocytes. J Appl Toxicol 2005;25:109–14.

[170] Besunder JB, Super DM, Anderson RL. Comparison of dimercaptosuccinic acid and calcium disodium ethylenediaminetetraacetic acid versus dimercaptopropanol and ethylenediaminetetraacetic acid in children with lead poisoning. J Pediatr 1997;130:966–71.

[171] American Academy of Pediatrics issues treatment guidelines for lead exposure in children. Am Fam Physician 1995;52:1022–3.

[172] Dietrich KN, Ware JH, Salganik M, et al. Effect of chelation therapy on the neuropsychological and behavioral development of lead-exposed children after school entry. Pediatrics 2004;114:19–26.

[173] Rogan WJ, Dietrich KN, Ware JH, et al. The effect of chelation therapy with succimer on neuropsychological development in children exposed to lead. N Engl J Med 2001;344: 1421–6.

[174] Hu H, Aro A, Payton M, et al. The relationship of bone and blood lead to hypertension. The normative aging study. JAMA 1996;275:1171–6.

[175] Maslinski PG, Loeb JA. Pica-associated cerebral edema in an adult. J Neurol Sci 2004; 225:149–51.

[176] Barats MS, Gonick HC, Rothenberg S, et al. Severe lead-induced peripheral neuropathy in a dialysis patient. Am J Kidney Dis 2000;35:963–8.

[177] Rabinowitz MB. Toxicokinetics of bone lead. Environ Health Perspect 1991;91:33–7.

[178] Magos L. Lead poisoning from retained lead projectiles: a critical review of case reports. Hum Exp Toxicol 1994;13:735–42.

[179] Hu H, Pepper L, Goldman R. Effect of repeated occupational exposure to lead, cessation of exposure, and chelation on levels of lead in bone. Am J Ind Med 1991;20:723–35.

ELSEVIER
SAUNDERS

Clin Lab Med 26 (2006) 99–125

CLINICS IN
LABORATORY
MEDICINE

Toxicity Associated with Carbon Monoxide

Louise W. Kao, MD[a,b,]*, Kristine A. Nañagas, MD[a,b]

[a]Department of Emergency Medicine, Indiana University School of Medicine,
Indianapolis, IN, USA
[b]Medical Toxicology of Indiana, Indiana Poison Center, Indianapolis, IN, USA

Carbon monoxide (CO) has been called a "great mimicker." The clinical presentations associated with CO toxicity may be diverse and nonspecific, including syncope, new-onset seizure, flu-like illness, headache, and chest pain. Unrecognized CO exposure may lead to significant morbidity and mortality. Even when the diagnosis is certain, appropriate therapy is widely debated.

Epidemiology and sources

CO is a colorless, odorless, nonirritating gas produced primarily by incomplete combustion of any carbonaceous fossil fuel. CO is the leading cause of poisoning mortality in the United States [1,2] and may be responsible for more than half of all fatal poisonings worldwide [3]. An estimated 5000 to 6000 people die in the United States each year as a result of CO exposure [2]. From 1968 to 1998, the Centers for Disease Control reported that non–fire-related CO poisoning caused or contributed to 116,703 deaths, 70.6% of which were due to motor vehicle exhaust and 29% of which were unintentional [4]. Although most accidental deaths are due to house fires and automobile exhaust, consumer products such as indoor heaters and stoves contribute to approximately 180 to 200 annual deaths [5]. Unintentional deaths peak in the winter months, when heating systems are being used and windows are closed [2].

Portions of this article were previously published in Holstege CP, Rusyniak DE: Medical Toxicology. 89:6, Med Clin North Am, 2005; with permission.

* Corresponding author. Department of Emergency Medicine, Indiana State University School of Medicine, 1701 North Senate Boulevard, Indianapolis, IN 46206.

E-mail address: lkao@clarian.org (L.W. Kao).

Environmental CO exposure is typically less than 0.001%, or 10 ppm [6], but it may be higher in urban areas [7]. The amount of CO absorbed by the body is dependent on minute ventilation, duration of exposure, and concentrations of CO and oxygen in the environment [8–11]. After cooking with a gas stove, indoor air concentrations of CO may reach 100 ppm [7]. A cigarette smoker is exposed to an estimated 400 to 500 ppm of CO while actively smoking [3]. Automobile exhaust may contain as much as 10% (100,000 ppm) CO [12]. Exposure to 70 ppm may lead to carboxyhemoglobin (CO-Hgb) levels of 10% at equilibrium (approximately 4 hours) [1,13], and exposure to 350 ppm may lead to CO-Hgb levels of 40% at equilibrium [3,13]. The current Occupational Safety and Health Administration permissible limit for CO exposure in workers is 50 ppm averaged over an 8-hour work day [14].

In addition to the above sources, CO poisoning has been reported in children riding in the back of pickup trucks [15], recreational boaters [16,17], factory workers operating propane-powered forklifts [18–20], and persons in an ice skating rink using propane-powered resurfacing machines [21,22]. Fatalities are reported in the cases of recreational boaters swimming underneath the swim platform near the boat exhaust [23] and campers using gas-powered stoves in outdoor tents [24]. In the winter, misuse of a gas stove or burning charcoal briquettes for heating purposes is predictive of high CO-Hgb levels [25–27]. Another source is methylene chloride, a solvent found in paint remover and aerosol propellants, which is converted by the liver to CO after exposure [28–30].

Endogenous production of CO occurs during heme catabolism by heme oxygenase but should not produce CO-Hgb levels in excess of 1%. However, in hemolytic anemia, CO-Hgb may increase to 3% to 4% [12,31,32]. Severe sepsis has also been shown to elevate endogenous CO production [33].

A patient who presents from a house fire or after a suicide attempt with automobile exhaust may not represent a diagnostic dilemma. However, a family presenting with symptoms of nausea and vomiting or a patient with a headache that is improving can easily be misdiagnosed and discharged back to the dangerous environment where they may subsequently suffer more serious exposures.

Pathophysiology

Hemoglobin binding

The pathophysiology of CO poisoning was initially thought to be due exclusively to the cellular hypoxia imposed by replacing oxyhemoglobin with CO-Hgb and producing a relative anemia [34]. CO binds to hemoglobin with an affinity more than 200 times that of oxygen [8,35,36]. It causes a leftward shift in the oxygen–hemoglobin dissociation curve, decreasing oxygen delivery to the tissues and resulting in tissue hypoxia [36].

Direct cellular toxicity

CO poisoning is much more complex than was initially presumed, and it clearly has mechanisms of toxicity beyond the formation of CO-Hgb. In a classic study, Goldbaum and colleagues [37] demonstrated that dogs breathing 13% CO died within 1 hour after achieving CO-Hgb levels from 54% to 90%. However, exchange transfusion with blood containing 80% CO-Hgb to otherwise healthy dogs resulted in no toxic effects, despite resultant CO-Hgb levels of 57% to 64%, suggesting that CO toxicity is not dependent on CO-Hgb formation. Other studies have corroborated the findings of morbidity and mortality due to CO poisoning independent of hypoxia or CO-Hgb formation [38–42].

The current understanding of the pathophysiology of CO poisoning relates its clinical effects to a combination of hypoxia/ischemia due to CO-Hgb formation and direct CO toxicity at the cellular level. This combination helps to explain why CO-Hgb levels do not correlate with the severity of clinical effects [43–47]. An outline of some of the proposed mechanisms is presented in Fig. 1.

Protein binding (cytochromes, myoglobin, guanylyl cyclase)

CO binds to many heme-containing proteins other than hemoglobin, including cytochromes, myoglobin, and guanylyl cyclase. CO binds to cytochrome a3 in vitro [48,49], and the disruption of oxidative metabolism may lead to the generation of oxygen free radicals [50,51]. Cellular respiration may also be impaired by inactivation of mitochondrial enzymes and impaired electron transport from oxygen radicals (ie, peroxynitrite) produced after CO exposure [50,52,53]. Cellular energy metabolism is inhibited even after normalization of CO-Hgb levels [47,54], which may explain the prolonged clinical effects after CO-Hgb levels decrease [9]. Binding to myoglobin may reduce oxygen availability in the heart and lead to arrhythmias and cardiac dysfunction [9,55,56]; it may also contribute to direct skeletal muscle toxicity and rhabdomyolysis [57–60]. CO also stimulates guanylyl cyclase, which increases cyclic guanylyl monophosphate, resulting in cerebral vasodilatation, which has been associated with loss of consciousness in an animal model of CO poisoning [61,62].

Nitric oxide

The role of nitric oxide (NO) and other oxygen free radicals has been extensively researched in the setting of CO poisoning. Many animal studies have shown cerebral vasodilatation after exposure to CO, which is temporally associated with loss of consciousness and increased NO levels [63–66]. This evidence has led to speculation that, clinically, syncope may be related to NO-mediated cerebral vessel relaxation and low blood flow. NO is also a peripheral vasodilator [67] and may result in systemic hypotension, although this effect has not been studied in the setting of CO poisoning. However, the presence of

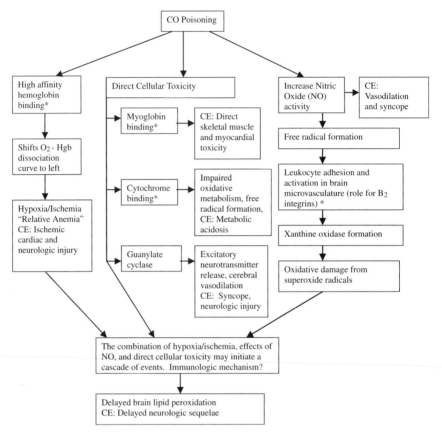

Fig. 1. Proposed pathophysiology of CO poisoning. *Potential hyperbaric oxygen therapy target. CE, clinical effect.

systemic hypotension in CO poisoning is correlated with the severity of cerebral lesions, particularly in watershed areas of perfusion (ie, basal ganglia, white matter, hippocampus) [9,46,68–71].

NO also appears to play a pivotal role in a cascade of events culminating in oxidative damage to the brain, which may be responsible for the clinical syndrome of delayed neurologic sequelae (DNS) [72]. NO may affect the adherence of neutrophils to the endothelium, potentially by affecting the function of neutrophil adhesion molecules such as B_2-integrin [52,72]. Neutrophil adherence to the microvasculature appears to lead to xanthine oxidase activation, oxidative radical formation, oxidative damage, and ultimately to brain lipid peroxidation, which is thought to be the underlying process responsible for the clinical syndrome of DNS [50,52,66,72–76].

Brain lipid peroxidation after CO exposure appears to be a postischemic reperfusion phenomenon, mediated by alterations in cerebral blood flow as well as oxidative free radical damage [50,51,66,73,76–78]. A period of hypotension and unconsciousness may be required for lipid peroxidation to occur [76]. Although the exact sequence of events is not known, the experimental administration of nitric oxide synthase inhibitors has been found to inhibit both cerebral vasodilatation [41] and oxidative damage [66]. Newer research has postulated an immune-mediated mechanism of DNS. Rats made immunologically tolerant to myelin basic protein (MBP) before CO poisoning did not suffer learning decrements, nor did they exhibit the typical degree of brain histologic changes seen in rats that were not immunologically tolerant. The authors hypothesize that CO poisoning induces biochemical and antigenic changes in MBP, which may react with products of lipid peroxidation to produce an immunologic cascade [79].

Other potential mechanisms of CO toxicity include excitotoxicity (ie, glutamate-mediated neuronal injury) [80–82], increased atherogenesis [83,84], involvement with cytochrome p450 [9,85], and apoptosis [80]. Further research is likely to continue to elucidate the complex pathophysiology of CO poisoning.

Clinical effects: acute

The clinical effects of CO poisoning are diverse and easily confused with other illnesses, such as nonspecific viral illness, benign headache, and various cardiovascular and neurologic syndromes [6,25,86–88]. Box 1 lists common signs and symptoms reported in the literature [1,6,89].

Initial symptoms after CO exposure include headache, nausea, and dizziness [90,91]. As exposure increases, patients develop more pronounced and severe symptoms, with oxygen-dependent organs (the brain and the heart) showing the earliest signs of injury.

Early neurologic manifestations include dizziness and headache. Increasing exposure may produce altered mental status, confusion, syncope, seizure, acute stroke-like syndromes, and coma. Isolated seizures have been reported in pediatric patients [92,93]. Abnormalities on neuroimaging studies, particularly bilateral globus pallidus lesions, are often seen in significant CO poisoning [94–97]. The presence of systemic hypotension in CO poisoning is correlated with the severity of central nervous system structural damage [9,46,68–71].

Early cardiovascular effects of CO poisoning are manifested by tachycardia in response to hypoxia [98]. More significant exposures result in hypotension, dysrhythmia, ischemia, infarction, and, in extreme cases, cardiac arrest. Early deaths after CO exposure may be due to cardiac dysrhythmias [45,50]. Hypotension may result from myocardial injury due to hypoxia/ischemia, direct myocardial depressant activity from myoglobin binding, peripheral vasodilatation, or a combination of these factors [78]. It may persist even after neurologic and metabolic symptoms have resolved [99].

CO poisoning exacerbates underlying cardiovascular disease, making this group of patients particularly susceptible to cardiovascular disturbances

---

Box 1. Clinical signs and symptoms associated with carbon monoxide poisoning

Mild
- Headache
- Nausea
- Vomiting
- Dizziness
- Blurred vision

Moderate
- Confusion
- Syncope
- Chest pain
- Dyspnea
- Weakness
- Tachycardia
- Tachypnea
- Rhabdomyolysis

Severe
- Palpitations
- Dysrhythmias
- Hypotension
- Myocardial ischemia
- Cardiac arrest
- Respiratory arrest
- Noncardiogenic pulmonary edema
- Seizures
- Coma

Data from Cobb N, Etzel RA. Unintentional carbon monoxide-related deaths in the United States, 1979 through 1988. JAMA 1991;266(5):659–63; and Forbes WH, Sargent F, Roughton FJW. The rate of carbon monoxide uptake by normal men. Am J Physiol 1945;143(4):594–608.

[100,101]. Low-level experimental CO exposures producing CO-Hgb levels from 2% to 6% in patients who had documented coronary artery disease have produced dysrhythmias and decreased latency to the development of cardiac ischemia during stress testing [102–104]. CO exposure lowers the threshold for malignant ventricular dysrhythmias [55]. In patients with undiagnosed underlying coronary artery disease, CO exposure may act as a stress test, much like anemia. Even in healthy volunteers, CO exposure has been found to result in nonspecific ECG changes [91]. Myocardial infarction has been reported in CO poisoning in the absence of underlying coronary disease [105].

CO poisoning may also result in rhabdomyolysis and acute renal failure, potentially as a direct toxic effect of CO on skeletal muscle [57–59]. Cutaneous blisters [106] and noncardiogenic pulmonary edema [107–109] have been reported in patients with severe CO poisoning. The "cherry red" skin color often discussed in textbooks is not commonly seen in practice [6,50,107].

CO binds more tightly to fetal than adult hemoglobin, making infants particularly vulnerable to its effects [110]. Occult CO poisoning may present as an acute life-threatening event in the infant [111]. Even older pediatric patients are more susceptible to the effects of CO because of their higher metabolic rate and oxygen uptake [112,113]. Symptoms in pediatric patients are often nonspecific, such as nausea and vomiting, and may easily be misdiagnosed as a viral illness [88,111]. An increased incidence of syncope and lethargy is reported in the pediatric population compared with adults [112].

CO exposure in the pregnant patient presents a unique scenario. CO crosses the placenta readily, and animal studies have shown that, with maternal CO exposure, fetal CO-Hgb levels reach a higher peak and eliminate more slowly than maternal CO-Hgb [114,115]. In humans, adverse fetal outcomes, such as stillbirth, anatomic malformations, and neurologic disability, are clearly associated with more severe maternal exposure [116–119]. However, even in mildly symptomatic mothers, the effects on the fetus may be severe, including anatomic malformations and fetal demise [117,120]. When autopsy is performed, fetal brain damage is generally apparent, particularly in the basal ganglia and globus pallidus [116,121]. Earlier gestational age of the fetus during CO exposure has been associated with anatomic malformations, whereas functional disturbances and poor neurologic development are reported after CO exposure at any gestational age [116,117,122,123].

Clinical effects: delayed

The effects of CO are not confined to the period immediately after exposure. Persistent or delayed neurologic effects have also been reported. Most intriguing is a syndrome of apparent recovery from acute CO poisoning followed by behavioral and neurologic deterioration after a latency period of 2 to 40 days. This syndrome, often referred to as DNS, may manifest as almost any conceivable neurologic or psychiatric symptom, including memory loss, confusion, ataxia, seizures, urinary and fecal incontinence, emotional lability, disorientation, hallucinations, parkinsonism, mutism, cortical blindness, psychosis, and gait and other motor disturbances [100,124–128].

The true prevalence of DNS is difficult to determine, with estimates ranging from less than 1% to 47% of patients after CO poisoning [44,108,125–127,129–131]. The large variability in prevalence is at least partially explained by a lack of consistency in defining DNS using clinical, subclinical (eg, neuropsychometric testing results), self-reported, or combination criteria.

The two largest case series are from Korea, where CO poisoning is common because of the use of coal stoves for cooking and heating [125,126]. Of 2360 victims of acute CO poisoning, DNS were diagnosed in 65 patients. Symptoms included mental deterioration, memory impairment, gait disturbance, urinary and fecal incontinence, and mutism. The rate of DNS in this series was 2.75% of all CO-poisoned patients and 11.8% of the subset of hospitalized patients. The lucid interval between recovery from the initial exposure and development of DNS was 2 to 40 days (mean 22.4 days). Of those patients who were followed, 75% recovered within 1 year. The incidence of DNS increased with the duration of unconsciousness experienced by the patient and with age greater than 30 [126]. Another large series reporting on 2967 patients who had CO poisoning had findings almost identical to the cohort already described. More than 90% of patients who developed DNS in this series were unconscious during the acute intoxication, and the incidence of DNS was disproportionally higher in older patients (50–79 years) and nonexistent in patients less than 30 years of age [125].

In general, patients who present with a more symptomatic initial clinical picture are the most likely to develop persistent or delayed neurologic sequelae. DNS occurs most frequently in patients who present comatose, in older patients, and perhaps in those with a prolonged exposure [19, 44,125,126,129,131–134]. Neuropsychometric testing abnormalities have been associated with decreased level of consciousness at presentation, particularly when the duration of unconsciousness exceeds 5 minutes [129,133].

Various definitions of DNS are used by investigators; the term may refer to clinical symptoms, neuropsychometric test abnormalities, or a combination of the two. Although using gross neurologic abnormalities to define DNS may underestimate subtle cognitive dysfunction, neuropsychometric testing may reveal subclinical and perhaps temporary cognitive dysfunction of unknown clinical and prognostic significance. Abnormalities found on neuropsychometric testing in CO-exposed patients may be partially explained by confounders. Patients who are acutely ill, suicidal, depressed, or have coingestion of other intoxicants may perform poorly on these tests [135–138]. In addition, these patients generally do not have a baseline for comparison [9,139]. Despite these limitations, neuropsychometric testing provides an objective measure of cognitive function that can be used to screen and follow CO-poisoned patients.

Clinical effects: chronic

Although some authors have hypothesized that chronic CO poisoning may be more pervasive and cause more morbidity and mortality than is currently recognized, the evidence to substantiate these claims is less than compelling, partially because of the inherent difficulties in quantifying both degree of exposure and degree of neurologic impairment [140–143]. Case reports and case series have been published that describe a syndrome of headache, nausea, lightheadedness, cerebellar dysfunction, and cognitive and mood disorders in association with chronic, low-level CO exposure. However, all these reports have uncontrolled confounding factors and lack data regarding the exposure [20,144–150]. These symptoms typically abate once the patient is removed from the environment [19,20,145,148,151]. Other problems that have been speculatively associated with chronic CO exposure include low birth weight [13,152–154], reduced exercise performance [98,155], and exacerbation of cardiac disease, although other risk factors, such as smoking, confound the picture [101,151,156]. In addition, chronic CO exposure has been associated with polycythemia and cardiomegaly, probably due to chronic hypoxia [98].

Diagnosis

A high index of suspicion is essential in making the diagnosis of occult CO poisoning. In prospective observational studies, patients presenting to the ED with winter flu–like syndrome were found to have CO-Hgb levels ranging from 3% to 24%; the possibility of CO exposure must be entertained in patients who have this ED presentation [25,86,87]. Important historical factors to elicit include the use of gas stoves for heating and cohabitants with similar symptoms [25,27,157]. In addition, patients whose symptoms are associated with particular environments (eg, workplace), activities (eg, boating), or appliances (eg, use of stove, fireplace) may be suffering from CO exposure.

Carboxyhemoglobin levels

Serum CO-Hgb levels should be obtained from patients suspected of CO exposure. A nonsmoker would be expected to have a baseline level of less than 1% to 3% from endogenous production and background environmental exposure, whereas smokers may have levels as high as 10%, perhaps slightly higher immediately after smoking [6,158]. Low CO-Hgb levels ($<15\%$–20%) are well correlated with mild symptoms, such as nausea and headache [25,90,91], and levels greater than 60% to 70% are usually rapidly fatal [9]. However, intermediate levels do not appear to correlate well with symptoms or with prognosis; therefore, treatment decisions cannot be based solely on CO-Hgb levels [31,50,95,159–161]. In one series, CO-Hgb levels ranged from 5% to 47% in minimally symptomatic or asymptomatic patients, 10% to 64% in patients who were found unconscious but awoke on hospital arrival, and 1% to 53% in patients who remained comatose [44]. The wide overlaps among blood levels and clinical symptoms underscore the difficulty of using levels alone to determine severity of exposure. The severity of clinical symptoms is related not only to the concentration of CO but also to the duration of exposure [31,89]. Therefore, a patient who attains a high CO-Hgb level after a brief, high-level exposure may not manifest any clinical toxicity [161], whereas a patient who attains the same CO-Hgb level after a prolonged lower-level exposure may be significantly symptomatic. It is also important to remember that, because CO-Hgb levels decline with time and with oxygen therapy, an initial CO-Hgb level may not accurately reflect the magnitude of a patient's exposure if it is drawn at a time that is remote from the exposure or after oxygen therapy has been instituted. Prehospital providers can be helpful by reporting CO air levels at the scene of exposure or by providing blood drawn shortly after exposure. In some circumstances, exhaled CO levels measured by using a Breathalyzer-type device may help to confirm the diagnosis, whether in the prehospital or hospital setting [19,162].

CO-Hgb levels should be measured with a co-oximeter, which measures total hemoglobin concentration, oxyhemoglobin, deoxyhemoglobin, and concentrations of abnormal hemoglobins, such as CO-Hgb and methemoglobin, by differentiating wavelength absorbance values [12]. Routine blood gas analyzers without co-oximeters calculate rather than measure oxyhemoglobin saturation and do not recognize the contribution of abnormal hemoglobins. Arterial sampling is not necessary, because prospective comparison of arterial and venous CO-Hgb levels in poisoned patients has shown a high degree of correlation [163]. In an animal model, the accuracy was maintained at CO-Hgb levels exceeding 60% [164].

Pulse oximetry

Pulse oximetry may be falsely elevated in the setting of significant CO poisoning, because CO-Hgb is difficult to distinguish from oxyhemoglobin by wavelength. The pulse oximetry gap, defined as the difference between the pulse oximetry measured by finger probe and the true pulse oximetry obtained spectrophotometrically with a co-oximeter, has been found to approximate the CO-Hgb level. Therefore, as the CO-Hgb level rises, the degree of pulse oximetry overestimation increases [165–167].

Other diagnostic testing

Other diagnostic testing in the CO-poisoned patient is dependent on the clinical scenario and may include complete blood count, arterial blood gas monitoring, electrolytes, cardiac markers, blood urea nitrogen, creatinine, creatine phosphokinase, chest radiography, ECG, neuropsychometric testing, and neuroimaging studies. The presence of metabolic acidosis, presumably from a combination of hypoxia, inhibition of cellular respiration, and increased metabolic demand, has been found to correlate with exposure duration, severity of clinical symptoms, and adverse sequelae after CO poisoning [108,109,160,168]. Lactate has been used as a marker for severe poisoning [160]. Chest radiography may show evidence of non-cardiogenic pulmonary edema in the severely poisoned patient. ECG may demonstrate nonspecific changes, dysrhythmias, or changes associated with myocardial ischemia. Cardiac markers and creatine phosphokinase may be elevated [169]. In the setting of smoke inhalation, concomitant cyanide toxicity may occur with CO poisoning [107,170]. In the setting of chronic CO poisoning, polycythemia may be seen as a response to chronic hypoxia. Fetal monitoring may be helpful to detect fetal compromise in the CO-poisoned pregnant patient [171]. Most recently, the role of biochemical markers of brain damage (neuron-specific enolase, S-100 beta) after CO poisoning has been investigated [172–174]. In one series of 38 CO-poisoned patients, S-100 beta levels correlated well with severity of illness [173].

Neuropsychometric testing

A battery of neuropsychometric tests has been developed specifically to screen for cognitive dysfunction as a result of CO poisoning [175]. The Carbon Monoxide Neuropsychological Screening Battery (CONSB) consists of six subtests assessing general orientation, digit span, trail making, digit symbol, aphasia, and block design. CO-poisoned patients without concomitant drug and alcohol ingestion were found to score worse than controls before hyperbaric oxygen therapy (HBOT) and to have improved scores after HBOT, particularly on the trail making test (Fig. 2) [175]. Volunteers exposed to CO were found to perform more poorly on the CONSB than controls without CO exposure [176].

The term neuropsychometric testing in the literature may refer to the CONSB or tests such as the Mini–Mental Status Exam, Weschler Adult Intelligence Scale—Revised, Weschler Memory Scale—Revised, and others. The utility of neuropsychometric testing in CO poisoning in the ED setting has yet to be determined, and significant controversy exists regarding its value. Although CO-poisoned patients have been shown to perform more poorly on neuropsychometric tests, abnormalities may not be explained exclusively by

Instructions: Draw a line from the number 1 to the letter A, from the number 2 to the letter B, and so on without lifting the pencil. The examiner may prompt the patient. The score is the total time in seconds for task completion.

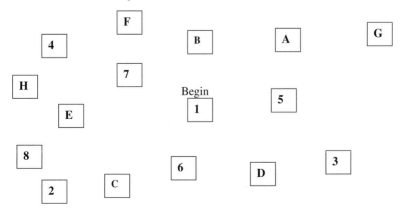

Fig. 2. Sample neuropsychometric trail-making test.

CO exposure. Patients attempting suicide by means other than CO perform as poorly on neuropsychometric tests as patients who attempt suicide with CO [177]. Improvement in neuropsychometric testing after HBOT in CO-poisoned patients is often cited as evidence for the effectiveness of HBOT. However, other factors could result in neuropsychometric test improvement, such as motivation, practice effect due to repetition of the test, improvement of overall mental status, and metabolism of coingestants or cointoxicants [43,135–138]. In addition, it is unknown whether neuropsychometric test abnormalities alone are associated with deleterious outcomes for patients with CO exposure. Despite these limitations, neuropsychometric testing provides an objective means of evaluating cognitive function. Some use these tests to assist in treatment decision making and to follow patients during recovery, although this practice is not uniform [43,127,136,178,179].

CT of the brain in patients who have severe CO exposure may show signs of cerebral infarction due to hypoxia, ischemia, and hypotension induced by severe CO exposure. However, an interesting and well-reported finding is bilateral globus pallidus low-density lesions (Fig. 3) [94–97]. The development of this lesion has been correlated with local low blood flow to the globus pallidus [71], metabolic acidosis, and hypotension [68,69].) during CO poisoning in animal models. Globus pallidus lesions may be delayed for as long as several days after initial presentation [180] and may resolve with time [133,181]. Concomitant white matter lesions may also be seen [94,97]. Although globus pallidus lesions are not pathognomonic for CO poisoning and may be seen in other intoxications, such as methanol or hydrogen sulfide poisoning, their presence should alert the clinician to the possibility of CO exposure. MRI in patients who have CO exposure may show diffuse,

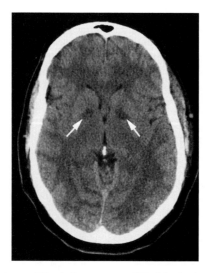

Fig. 3. Bilateral globus pallidus lesions seen on CT of the brain after CO poisoning.

symmetric white matter lesions, predominantly in the periventricular areas, although the centrum semiovale, deep subcortical white matter, thalamus, basal ganglia, and hippocampus may also be affected [133,150,182,183].

Patients who have abnormal neuroimaging findings after CO exposure are more likely to have poorer outcomes, such as death or persistent functional neurologic impairment, than are those with normal neuroimaging studies [94,95,97,128,133,150]. However, exceptions exist, and the results of neuroimaging studies do not always accurately predict outcome [128,150].

Single photon emission computed tomography (SPECT) scanning, electroencephalography, and quantitative MRI have been studied as adjunctive diagnostic tests in CO-exposed patients but are not widely available [183–185]. SPECT scanning in particular may correlate better than other neuroimaging findings with the development of delayed neurologic sequelae [186].

Treatment

Treatment of the CO-poisoned patient begins with supplemental oxygen and aggressive supportive care, including airway management, blood pressure support, and stabilization of cardiovascular status. When occult CO poisoning is discovered, other patients may remain at the scene and should be warned and evacuated until the source is identified and the environment is safe.

High-flow oxygen therapy should be administered immediately to treat hypoxia due to CO poisoning and also to accelerate elimination of CO from the body. Whether this oxygen should be given under increased pressure with HBOT or under ambient pressures (ie, normobaric oxygen [NBO]) is a subject of much debate. HBOT is neither universally available nor entirely risk free. However, HBOT may have a role in preventing adverse neurologic sequelae in the setting of CO poisoning and is indicated for selected patients. HBOT consists of the delivery of 100% oxygen within a pressurized chamber, resulting in a manifold increase in the dissolved oxygen in the body (PaO_2 up to 2000 mm Hg). One hundred percent oxygen at ambient pressure provides 2.09 vol%—one third of the body's requirement—whereas 2.5 atmospheres absolute (ATA) provides 5.62 vol% [187,188]. Interestingly, HBOT at 3.0 ATA was found in a porcine study to provide enough dissolved oxygen to supply the body's needs in the near-absence of hemoglobin [189]. Increasing the partial pressure of oxygen decreases the half life of CO-Hgb. The reported half life of CO-Hgb is 240 to 320 minutes at room air (21% oxygen), 40 to 80 minutes at 100% oxygen, and approximately 20 minutes at 100% HBOT at 2.5 to 3.0 ATA [8,190–192]. Wide individual variation exists, however, and prolonged exposures may result in prolonged half life [190,193].

HBOT for CO poisoning was first discussed by Haldane in the 1890s and first used in the 1960s [194]. Because CO toxicity was initially thought to result entirely from the relative anemia imposed by the formation of

CO-Hgb, HBOT was thought to be beneficial merely by accelerating the dissociation of CO from hemoglobin. However, as our understanding of the pathophysiology of CO poisoning and of HBOT has evolved, it appears that HBOT has other effects. HBOT has been shown in CO-poisoned animals not only to reduce CO binding to hemoglobin [190,195] but also to reduce CO binding to other heme-containing proteins, such as cytochrome a3, that affect cellular metabolism [196,197]. HBOT may also alter neutrophil adhesion to endothelium [198,199], decrease free radical–mediated oxidative damage [196,198], reduce neurologic deficits [75], and reduce overall mortality [65,200] when compared with NBO. Other animal studies have found that HBOT does not prevent neuronal injury in the setting of CO poisoning [75,201], and oxygen has the potential to increase oxidative damage owing to increased generation of free radicals [51,188,198].

Six prospective randomized controlled trials compare HBOT with NBO for CO poisoning [130,185,203–206]. Four of these studies show a benefit for HBOT; two do not. The data and conclusions drawn from these studies are conflicting and highlight the controversy surrounding the utility of HBOT. Because of significant variations in study design, HBOT and NBO protocols used, outcomes measured, and patient population included, it is difficult to draw firm conclusions based on the weight of the evidence. Development of a consensus on the definition of DNS and validation of diagnostic parameters for DNS would strengthen future investigations [137,207,208]. A recent Cochrane review [209] including three of these trials [130,203,205] concluded that the overall odds ratio (OR) for benefit of HBOT was 0.82 (95% confidence interval [CI], 0.41–1.66) using an outcome measure of symptoms at 1 month. The study by Weaver and colleagues [206], considered by many to be the most methodologically rigorous [137,202,210], was published after the Cochrane review.

Although more research is needed in this area, the unwillingness of some authors to advocate further randomized controlled trials underscores the considerable controversy regarding HBOT for CO poisoning. Some believe that withholding HBOT from CO-poisoned patients in future trials would be unethical, because of their firm belief in the efficacy of this treatment [45,211,214]. Others believe that further trials would be unethical because the paucity of data on the effectiveness of HBOT therapy does not justify the risk and expense of transferring patients to HBOT treatment facilities [212]. Still others have expressed concern that HBOT supporters appear to be located in facilities that offer HBOT [211,213].

No widespread agreement exists regarding selection of patients for HBOT in the setting of CO poisoning [188,211], and no reliable method of identifying patients at high risk for neurologic sequelae is available [137,202,215]. Based on the available knowledge regarding the pathophysiology of CO poisoning and the current clinical data, broad criteria for recommending HBOT for CO poisoning have included any history of LOC, neurologic symptoms, cardiovascular dysfunction, metabolic acidosis, abnormalities on neuropsychometric testing, pregnancy with an elevated (>15%–20%) CO-Hgb level, persistent symptoms despite NBO, and a significantly high CO-Hgb level. Many practitioners use a CO-Hgb level greater than 25% as criterion for HBOT [8,137,188,210,215–217]. A survey of hyperbaric centers revealed that more than three fourths of the responders use HBOT for coma, focal neurologic deficits, ischemic changes on EKG, abnormal psychometric testing, and transient LOC [179]. Because CO exacerbates underlying heart disease, cardiac dysfunction in the setting of CO poisoning should be treated with standard therapy (eg, antidysrhythmics, aspirin, nitrates), high-flow oxygen, and consideration of HBOT [1].

Although they acknowledge the lack of data to substantiate various criteria and treatment protocols, the members of the Undersea and Hyperbaric Medical Society [137] recommend HBOT therapy for CO-poisoned patients with LOC (transient or prolonged), neurologic signs, cardiovascular dysfunction, or severe metabolic acidosis. They recognize that many practitioners use abnormal neuropsychometric testing and absolute CO-Hgb levels (typically >25%) to guide treatment decisions. Although they could not absolutely define a high-risk population for neurologic sequelae, they believe that patients at the extremes of age and those with neurologic abnormalities, LOC, or a CO-Hgb level greater than 25% "require special consideration." Although the efficacy of one HBOT treatment protocol over another has not been determined [139,202,210,218–220], one session of HBOT at 2.5 to 3.0 ATA is recommended initially, with further sessions considered if symptoms persist [137,208,215]. Physicians treating CO-poisoned patients who do not meet criteria for HBOT should consider administration of 100% oxygen for 6 to 12 hours delivered by tight-fitting face mask [9,137,202,212,219,221]. Infants and children receive the same HBOT protocols as adults [222]. The safety of HBOT in pregnancy has been questioned, but many authors recommend HBOT for the pregnant patient in the setting of CO poisoning, because of the potential benefit to both mother and fetus and the difficulty of assessing intrauterine hypoxia [118,120,123,171,223,224]. A maternal CO-Hgb level greater than 15% to 20%, evidence of fetal distress, or other standard criteria for HBOT in CO poisoning are often cited as indications for HBOT in the CO-poisoned pregnant patient [1,171,215]. Pregnant women may require longer treatment with oxygen than the nonpregnant patient [114,115,119,223,225]. Box 2 lists suggested indications for HBOT in CO poisoning.

HBOT is not entirely risk free. Most commonly, patients complain of painful barotrauma affecting the ears and sinuses, and patients with claustrophobia are often unable to tolerate the close confines of a monoplace hyperbaric chamber (ie, sized for a single individual). Other, less common risks include oxygen toxicity seizures, pulmonary edema and hemorrhage, decompression sickness, including pneumothorax and nitrogen emboli, and fire hazard [44,226–228]. The only absolute contraindication to HBOT is an untreated pneumothorax [215]. Relative contraindications include

---

Box 2. Suggested indications for hyperbaric oxygen therapy in carbon monoxide poisoning

Strongly consider for
(1) Neurologic findings
    (a) Altered mental status
    (b) Coma
    (c) Focal neurologic deficits
    (d) Seizures
(2) Pregnancy with CO-Hgb levels >15%
(3) History of loss of consciousness

Possibly consider for
Cardiovascular compromise (ischemia, infarction, dysrhythmia)
Metabolic acidosis
Extremes of age
Abnormal neuropsychometric testing results
Persistent symptoms despite normobaric oxygen

Data from Tomaszewski C. Carbon monoxide. In: Goldfrank LR, Flomenbaum NE, Lewin NA, et al, editors. Goldfrank's toxicologic emergencies. 7th edition. New York: McGraw-Hill; 2002. p. 1478–97; and Hampson NB, Mathieu D, Piantadosi CA, et al. Carbon monoxide poisoning: interpretation of randomized clinical trials and unresolved treatment issues. Undersea Hyperb Med 2001; 28(3):157–64.

---

claustrophobia, otosclerosis or other scarring of middle ear, bowel obstruction, significant chronic obstructive pulmonary disease, particularly with bullae formation, and requirement of care beyond what may be provided in a monoplace chamber (eg, tracheal suctioning in burns). In addition, if the patient requires emergency intervention (eg, defibrillation) while undergoing HBOT, several minutes are required to decompress the patient safely before interventions may proceed [188]. One retrospective series of 297 patients, 41 of whom had serious cardiovascular complications, showed that all but one manifested their cardiovascular distress before HBOT. Few complications occurred during HBOT. The authors concluded that most patients at risk for emergent cardiovascular decompensation can be identified before they enter the HBOT chamber [229]. Because of the significant controversy still surrounding the appropriate treatment for CO-poisoned patients, a standard of care regarding HBOT for these patients is difficult to define. A risk-benefit analysis should be considered for each individual patient, depending on other concomitant medical needs, and discussed with the patient or family.

Other treatments tried for CO poisoning in the past have included hyperventilation, hypothermia, osmotherapy, fluid restriction, and glucocorticoids, none of which were found effective [109,230]. Ongoing research is being performed to delineate the possible roles of free radical scavengers, mono-amine oxidase inhibitors [54], and N-methyl D-aspartate (NMDA) blockers [82].

Prevention

The widespread use of catalytic converters on automobiles and improved emissions policies have resulted in a significant decline in accidental CO poisoning deaths [4,231]. Prevention of high indoor concentrations of CO is optimal and can be accomplished by frequent inspection and maintenance of furnaces, stoves, and fireplaces, avoidance of indoor unvented combustion sources such as grills and space heaters, careful use of gas stoves, and installation of CO detectors [3]. In the United States, CO alarms are designed to activate within 189 minutes of 70 ppm exposure, 50 minutes of 150 ppm exposure, or 15 minutes of 400 ppm exposure [3]. Although the effectiveness of CO detectors may be limited in the significant proportion of victims of fatal CO poisoning who succumb while asleep or under the influence of alcohol, appropriate and widespread use is likely to decrease the incidence of occult indoor CO poisoning [232].

Summary

CO is an ubiquitous poison with many sources of exposure. CO poisoning produces diverse signs and symptoms that are often subtle and may be easily misdiagnosed. Failure to diagnose CO poisoning may result in significant morbidity and mortality and permit continued exposure to a dangerous environment.

Treatment of CO poisoning begins with inhalation of supplemental oxygen and aggressive supportive care. HBOT accelerates dissociation of CO from hemoglobin and may also prevent DNS. Absolute indications for HBOT for CO poisoning remain controversial, although most authors would agree that HBOT is indicated in patients who are comatose or neurologically abnormal, have a history of LOC with their exposure, or have cardiac dysfunction. Pregnancy with an elevated CO-Hgb level (>15%–20%) is also widely considered an indication for treatment. HBOT may be considered in patients who have persistent symptoms despite NBO, metabolic acidosis, abnormalities on neuropsychometric testing, or significantly elevated levels. The ideal regimen of oxygen therapy has yet to be determined, and significant controversy exists regarding HBOT treatment protocols. Often the local medical toxicologist, poison control center, or hyperbaric unit may assist the treating physician with decisions regarding therapy.

References

[1] Tomaszewski C. Carbon monoxide. In: Goldfrank LR, Flomenbaum NE, Lewin NA, et al, editors. Goldfrank's toxicologic emergencies. 7th edition. New York: McGraw-Hill; 2002. p. 1478–97.

[2] Cobb N, Etzel RA. Unintentional carbon monoxide-related deaths in the United States, 1979 through 1988. JAMA 1991;266(5):659–63.

[3] Raub JA, Mathieu-Nolf M, Hampson NB, et al. Carbon monoxide poisoning—a public health perspective. Toxicology 2000;145(1):1–14.

[4] Mott JA, Wolfe MI, Alverson CJ, et al. National vehicle emissions policies and practices and declining US carbon monoxide–related mortality. JAMA 2002;288(8): 988–95.

[5] Mah JC. Non-fire carbon monoxide deaths and injuries associated with the use of consumer products: annual estimates—1998. US Consumer Product Safety Commission (Bethesda, MD). Available at: http://www.cpsc.gov/library/data.html. Accessed February 4, 2005.

[6] Ernst A, Zibrak JD. Carbon monoxide poisoning. N Engl J Med 1998;339(22):1603–8.

[7] Abelsohn A, Sanborn MD, Jessiman BJ, et al. Identifying and managing adverse environmental health effects. 6. Carbon monoxide poisoning. CMAJ 2002;166(13): 1685–90.

[8] Ilano AL, Raffin TA. Management of carbon monoxide poisoning. Chest 1990;97(1): 165–9.

[9] Olson KR. Carbon monoxide poisoning: mechanisms, presentation, and controversies in management. J Emerg Med 1984;1(3):233–43.

[10] Forbes WH, Sargent F, Roughton FJW. The rate of carbon monoxide uptake by normal men. Am J Physiol 1945;143(4):594–608.

[11] Roughton FJW. The kinetics of the reaction $CO + O_2Hb <-> O_2 + COHb$ in human blood at body temperature. Am J Physiol 1945;143(4):609–20.

[12] Widdop B. Analysis of carbon monoxide. Ann Clin Biochem 2002;39(4):378–91.

[13] Raub JA, Benignus VA. Carbon monoxide and the nervous system. Neurosci Biobehav Rev 2002;26(8):925–40.

[14] Administration OSHA. Occupational safety and health guidelines for carbon monoxide. Available at: http://www.osha.gov/SLTC/healthguidelines/carbonmonoxide/recognition. html. Accessed February 4, 2005.

[15] Hampson NB, Norkool DM. Carbon monoxide poisoning in children riding in the back of pickup trucks. JAMA 1992;267(4):538–40.

[16] Anonymous. Carbon-monoxide poisoning resulting from exposure to ski-boat exhaust—Georgia, June 2002. MMWR Morbid Mortal Wkly Rep 2002;51(37):829–30.

[17] Silvers SM, Hampson NB. Carbon monoxide poisoning among recreational boaters. JAMA 1995;274(20):1614–6.

[18] Anonymous. From the Centers for Disease Control and Prevention. Carbon monoxide poisoning associated with use of LPG-powered (propane) forklifts in industrial settings—Iowa, 1998. JAMA 2000;283(3):331–2.

[19] Ely EW, Moorehead B, Haponik EF. Warehouse workers' headache: emergency evaluation and management of 30 patients with carbon monoxide poisoning. Am J Med 1995;98(2): 145–55.

[20] Fawcett TA, Moon RE, Fracica PJ, et al. Warehouse workers' headache. Carbon monoxide poisoning from propane-fueled forklifts. J Occup Med 1992;34(1):12–5.

[21] Pelham TW, Holt LE, Moss MA. Exposure to carbon monoxide and nitrogen dioxide in enclosed ice arenas. Occup Environ Med 2002;59(4):224–33.

[22] Anonymous. Carbon monoxide poisoning at an indoor ice arena and bingo hall—Seattle, 1996. From the Centers for Disease Control and Prevention. JAMA 1996;275(19): 1468–9.

[23] Anonymous. From the Centers for Disease Control and Prevention. Houseboat-associated carbon monoxide poisonings on Lake Powell—Arizona and Utah, 2000. JAMA 2001; 285(5):530–2.

[24] Anonymous. From the Centers for Disease Control and Prevention. Carbon monoxide poisoning deaths associated with camping—Georgia, March 1999. JAMA 1999;282(14): 1326.

[25] Heckerling PS, Leikin JB, Maturen A, et al. Predictors of occult carbon monoxide poisoning in patients with headache and dizziness. Ann Intern Med 1987;107(2): 174–6.

[26] Hampson NB, Kramer CC, Dunford RG, et al. Carbon monoxide poisoning from indoor burning of charcoal briquets. JAMA 1994;271(1):52–3.

[27] Wrenn K, Connors GP. Carbon monoxide poisoning during ice storms: a tale of two cities. J Emerg Med 1997;15(4):465–7.

[28] Rioux JP, Myers RA. Hyperbaric oxygen for methylene chloride poisoning: report on two cases. Ann Emerg Med 1989;18(6):691–5.

[29] Nager EC, O'Connor RE. Carbon monoxide poisoning from spray paint inhalation. Acad Emerg Med 1998;5(1):84–6.

[30] Langehennig PL, Seeler RA, Berman E. Paint removers and carboxyhemoglobin. N Engl J Med 1976;295(20):1137.

[31] Piantadosi CA. Diagnosis and treatment of carbon monoxide poisoning. Respir Care Clin N Am 1999;5(2):183–202.

[32] Naik JS, O'Donaughy TL, Walker BR. Endogenous carbon monoxide is an endothelial-derived vasodilator factor in the mesenteric circulation. Am J Physiol Heart Circ Physiol 2003;284(3):H838–45.

[33] Zegdi R, Perrin D, Burdin M, et al. Increased endogenous carbon monoxide production in severe sepsis. Intensive Care Med 2002;28(6):793–6.

[34] Haldane J. Medicolegal contributions of historical interest. The action of carbonic oxide on man. Forensic Sci 1972;1(4):451–83.

[35] Sendroy J, Liu SH, Van Slyke DO. The gasometric estimation of the relative affinity constant for carbon monoxide and oxygen in whole blood at 38C. Am J Physiol 1929;90: 511–2.

[36] Roughton FJW, Darling RC. The effect of carbon monoxide on the oxyhemoglobin dissociation curve. Am J Physiol 1944;141:17–31.

[37] Goldbaum LR, Ramirez RG, Absalon KB. What is the mechanism of carbon monoxide toxicity? Aviat Space Environ Med 1975;46(10):1289–91.

[38] Goldbaum LR, Orellano T, Dergal E. Mechanism of the toxic action of carbon monoxide. Ann Clin Lab Sci 1976;6(4):372–6.

[39] Orellano T, Dergal E, Alijani M, et al. Studies on the mechanism of carbon monoxide toxicity. J Surg Res 1976;20(5):485–7.

[40] Ramirez RG, Albert SN, Agostin JC, et al. Lack of toxicity of transfused carboxyhemo-globin. Surg Forum 1974;25:165–8.

[41] Meilin S, Rogatsky GG, Thom SR, et al. Effects of carbon monoxide on the brain may be mediated by nitric oxide. J Appl Physiol 1996;81(3):1078–83.

[42] Mendelman A, Zarchin N, Meilin S, et al. Blood flow and ionic responses in the awake brain due to carbon monoxide. Neurol Res 2002;24(8):765–72.

[43] Rottman SJ. Carbon monoxide screening in the ED. Am J Emerg Med 1991;9(2): 204–5.

[44] Norkool DM, Kirkpatrick JN. Treatment of acute carbon monoxide poisoning with hyperbaric oxygen: a review of 115 cases. Ann Emerg Med 1985;14(12):1168–71.

[45] Myers RA. Carbon monoxide poisoning. J Emerg Med 1984;1(3):245–8.

[46] Okeda R, Funata N, Takano T, et al. The pathogenesis of carbon monoxide encephalopathy in the acute phase—physiological and morphological correlation. Acta Neuropathol (Berl) 1981;54(1):1–10.

[47] Brown SD, Piantadosi CA. Recovery of energy metabolism in rat brain after carbon monoxide hypoxia. J Clin Invest 1992;89(2):666–72.

[48] Hill BC. The pathway of CO binding to cytochrome c oxidase. Can the gateway be closed? FEBS Lett 1994;354(3):284–8.

[49] Chance B, Erecinska M, Wagner M. Mitochondrial responses to carbon monoxide toxicity. Ann N Y Acad Sci 1970;174(1):193–204.

[50] Hardy KR, Thom SR. Pathophysiology and treatment of carbon monoxide poisoning. J Toxicol Clin Toxicol 1994;32(6):613–29.

[51] Zhang J, Piantadosi CA. Mitochondrial oxidative stress after carbon monoxide hypoxia in the rat brain. J Clin Invest 1992;90(4):1193–9.

[52] Thom SR, Ohnishi ST, Ischiropoulos H. Nitric oxide released by platelets inhibits neutrophil B2 integrin function following acute carbon monoxide poisoning. Toxicol Appl Pharmacol 1994;128(1):105–10.

[53] Radi R, Rodriguez M, Castro L, et al. Inhibition of mitochondrial electron transport by peroxynitrite. Arch Biochem Biophys 1994;308(1):89–95.

[54] Piantadosi CA, Tatro L, Zhang J. Hydroxyl radical production in the brain after CO hypoxia in rats. Free Rad Biol Med 1995;18(3):603–9.

[55] DeBias DA, Banerjee CM, Birkhead NC, et al. Effects of carbon monoxide inhalation on ventricular fibrillation. Arch Environ Health 1976;31(1):42–6.

[56] Sangalli BC, Bidanset JH. A review of carboxymyoglobin formation: a major mechanism of carbon monoxide toxicity. Vet Hum Toxicol 1990;32(5):449–53.

[57] Florkowski CM, Rossi ML, Carey MP, et al. Rhabdomyolysis and acute renal failure following carbon monoxide poisoning: two case reports with muscle histopathology and enzyme activities. J Toxicol Clin Toxicol 1992;30(3):443–54.

[58] Wolff E. Carbon monoxide poisoning with severe myonecrosis and acute renal failure. Am J Emerg Med 1994;12(3):347–9.

[59] Herman GD, Shapiro AB, Leikin J. Myonecrosis in carbon monoxide poisoning. Vet Hum Toxicol 1988;30(1):28–30.

[60] Richardson RS, Noyszewski EA, Saltin B, et al. Effect of mild carboxy-hemoglobin on exercising skeletal muscle: intravascular and intracellular evidence. Am J Physiol 2002; 283(5):R1131–9.

[61] Barinaga M. Carbon monoxide: killer to brain messenger in one step. Science 1993; 259(5093):309.

[62] Verma A, Hirsch DJ, Glatt CE, et al. Carbon monoxide: a putative neural messenger. Science 1993;259(5093):381–4.

[63] Meyer-Witting M, Helps S, Gorman DF. Acute carbon monoxide exposure and cerebral blood flow in rabbits. Anaesth Intensive Care 1991;19(3):373–7.

[64] Sinha AK, Klein J, Schultze P, et al. Cerebral regional capillary perfusion and blood flow after carbon monoxide exposure. J Appl Physiol 1991;71(4):1196–200.

[65] Jiang J, Tyssebotn I. Cerebrospinal fluid pressure changes after acute carbon monoxide poisoning and therapeutic effects of normobaric and hyperbaric oxygen in conscious rats. Undersea Hyperb Med 1997;24(4):245–54.

[66] Ischiropoulos H, Beers MF, Ohnishi ST, et al. Nitric oxide production and perivascular tyrosine nitration in brain after carbon monoxide poisoning in the rat. J Clin Invest 1996; 97(10):2260–7.

[67] Landry DW, Oliver JA. The pathogenesis of vasodilatory shock. N Engl J Med 2001;345(8): 588–95.

[68] Ginsberg MD, Myers RE, McDonagh BF. Experimental carbon monoxide encephalopathy in the primate. II. Clinical aspects, neuropathology, and physiologic correlation. Arch Neurol 1974;30(3):209–16.

[69] Koehler RC, Jones MD Jr, Traystman RJ. Cerebral circulatory response to carbon monoxide and hypoxic hypoxia in the lamb. Am J Physiol 1982;243(1):H27–32.

[70] Okeda R, Funata N, Song SJ, et al. Comparative study on pathogenesis of selective cerebral lesions in carbon monoxide poisoning and nitrogen hypoxia in cats. Acta Neuropathol (Berl) 1982;56(4):265–72.

[71] Song SY, Okeda R, Funata N, et al. An experimental study of the pathogenesis of the selective lesion of the globus pallidus in acute carbon monoxide poisoning in cats. Acta Neuropathol (Berl) 1983;61:232–8.

[72] Thom SR, Kang M, Fisher D, et al. Release of glutathione from erythrocytes and other markers of oxidative stress in carbon monoxide poisoning. J Appl Physiol 1997;82(5): 1424–32.

[73] Thom SR. Leukocytes in carbon monoxide–mediated brain oxidative injury. Toxicol Appl Pharmacol 1993;123(2):234–47.

[74] Thom SR, Fisher D, Manevich Y. Roles for platelet-activating factor and *NO-derived oxidants causing neutrophil adherence after CO poisoning. Am J Physiol Heart Circ Physiol 2001;281(2):H923–30.

[75] Tomaszewski C, Rosenberg N, Wanthen J, et al. Prevention of neurological sequelae from carbon monoxide by hyperbaric oxygen in rats. Neurology 1992;42(Suppl 3):196.

[76] Thom SR. Carbon monoxide–mediated brain lipid peroxidation in the rat. J Appl Physiol 1990;68(3):997–1003.

[77] Thom SR. Dehydrogenase conversion to oxidase and lipid peroxidation in brain after carbon monoxide poisoning. J Appl Physiol 1992;73(4):1584–9.

[78] Penney DG. Acute carbon monoxide poisoning: animal models: a review. Toxicology 1990; 62(2):123–60.

[79] Thom SR, Bhopale VM, Fisher D, et al. Delayed neuropathology after carbon monoxide poisoning is immune-mediated. Proc Natl Acad Sci U S A 2004;101(37):13660–5.

[80] Piantadosi CA, Zhang J, Levin ED, et al. Apoptosis and delayed neuronal damage after carbon monoxide poisoning in the rat. Exp Neurol 1997;147(1):103–14.

[81] Penney DG, Chen K. NMDA receptor–blocker ketamine protects during acute carbon monoxide poisoning, while calcium channel–blocker verapamil does not. J Appl Toxicol 1996;16(4):297–304.

[82] Ishimaru H, Katoh A, Suzuki H, et al. Effects of N-methyl-D-aspartate receptor antagonists on carbon monoxide–induced brain damage in mice. J Pharmacol Exp Ther 1992;261(1):349–52.

[83] Lightfoot NF. Chronic carbon monoxide exposure. Proc R Soc Med 1972;65(9):798–9.

[84] Thom SR, Fisher D, Xu YA, et al. Role of nitric oxide–derived oxidants in vascular injury from carbon monoxide in the rat. Am J Physiol 1999;276(3 Pt 2):H984–92.

[85] Estabrook RW, Franklin MR, Hildebrandt AG. Factors influencing the inhibitory effect of carbon monoxide on cytochrome P-450–catalyzed mixed function oxidation reactions. Ann N Y Acad Sci 1970;174(1):218–32.

[86] Dolan MC, Haltom TL, Barrows GH, et al. Carboxyhemoglobin levels in patients with flu-like symptoms. Ann Emerg Med 1987;16(7):782–6.

[87] Heckerling PS. Occult carbon monoxide poisoning: a cause of winter headache. Am J Emerg Med 1987;5:201–4.

[88] Baker MD, Henretig FM, Ludwig S. Carboxyhemoglobin levels in children with nonspecific flu-like symptoms. J Pediatr 1988;113(3):501–4.

[89] Burney RE, Wu SC, Nemiroff MJ. Mass carbon monoxide poisonings: clinical effects and results of treatment in 184 victims. Ann Emerg Med 1982;11(8):394–9.

[90] Stewart RD, Peterson JE, Baretta ED, et al. Experimental human exposure to carbon monoxide. Arch Environ Health 1970;21(2):154–64.

[91] Stewart RD, Peterson JE, Fisher TN, et al. Experimental human exposure to high concentrations of carbon monoxide. Arch Environ Health 1973;26(1):1–7.

[92] Herman LY. Carbon monoxide poisoning presenting as an isolated seizure. J Emerg Med 1998;16(3):429–32.

[93] Mori T, Nagai K. Carbon-monoxide poisoning presenting as an afebrile seizure. Pediatr Neurol 2000;22(4):330–1.

[94] Silver DA, Cross M, Fox B, et al. Computed tomography of the brain in acute carbon monoxide poisoning. Clin Radiol 1996;51(7):480–3.

[95] Jones JS, Lagasse J, Zimmerman G. Computed tomographic findings after acute carbon monoxide poisoning. Am J Emerg Med 1994;12(4):448–51.

[96] Miura T, Mitomo M, Kawai R, et al. CT of the brain in acute carbon monoxide intoxication: characteristic features and prognosis. AJNR Am J Neuroradiol 1985;6(5):739–42.

[97] Sawada Y, Takahashi M, Ohashi N, et al. Computerised tomography as an indication of long-term outcome after acute carbon monoxide poisoning. Lancet 1980;1(8172):783–4.

[98] Penney DG. Hemodynamic response to carbon monoxide. Environ Health Perspect 1988; 77:121–30.

[99] Yanir Y, Shupak A, Abramovich A, et al. Cardiogenic shock complicating acute carbon monoxide poisoning despite neurologic and metabolic recovery. Ann Emerg Med 2002; 40(4):420–4.

[100] Thom SR, Keim LW. Carbon monoxide poisoning: a review. Epidemiology, pathophysiology, clinical findings, and treatment options including hyperbaric oxygen therapy. J Toxicol Clin Toxicol 1989;27(3):141–56.

[101] Atkins EH, Baker EL. Exacerbation of coronary artery disease by occupational carbon monoxide exposure: a report to two fatalities and a review of the literature. Am J Ind Med 1985;7(1):73–9.

[102] Aronow WS, Isbell MW. Carbon monoxide effect on exercise-induced angina pectoris. Ann Intern Med 1973;79(3):392–5.

[103] Sheps DS, Herbst MC, Hinderliter AL, et al. Production of arrhythmias by elevated carboxyhemoglobin in patients with coronary artery disease. Ann Intern Med 1990;113(5): 343–51.

[104] Allred EN, Bleecker ER, Chaitman BR, et al. Short-term effects of carbon monoxide exposure on the exercise performance of subjects with coronary artery disease. N Engl J Med 1989;321(21):1426–32.

[105] Marius-Nunez AL. Myocardial infarction with normal coronary arteries after acute exposure to carbon monoxide. Chest 1990;97(2):491–4.

[106] Myers RA, Snyder SK, Majerus TC. Cutaneous blisters and carbon monoxide poisoning. Ann Emerg Med 1985;14(6):603–6.

[107] Thom SR. Smoke inhalation. Emerg Med Clin North Am 1989;7(2):371–87.

[108] Goulon M, Barois A, Rapin M, et al. Carbon monoxide poisoning and acute anoxia due to breathing coal tar gas and hydrocarbons. Journal of Hyperbaric Medicine 1986;1(1):23–41.

[109] Krantz T, Thisted B, Strom J, et al. Acute carbon monoxide poisoning. Acta Anaesthesiol Scand 1988;32(4):278–82.

[110] Vreman HJ, Mahoney JJ, Stevenson DK. Carbon monoxide and carboxyhemoglobin. Adv Pediatr 1995;42:303–34.

[111] Foster M, Goodwin SR, Williams C, et al. Recurrent acute life-threatening events and lactic acidosis caused by chronic carbon monoxide poisoning in an infant. Pediatrics 1999;104(3): e34.

[112] Crocker PJ, Walker JS. Pediatric carbon monoxide toxicity. J Emerg Med 1985;3(6):443–8.

[113] Liebelt EL. Hyperbaric oxygen therapy in childhood carbon monoxide poisoning. Curr Opin Pediatr 1999;11(3):259–64.

[114] Longo LD, Hill EP. Carbon monoxide uptake and elimination in fetal and maternal sheep. Am J Physiol 1977;232(3):H324–30.

[115] Longo LD. Carbon monoxide in the pregnant mother and fetus and its exchange across the placenta. Ann N Y Acad Sci 1970;174(1):312–41.

[116] Norman CA, Halton DM. Is carbon monoxide a workplace teratogen? Ann Occup Hyg 1990;34(4):335–47.

[117] Caravati EM, Adams CJ, Joyce SM, et al. Fetal toxicity associated with maternal carbon monoxide poisoning. Ann Emerg Med 1988;17(7):714–7.

[118] Koren G, Sharav T, Pastuszak A, et al. A multicenter, prospective study of fetal outcome following accidental carbon monoxide poisoning in pregnancy. Reprod Toxicol 1991;5(5): 397–403.

[119] Farrow JR, Davis GJ, Roy TM, et al. Fetal death due to nonlethal maternal carbon monoxide poisoning. J Forensic Sci 1990;35(6):1448–52.

[120] Cramer CR. Fetal death due to accidental maternal carbon monoxide poisoning. J Toxicol Clin Toxicol 1982;19(3):297–301.

[121] Ginsberg MD, Myers RE. Fetal brain injury after maternal carbon monoxide intoxication. Clinical and neuropathologic aspects. Neurology 1976;26(1):15–23.

[122] Woody RC, Brewster MA. Telencephalic dysgenesis associated with presumptive maternal carbon monoxide intoxication in the first trimester of pregnancy. J Toxicol Clin Toxicol 1990;28(4):467–75.

[123] Elkharrat D, Raphael JC, Korach JM, et al. Acute carbon monoxide intoxication and hyperbaric oxygen in pregnancy. Intensive Care Med 1991;17(5):289–92.

[124] Garland H, Pearce J. Neurological complications of carbon monoxide poisoning. Q J Med 1967;36(144):445–55.

[125] Min SK. A brain syndrome associated with delayed neuropsychiatric sequelae following acute carbon monoxide intoxication. Acta Psychiatr Scand 1986;73(1):80–6.

[126] Choi IS. Delayed neurologic sequelae in carbon monoxide intoxication. Arch Neurol 1983; 40(7):433–5.

[127] Myers RA, Snyder SK, Emhoff TA. Subacute sequelae of carbon monoxide poisoning. Ann Emerg Med 1985;14(12):1163–7.

[128] Lee MS, Marsden CD. Neurological sequelae following carbon monoxide poisoning: clinical course and outcome according to the clinical types and brain computed tomography scan findings. Mov Disord 1994;9(5):550–8.

[129] Smith JS, Brandon S. Morbidity from acute carbon monoxide poisoning at three-year follow-up. BMJ 1973;1(5849):318–21.

[130] Raphael JC, Elkharrat D, Jars-Guincestre MC, et al. Trial of normobaric and hyperbaric oxygen for acute carbon monoxide intoxication. Lancet 1989;2(8660):414–9.

[131] Shillito FH, Drinker CK, Shaughnessy TJ. The problem of nervous and mental sequelae in carbon monoxide poisoning. JAMA 1936;106(9):669–74.

[132] Kim JK, Coe CJ. Clinical study on carbon monoxide intoxication in children. Yonsei Med J 1987;28(4):266–73.

[133] Parkinson RB, Hopkins RO, Cleavinger HB, et al. White matter hyperintensities and neuropsychological outcome following carbon monoxide poisoning. Neurology 2002; 58(10):1525–32.

[134] Mathieu D, Nolf M, Durocher A, et al. Acute carbon monoxide poisoning. Risk of late sequelae and treatment by hyperbaric oxygen. J Toxicol Clin Toxicol 1985;23(4–6): 315–24.

[135] Schiltz KL. Failure to assess motivation, need to consider psychiatric variables, and absence of comprehensive examination: a skeptical review of neuropsychologic assessment in carbon monoxide research. Undersea Hyperb Med 2000;27(1):48–50.

[136] Seger D, Welch L. Carbon monoxide controversies: neuropsychologic testing, mechanism of toxicity, and hyperbaric oxygen. Ann Emerg Med 1994;24(2):242–8.

[137] Hampson NB, Mathieu D, Piantadosi CA, et al. Carbon monoxide poisoning: interpretation of randomized clinical trials and unresolved treatment issues. Undersea Hyperb Med 2001;28(3):157–64.

[138] Deschamps D, Geraud C, Julien H, et al. Memory one month after acute carbon monoxide intoxication: a prospective study. Occup Environ Med 2003;60(3):212–6.

[139] Gorman D, Drewry A, Huang YL, et al. The clinical toxicology of carbon monoxide. Toxicology 2003;187(1):25–38.

[140] Watkins CG, Strope GL. Chronic carbon monoxide poisoning as a major contributing factor in the sudden infant death syndrome. Am J Dis Child 1986;140(7):619.

[141] Halpern JS. Chronic occult carbon monoxide poisoning. J Emerg Nurs 1989;15(2 Pt 1): 107–11.

[142] Manuel J. A healthy home environment? Environ Health Perspect 1999;107(7):A352–7.

[143] Wright J. Chronic and occult carbon monoxide poisoning: we don't know what we're missing. Emerg Med J 2002;19(5):386–90.

[144] Devine SA, Kirkley SM, Palumbo CL, et al. MRI and neuropsychological correlates of carbon monoxide exposure: a case report. Environ Health Perspect 2002;110(10):1051–5.

[145] Gilbert GJ, Glaser GH. Neurologic manifestations of chronic carbon monoxide poisoning. N Engl J Med 1959;261(24):1217–20.

[146] Thorpe M. Chronic carbon monoxide poisoning. Can J Psychiatry 1994;39(1):59–61.

[147] Khan K, Sharief N. Chronic carbon monoxide poisoning in children. Acta Paediatr 1995; 84(7):742.

[148] Myers RA, DeFazio A, Kelly MP. Chronic carbon monoxide exposure: a clinical syndrome detected by neuropsychological tests. J Clin Psychol 1998;54(5):555–67.

[149] Knobeloch L, Jackson R. Recognition of chronic carbon monoxide poisoning. Wis Med J 1999;98(6):26–9.

[150] Pavese N, Napolitano A, De Iaco G, et al. Clinical outcome and magnetic resonance imaging of carbon monoxide intoxication. A long-term follow-up study. Ital J Neurol Sci 1999;20(3):171–8.

[151] Townsend CL, Maynard RL. Effects on health of prolonged exposure to low concentrations of carbon monoxide. Occup Environ Med 2002;59(10):708–11.

[152] Ritz B, Yu F, Chapa G, et al. Effect of air pollution on preterm birth among children born in Southern California between 1989 and 1993 2000;11(5):502–11.

[153] Ritz B, Yu F, Fruin S, et al. Ambient air pollution and risk of birth defects in Southern California. Am J Epidemiol 2002;155(1):17–25.

[154] Fechter LD, Karpa MD, Proctor B, et al. Disruption of neostriatal development in rats following perinatal exposure to mild, but chronic carbon monoxide. Neurotoxicol Teratol 1987;9(4):277–81.

[155] Weir FW, Fabiano VL. Re-evaluation of the role of carbon monoxide in production or aggravation of cardiovascular disease processes. J Occup Med 1982;24(7):519–25.

[156] Morris RD, Naumova EN, Munasinghe RL. Ambient air pollution and hospitalization for congestive heart failure among elderly people in seven large US cities. Am J Public Health 1995;85(10):1361–5.

[157] Heckerling PS, Leikin JB, Terzian CG, et al. Occult carbon monoxide poisoning in patients with neurologic illness. J Toxicol Clin Toxicol 1990;28(1):29–44.

[158] Stewart RD, Baretta ED, Platte LR, et al. Carboxyhemoglobin levels in American blood donors. JAMA 1974;229(9):1187–95.

[159] Benignus VA, Kafer ER, Muller KE, et al. Absence of symptoms with carboxyhemoglobin levels of 16–23%. Neurotoxicol Teratol 1987;9(5):345–8.

[160] Sokal JA, Kralkowska E. The relationship between exposure duration, carboxyhemoglobin, blood glucose, pyruvate and lactate and the severity of intoxication in 39 cases of acute carbon monoxide poisoning in man. Arch Toxicol 1985;57(3):196–9.

[161] Davis SM, Levy RC. High carboxyhemoglobin level without acute or chronic findings. J Emerg Med 1984;1(6):539–42.

[162] Kurt TL, Anderson RJ, Reed WG. Rapid estimation of carboxyhemoglobin by breath sampling in an emergency setting. Vet Hum Toxicol 1990;32(3):227–9.

[163] Touger M, Gallagher EJ, Tyrell J. Relationship between venous and arterial carboxyhemoglobin levels in patients with suspected carbon monoxide poisoning. Ann Emerg Med 1995;25(4):481–3.

[164] Lopez DM, Weingarten-Arams JS, Singer LP, et al. Relationship between arterial, mixed venous, and internal jugular carboxyhemoglobin concentrations at low, medium, and high concentrations in a piglet model of carbon monoxide toxicity. Crit Care Med 2000;28(6): 1998–2001.

[165] Bozeman WP, Myers RA, Barish RA. Confirmation of the pulse oximetry gap in carbon monoxide poisoning. Ann Emerg Med 1997;30(5):608–11.

[166] Buckley RG, Aks SE, Eshom JL, et al. The pulse oximetry gap in carbon monoxide intoxication. Ann Emerg Med 1994;24(2):252–5.

[167] Hampson NB. Pulse oximetry in severe carbon monoxide poisoning. Chest 1998;114(4): 1036–41.

[168] Larkin JM, Brahos GJ, Moylan JA. Treatment of carbon monoxide poisoning: prognostic factors. J Trauma 1976;16(2):111–4.

[169] Holstege CP, Baer AB, Eldridge DL, et al. Case series of elevated troponin I following carbon monoxide poisoning. J Toxicol Clin Toxicol 2004;42(5):742–3.

[170] Shusterman D, Alexeeff G, Hargis C, et al. Predictors of carbon monoxide and hydrogen cyanide exposure in smoke inhalation patients. J Toxicol Clin Toxicol 1996; 34(1):61–71.

[171] Van Hoesen KB, Camporesi EM, Moon RE, et al. Should hyperbaric oxygen be used to treat the pregnant patient for acute carbon monoxide poisoning? A case report and literature review. JAMA 1989;261(7):1039–43.

[172] Rasmussen LS, Poulsen MG, Christiansen M, et al. Biochemical markers for brain damage after carbon monoxide poisoning. Acta Anaesthesiol Scand 2004;48(4): 469–73.

[173] Brvar M, Mozina H, Osredkar J, et al. S100B protein in carbon monoxide poisoning: a pilot study. Resuscitation 2004;61(3):357–60.

[174] Brvar M, Mozina H, Osredkar J, et al. The potential value of the protein S-100B level as a criterion for hyperbaric oxygen treatment and prognostic marker in carbon monoxide poisoned patients. Resuscitation 2003;56(1):105–9.

[175] Messier LD, Myers RA. A neuropsychological screening battery for emergency assessment of carbon-monoxide-poisoned patients. J Clin Psychol 1991;47(5):675–84.

[176] Amitai Y, Zlotogorski Z, Golan-Katzav V, et al. Neuropsychological impairment from acute low-level exposure to carbon monoxide. Arch Neurol 1998;55(6):845–8.

[177] Hay PJ, Denson LA, van Hoof M, et al. The neuropsychiatry of carbon monoxide poisoning in attempted suicide: a prospective controlled study. J Psychosom Res 2002; 53(2):699–708.

[178] Myers RA, Britten JS. Are arterial blood gases of value in treatment decisions for carbon monoxide poisoning? Crit Care Med 1989;17(2):139–42.

[179] Hampson NB, Dunford RG, Kramer CC, et al. Selection criteria utilized for hyperbaric oxygen treatment of carbon monoxide poisoning. J Emerg Med 1995;13(2): 227–31.

[180] Hart IK, Kennedy PG, Adams JH, et al. Neurological manifestation of carbon monoxide poisoning. Postgrad Med J 1988;64(749):213–6.

[181] Vieregge P, Klostermann W, Blumm RG, et al. Carbon monoxide poisoning: clinical, neurophysiological, and brain imaging observations in acute disease and follow-up. J Neurol 1989;236(8):478–81.

[182] Zagami AS, Lethlean AK, Mellick R. Delayed neurological deterioration following carbon monoxide poisoning: MRI findings. J Neurol 1993;240(2):113–6.

[183] Gale SD, Hopkins RO, Weaver LK, et al. MRI, quantitative MRI, SPECT, and neuropsychological findings following carbon monoxide poisoning. Brain Inj 1999;13(4): 229–43.

[184] Denays R, Makhoul E, Dachy B, et al. Electroencephalographic mapping and 99mTc HMPAO single-photon emission computed tomography in carbon monoxide poisoning. Ann Emerg Med 1994;24(5):947–52.

[185] Ducasse JL, Celsis P, Marc-Vergnes JP. Non-comatose patients with acute carbon monoxide poisoning: hyperbaric or normobaric oxygenation? Undersea Hyperb Med 1995; 22(1):9–15.

[186] Choi IS, Kim SK, Lee SS, et al. Evaluation of outcome of delayed neurologic sequelae after carbon monoxide poisoning by technetium-99m hexamethylpropylene amine oxime brain single photon emission computed tomography. Eur Neurol 1995;35(3):137–42.

[187] Winter PM, Miller JN. Carbon monoxide poisoning. JAMA 1976;236(13):1502.

[188] Thom SR. Antidotes in depth: hyperbaric oxygen. In: Goldfrank LR, Flomenbaum NE, Lewin NA, et al, editors. Goldfrank's toxicologic emergencies. 7th edition. New York: McGraw-Hill; 2002. p. 1492–7.
[189] Boerema I, Meyne NG, Brummelkamp WH, et al. Life without blood. Arch Chir Neerl 1959;11:70.
[190] Pace N, Stajman E, Walker EL. Acceleration of carbon monoxide elimination in man by high pressure oxygen. Science 1950;111:652–4.
[191] Jay GD, McKindley DS. Alterations in pharmacokinetics of carboxyhemoglobin produced by oxygen under pressure. Undersea Hyperb Med 1997;24(3):165–73.
[192] Araki R, Nashimoto I, Takano T. The effect of hyperbaric oxygen on cerebral hemoglobin oxygenation and dissociation rate of carboxyhemoglobin in anesthetized rats: spectroscopic approach. Adv Exp Med Biol 1988;222:375–81.
[193] Peterson JE, Stewart RD. Absorption and elimination of carbon monoxide by inactive young men. Arch Environ Health 1970;21(2):165–71.
[194] Smith G. The treatment of carbon monoxide poisoning with oxygen at two atmospheres absolute. Ann Occup Hyg 1962;5:259–63.
[195] End E, Long CW. Oxygen under pressure in carbon monoxide poisoning. J Ind Hyg Toxicol 1942;24(10):302–6.
[196] Thom SR. Antagonism of carbon monoxide–mediated brain lipid peroxidation by hyperbaric oxygen. Toxicol Appl Pharmacol 1990;105(2):340–4.
[197] Brown SD, Piantadosi CA. Reversal of carbon monoxide–cytochrome c oxidase binding by hyperbaric oxygen in vivo. Adv Exp Med Biol 1989;248:747–54.
[198] Thom SR. Functional inhibition of leukocyte B2 integrins by hyperbaric oxygen in carbon monoxide–mediated brain injury in rats. Toxicol Appl Pharmacol 1993;123(2):248–56.
[199] Thom SR, Mendiguren I, Nebolon M. Temporary inhibition of human neutrophil B2 integrin function by hyperbaric oxygen (HBO). Clin Res 1994;42:130A.
[200] Jiang J, Tyssebotn I. Normobaric and hyperbaric oxygen treatment of acute carbon monoxide poisoning in rats. Undersea Hyperb Med 1997;24(2):107–16.
[201] Gilmer B, Kilkenny J, Tomaszewski C, et al. Hyperbaric oxygen does not prevent neurologic sequelae after carbon monoxide poisoning. Acad Emerg Med 2002;9(1):1–8.
[202] Piantadosi CA. Carbon monoxide poisoning. N Engl J Med 2002;347(14):1054–5.
[203] Thom SR, Taber RL, Mendiguren II, et al. Delayed neuropsychologic sequelae after carbon monoxide poisoning: prevention by treatment with hyperbaric oxygen. Ann Emerg Med 1995;25(4):474–80.
[204] Mathieu D, Wattel F, Mathieu-Nolf M, et al. Randomized prospective study comparing the effect of HBO versus 12 hours NBO in non comatose CO poisoned patients: results of the interim analysis. Undersea Hyperb Med 1996;23:7–8.
[205] Scheinkestel CD, Bailey M, Myles PS, et al. Hyperbaric or normobaric oxygen for acute carbon monoxide poisoning: a randomised controlled clinical trial. Med J Aust 1999;170(5):203–10.
[206] Weaver LK, Hopkins RO, Chan KJ, et al. Hyperbaric oxygen for acute carbon monoxide poisoning. N Engl J Med 2002;347(14):1057–67.
[207] Weaver LK, Hopkins RO, Larson-Lohr V. Carbon monoxide poisoning: a review of human outcome studies comparing normobaric oxygen with hyperbaric oxygen. Ann Emerg Med 1995;25(2):271–2.
[208] Tibbles PM, Perrotta PL. Treatment of carbon monoxide poisoning: a critical review of human outcome studies comparing normobaric oxygen with hyperbaric oxygen. Ann Emerg Med 1994;24(2):269–76.
[209] Juurlink DN, Stanbrook MB, McGuigan MA. Hyperbaric oxygen for carbon monoxide poisoning. Cochrane Database Syst Rev 2000;2:CD002041.
[210] Thom SR. Hyperbaric-oxygen therapy for acute carbon monoxide poisoning. N Engl J Med 2002;347(14):1105–6.

[211] Olson KR, Seger D. Hyperbaric oxygen for carbon monoxide poisoning: does it really work? Ann Emerg Med 1995;25(4):535–7.

[212] Scheinkestel CD, Tuxen DV, Bailey M, et al. Hyperbaric oxygen in carbon monoxide poisoning. Authors of study clarify points that they made. BMJ 2000;321(7253):109–10 [author reply: 110–1].

[213] Unsworth IP. Hyperbaric or normobaric oxygen for acute carbon monoxide poisoning: a randomised controlled clinical trial. Was the best treatment protocol used? Med J Aust 1999;170(11):564–5.

[214] Kindwall EP. Hyperbaric treatment of carbon monoxide poisoning. Ann Emerg Med 1985; 14(12):1233–4.

[215] Tomaszewski CA, Thom SR. Use of hyperbaric oxygen in toxicology. Emerg Med Clin North Am 1994;12(2):437–59.

[216] Myers RA, Snyder SK, Linberg S, et al. Value of hyperbaric oxygen in suspected carbon monoxide poisoning. JAMA 1981;246(21):2478–80.

[217] Myers RAM, Thom SR. Carbon monoxide and cyanide poisoning. In: Kindwall EP, editor. Hyperbaric medicine practice. Flagstaff (AZ): Best Publishing; 1994. p. 357.

[218] Van Meter KW, Weiss L, Harch PG, et al. Should the pressure be off or on in the use of oxygen in the treatment of carbon monoxide–poisoned patients? Ann Emerg Med 1994; 24(2):283–8.

[219] Tibbles PM, Edelsberg JS. Hyperbaric oxygen therapy. N Engl J Med 1996;334(25): 1642–8.

[220] Geiderman JM, Ault MJ. Hyperbaric-oxygen therapy. N Engl J Med 1996;335(22):1684 [author reply: 1685–6].

[221] Finnerty JP. Hyperbaric oxygen for acute carbon monoxide poisoning. N Engl J Med 2003; 348(6):557–60 [author reply: 557–60].

[222] Rudge FW. Carbon monoxide poisoning in infants: treatment with hyperbaric oxygen. South Med J 1993;86(3):334–7.

[223] Margulies JL. Acute carbon monoxide poisoning during pregnancy. Am J Emerg Med 1986;4(6):516–9.

[224] Brown DB, Mueller GL, Golich FC. Hyperbaric oxygen treatment for carbon monoxide poisoning in pregnancy: a case report. Aviat Space Environ Med 1992;63(11):1011–4.

[225] Hill EP, Hill JR, Power GG, et al. Carbon monoxide exchanges between the human fetus and mother: a mathematical model. Am J Physiol 1977;232(3):H311–23.

[226] Gabb G, Robin ED. Hyperbaric oxygen. A therapy in search of diseases. Chest 1987;92(6): 1074–82.

[227] Weaver LK, Hopkins RO, Elliott G. Carbon monoxide poisoning. N Engl J Med 1999; 340(16):1290 [author reply: 1292].

[228] Hampson NB, Simonson SG, Kramer CC, et al. Central nervous system oxygen toxicity during hyperbaric treatment of patients with carbon monoxide poisoning. Undersea Hyperb Med 1996;23(4):215–9.

[229] Sloan EP, Murphy DG, Hart R, et al. Complications and protocol considerations in carbon monoxide–poisoned patients who require hyperbaric oxygen therapy: report from a ten-year experience. Ann Emerg Med 1989;18(6):629–34.

[230] Pierce EC II, Zacharias A, Alday JM Jr, et al. Carbon monoxide poisoning: experimental hypothermic and hyperbaric studies. Surgery 1972;72(2):229–37.

[231] Vossberg B, Skolnick J. The role of catalytic converters in automobile carbon monoxide poisoning: a case report. Chest 1999;115(2):580–1.

[232] Yoon SS, Macdonald SC, Parrish RG. Deaths from unintentional carbon monoxide poisoning and potential for prevention with carbon monoxide detectors. JAMA 1998; 279(9):685–7.

ELSEVIER
SAUNDERS

CLINICS IN
LABORATORY
MEDICINE

Clin Lab Med 26 (2006) 127–146

Cocaine-Induced Chest Pain

James H. Jones, MD*, William B. Weir, MD

*Department of Emergency Medicine, Indiana University School of Medicine,
Indianapolis, IN, USA*

It is estimated that as many as 25 million people in the United States have used cocaine at least once, 3.7 million people have used in the past year, and 1.5 million could be classified as abusers of cocaine [1]. According to the National Institute on Drug Abuse in 2002, the lifetime prevalence rate of cocaine use is 2.7% [2]. Cocaine is implicated as the cause of nontraumatic chest pain in 14% to 25% of patients in urban centers and 7% of those in suburban areas [3]. Chest pain is the most common complaint associated with cocaine use. As many as 25% of acute myocardial infarctions (AMI) in patients 18 to 45 years of age may be attributed to cocaine use [4]. Many of these patients (60%) will continue to use cocaine, and some 75% of these patients will develop recurrent chest pain [5].

History

The use of the erythroxylon coca plant, from which cocaine is derived, dates back to early recorded history. Archaeological evidence suggests that chewing of coca leaves was practiced among South American people 5000 years ago [6]. Incans purportedly used cocaine to relieve thirst and hunger and also used it as a local anesthetic during ritual skull trephination [6].

Cocaine, the alkaloid extract of coca leaves, was first described by Albert Niemann in 1859 [6]. An ophthalmologist, Koller, reported the use of cocaine in surgery in 1884, and cocaine's combined vasoconstrictive and local anesthetic properties made it a welcome adjunct for invasive procedures [6]. Halsted used cocaine as a nerve block agent and became addicted secondary to self-experimentation [6]. Freud advocated cocaine use to treat depression,

---

Portions of this article were previously published in Holstege CP, Rusyniak DE: Medical Toxicology. 89:6, Med Clin North Am, 2005; with permission.

* Corresponding author. Department of Emergency Medicine, Indiana University School of Medicine, 1050 Wishard Boulevard, R2200, Indianapolis, IN 46202.

E-mail address: jhjones@iupui.edu (J.H. Jones).

cachexia, and asthma and to overcome morphine addiction [6]. In response to reports of addiction, the Harrison Narcotic Act of 1914 banned cocaine importation except for medicinal use [6]. The Controlled Substance Act of 1970 prohibited manufacture, distribution, and possession of cocaine except for restricted medical purposes [6]. Despite legislative and drug enforcement efforts, cocaine use remains prevalent. Of the more than 600,000 drug-related emergency department (ED) presentations in 2000, cocaine was second only to alcohol in prevalence and was associated with 29% of these patient visits [7].

Pathogenesis

The pathophysiology of cocaine-induced cardiac chest pain is multifactorial and may be best understood in terms of the timeframe of cocaine's effects. One of the most concerning manifestations of cocaine-induced chest pain is AMI. The typical patient who has cocaine-induced chest pain is a young man with minimal or absent coronary artery disease risk factors. AMI is equally likely regardless of the dose, route, or frequency of cocaine use [8]. Often chest pain develops minutes after cocaine use, but AMI has been reported up to 15 hours afterward [8]. A systematic literature review stated that the onset of cocaine-induced ischemia ranged from 1 minute to 4 days after use [5].

Coronary artery tone is mediated by both local metabolic and neural factors. Among the chemical mediators of coronary artery caliber are adenosine, vasopressin, angiotensin II, and endothelial-derived relaxing factor [9]. Neural control is mediated by the balance between the sympathetic nervous system and the parasympathetic nervous system. Even within the sympathetic nervous system, norepinephrine causes vasoconstriction by means of alpha-1 receptors and vasodilatation with its effects on beta-2 receptors. The parasympathetic system causes only vasodilatation, mediated by M3 cholinergic receptors. Myocardial oxygen delivery is largely mediated by the aforementioned mechanisms that alter coronary artery diameter and thus affect coronary blood flow [9].

Vasoconstriction

Animal investigations have demonstrated vasodilatation within the first 1 to 2 minutes of cocaine administration [9]. This vasodilatation was quickly followed by vasoconstriction some 5 minutes later. It has been hypothesized that this early vasodilatory effect may be the result of local sodium channel blockade mediated by cocaine. Several animal models have quantified the magnitude of cocaine-induced vasoconstriction. With a cocaine dose of 2 mg/kg (a commonly used dose for otorhinolaryngologic procedures), a decrease in coronary artery diameter of as much as 19% has been observed in anesthetized healthy dogs [10]. It was also demonstrated that pretreatment with phentolamine prevented the cocaine-induced vasoconstriction and that propranolol administration increased vasoconstriction, presumably because of the blockade of vasodilatory effects from beta-2 receptors. Higher doses of cocaine, similar to those used recreationally by humans (3 to 9 mg/kg), resulted in decreased coronary diameters of 33% to 46% in a study by Hayes and colleagues [11]. Investigators in two studies with denuded and atherosclerotic coronary endothelial models observed further decreases in the diameters of diseased arteries versus those of healthy arteries [12,13].

In humans, coronary vasoconstriction has been the most commonly observed response. A study by Lange and colleagues [14] demonstrated that phentolamine decreased the amount of vasoconstriction following intranasal (IN) cocaine administration. Using IN cocaine, Flores and colleagues [15] demonstrated that coronary arteries with 50% atherosclerotic stenosis were subject to greater cocaine-induced vasoconstriction than were nondiseased arteries (29% versus 13%). Cigarette smoking may cause a synergistic vasoconstriction with IN cocaine; investigators recorded a 19% decrease in coronary artery diameter among cigarette smokers who used cocaine versus 7% in those who used cocaine alone [16]. Vasoconstriction is not the sole mediator of cocaine-induced myocardial ischemia. A study by Majid and colleagues [17] evaluating typical recreational intravenous cocaine doses (8 mg, 16 mg, and 32 mg) did not result in appreciable coronary artery diameter change nor in ischemia on the basis of echocardiography. Using intracoronary (IC) cocaine, a similar study by Daniel and colleagues [18] showed that diseased coronary arteries did not constrict to a greater extent than native arteries. In a classic study, Lange and colleagues [19] examined the coronary arterial blood flow, coronary artery dimensions, and myocardial oxygen demand in 29 patients referred for cardiac catheterization to evaluate chest pain. Left coronary angiography and hemodynamic monitoring were performed at baseline and 15 minutes after IN cocaine (2 mg/kg) was administered. A significant rise in heart rate and blood pressure with a concomitant decrease in coronary sinus blood flow was noted after cocaine administration. Left coronary arterial diameters shrank 8% to 12%. None of the subjects developed chest pain or ECG changes reflective of ischemia. It is apparent that cocaine is a potent sympathetic agent, given the hemodynamic effects after a small dose as demonstrated in this study.

Multiple case reports of individuals who have sporadic ST-segment elevations and normal coronary arteries on catheterization suggest that vasoconstriction contributes to the development of myocardial infarctions [8]. It is important to note that the pathophysiology of cocaine-induced coronary vasospasm differs from that of Prinzmetal's angina. The ergonovine challenge test, which causes vasoconstriction in 90% of Prinzmetal's angina patients, does not do so in cocaine users [8]. This finding suggests that there are other mediators of cocaine-induced vasoconstriction.

Vasoconstriction may be a result of both alpha-adrenergic stimulation and a direct smooth muscle effect of cocaine. Evidence that cocaine-induced coronary vasoconstriction is alpha-mediated is derived from observations that vasospasm is reversed by phentolamine and exacerbated by non-selective beta-blockers, such as propranolol [14,19]. Other studies demonstrate that vasoconstriction is most severe at sites of atherosclerotic plaques and may be reversed with nitroglycerine [15,20]. Additional studies show that cocaine may directly constrict smooth muscle or act by a calcium-mediated mechanism [8]. Kuhn and colleagues [12] studied an endothelial denuded dog coronary artery model that showed that endothelial injury did not potentiate cocaine-induced vasospasm. Similar results were obtained in a model using human umbilical arteries, which lack sympathetic innervation [21]. It was therefore hypothesized that the sodium-channel blocking properties of cocaine decrease intracellular calcium by reducing the number of sodium ions available for sodium–calcium ion pump exchange [22].

Although most myocardial ischemia occurs within 1 hour of cocaine use, reports of delayed tachycardia and hypertension several hours after use suggest an additional effect of cocaine. A cardiac catheterization study of 10 patients consisted of left coronary angiography at baseline, followed by measurements at 30, 60, and 90 minutes after IN cocaine, 2 mg/kg dose [20]. As in prior experiments, a statistically significant decrease in left anterior descending and left circumflex coronary artery diameters was noted 30 minutes after cocaine administration. This decrease corresponded to the peak blood concentration of cocaine. At 60 minutes after cocaine administration, a return to baseline diameter in the left coronary arteries was observed. Recurrent vasoconstriction was noted in all subjects at 90 minutes, despite further decrease in cocaine blood concentration. This recrudescence of vasoconstriction accompanied a rise in the major active metabolites of cocaine: benzoylecgonine and ethyl methyl ecgonine. Such recurrent or "delayed" coronary vasospasm associated with cocaine use appears to be mediated by these two metabolites [23].

Left ventricular function

A study by Pitts and colleagues [24] suggests that, in addition to the sympathomimetic effects of cocaine, cardiac left ventricular function decreases from cocaine exposure. Twenty patients (aged 39 to 72 years, 14 male) who underwent cardiac catheterization for evaluation of chest pain were given either IC cocaine (n = 10) or saline control (n = 10). Left ventricular pressures and derivative (LV dP/dt), volumes, and ejection fraction were measured at baseline, then every 2 minutes during infusion of cocaine or control. Cocaine levels within the coronary sinus approached those of patients with fatal cocaine intoxications. In this study, cocaine did not significantly change heart rate, LV dP/dt, or LV end-diastolic volume. However, patients who received cocaine did manifest an increase in systolic and mean arterial pressures (MAP), LV end-diastolic pressures, and LV end-systolic volume and a decrease in LV ejection fraction as measured during cardiac catheterization.

Hemodynamic responses to cocaine were further elucidated in a study by Baumann and colleagues [25]. In this study, ED patients who had a chief complaint of chest pain and a history of cocaine use within 24 hours before presentation were placed on a previously validated noninvasive trans-thoracic cardiac output monitor. Twenty-seven patients, 74% male with a median age of 37 years, were enrolled. Most patients used crack cocaine (67%), smoked tobacco (82%), and had prior cocaine-associated chest pain (67%), although only 33% had known prior myocardial infarction. Hemodynamic results included a mean MAP of 92 mm Hg, a mean heart rate of 83 per minute, cardiac output of 6.9 L/min, a cardiac index of 3.2 L/min/m^2, and a stroke volume of 78 mL/beat. The authors concluded that cocaine used in recreational (uncontrolled) doses does not result in myocardial depression, as described in some animal models.

Myocardial demand

Cocaine increases heart rate and systemic arterial pressure in a dose-dependent fashion [23]. The increased chronotropy and afterload thereby elevate the myocardial oxygen demand to meet the increased cardiac workload. Another mechanism by which cocaine increases myocardial oxygen demand is that of decreased contractility [26]. In vitro human myocardium exposure to cocaine resulted in negative inotropy, which was thought to be mediated by a decrease in myofilament response through cyclic AMP [27] or protein kinase C [28]. Methylecgonidine, an active metabolite of cocaine, has been shown to be a negative inotrope in both an animal model and in vitro human myocardium [29].

Thrombogenesis

Cocaine promotes platelet aggregation and affects endothelial cell function, which may potentiate endothelial damage and thrombosis at sites of cocaine-induced vasospasm [8]. In vitro studies have demonstrated that cocaine increases platelet activation (by means of enhanced platelet calcium membrane binding and increased calcium influx), enhances platelet aggregation, and augments thromboxane production [30,31]. Other procoagulant effects of cocaine, besides increased platelet activation and aggregation, include increased production of plasminogen-activator in-hibitor [32]. Cocaine activates platelets by means of fibrinogen binding to the platelet's surface mediated by release of alpha-granule content in whole blood studies. In a study referenced by Mouhaffel and colleagues [8], patients who had cocaine-related arterial thromboses demonstrated de-creased antithrombin III and combined protein C. This study suggests that cocaine may alter clotting factor function, as described by Mouhaffel and colleagues [8]. Their assertion is supported by the normalization of these factors following cessation of cocaine use. Cocaine induces platelet activation through degranulation of alpha-granules and P-selectin expression as well as through increased epinephrine and blockade of serotonin uptake by platelets [33].

Chronic use: elevated catecholamines, atherogenesis, cardiomyopathy

Long-term cocaine use is associated with chronically elevated catecholamine levels, accelerated atherosclerosis, and myocardial remodeling. Chronic cocaine use may cause alterations in catecholamine levels and result in an increase in myocardial oxygen demand several weeks after cocaine cessation [34]. In a study by Nademanee and colleagues [35], ambulatory electrocardiographic monitoring among patients who were withdrawing from cocaine demonstrated spontaneous ischemic episodes. These were thought to be due to a relatively dopamine-deficient milieu that predisposes recovering cocaine users to coronary vasospasm.

Long-term users of cocaine exhibit accelerated atherosclerosis independent of other known risk factors. Among young adult users of cocaine, intimal hyperplasia and large atherosclerotic lesions have been noted in epicardial coronary arteries on autopsy after AMI [8]. In another postmortem study, increased aortic and right coronary atherosclerosis was noted among cocaine users [36]. Endothelial-cell barrier changes in response to cocaine enhance permeability to low-density lipoprotein, based on in vitro models [37]. Cocaine further accelerates atherosclerosis by expression of endothelial adhesion molecules and leukocyte migration [38]. Additional evidence supporting cocaine-induced atherogenesis is the electron-beam computed tomography study by Lai and colleagues [39]. This study used electron-beam and high-speed spiral CT technology to quantify calcium deposition as a surrogate marker of atherosclerosis. This methodology is commonly used to detect calcium deposits within subclinical atherosclerotic plaques. The authors examined data from an ongoing study of African American patients aged 25 to 45 years with a history of intravenous drug use. Multiple regression analysis to adjust for age and gender demonstrated that cocaine was independently associated with an increase in coronary calcium deposition.

Chronic cocaine use has been associated with left ventricular hypertrophy and systolic dysfunction. In addition, a dilated cardiomyopathy may ensue after long-term cocaine abuse [23]. One possible mechanism of myocardial damage induced by cocaine may be contraction band myonecrosis [34]. Elevated levels of catecholamines are associated with a hypercontracted sarcomere and myofibrillary disruption [40]. Karch and Billingham [40] hypothesized that contraction band necrosis may represent reperfusion injury. Contraction band necrosis has been found with greater prevalence among fatal cocaine-induced myocardial infarctions in some but not all studies [34]. Aside from contraction band necrosis, cocaine-induced myocardial infarction may result in dilated cardiomyopathy from binge use or repeated exposure [41–43]. Adulterant agents taken with cocaine have been implicated in myocarditis [23]. Finally, animal studies have revealed that cocaine deranges cytokine production from endothelial cells and leukocytes, which induces transcription of myosin and collagen and thereby alters myocardial structure [44–46]. Myocyte apoptosis by such a mechanism has been linked to cocaine use.

Coexisting coronary artery disease

Although patients with normal coronary arteries may suffer myocardial infarction following cocaine use, cocaine-induced myocardial infarction is more likely to occur among patients with coronary artery disease. Kontos and colleagues [47] described a 50% prevalence of significant coronary artery disease among 90 patients with cocaine-associated chest pain who underwent coronary angiography. Of these patients who sustained myocardial infarctions, 77% had significant coronary artery disease. This finding is similar to data presented by Hollander and Hoffman [48], in which the percentage of cocaine users undergoing angiography with thrombotic occlusion or critical stenosis was 34 of 54 (55%) in one study and 42 of 63 (67%) in another multicenter study. Single-vessel disease was the most prevalent type of coronary atherosclerosis among patients described by Kontos and colleagues [47]. Immediate effects of cocaine that can induce cardiac ischemia include increased myocardial workload, coronary artery vasoconstriction, and potentiation of coronary thrombosis (Table 1). It has been estimated that, among otherwise healthy patients, myocardial infarction risk increases 24 times for cocaine users versus nonusers [49].

Cocaethylene

Consumption of ethanol along with cocaine is common [50] and results in the formation of a toxic compound, cocaethylene, by hepatic transesterification [23]. Cocaethylene, like cocaine, prevents reuptake of dopamine, which further exacerbates the sympathomimetic effects of cocaine [51]. In animal models, cocaethylene is deadlier than cocaine or ethanol alone [52]. A study by Pirwitz and colleagues [53] portrayed the vasoconstrictive effects of cocaethylene on coronary arteries and also demonstrated increased myocardial oxygen demand in human subjects.

Differential diagnosis

As in the case of almost all patients who present with chest pain, immediate evaluation for myocardial ischemia and infarction is mandatory in patients with cocaine-associated chest pain. However, other diagnostic

Table 1
Mechanisms of cocaine-induced myocardial ischemia

Time line of cocaine use	Pathophysiologic effects	Pathogenesis
Immediate	Increased cardiac oxygen demand	Sympathomimetic effects (increased chronotropy, inotropy, and peripheral vascular resistance)
	Compromised coronary blood flow	Coronary vasoconstriction
Immediate	Thrombogenesis	Increased platelet activation and aggregation, enhanced fibrin deposition, altered clotting factor function, endothelial dysfunction
Intermediate	Prolonged (or recurrent) systemic and coronary artery vasoconstriction	Active metabolites of cocaine
		Cocaethylene
Long-term	Accelerated atherosclerosis	Increased low-density lipoprotein deposition, altered endothelial function, endothelial injury
Long-term	Cardiomyopathy	Deranged myocardial structure and function

possibilities must be kept in mind. Insufflation and inhalation of cocaine may result in pneumothorax, pneumomediastinum, or pneumopericardium. Intravenous use may lead to the development of endocarditis. Aortic dissection has been described in this setting [54,55]. Infectious, traumatic, and other causes of chest pain must still be considered (Box 1). The differential diagnosis must initially be broad, and it is incumbent on the evaluating physician to consider a host of possibilities.

Diagnostic evaluation

Unfortunately for the evaluating physician, patients with cocaine-associated chest pain may not be forthcoming about their recent drug use [3] or may present hours after the initial symptoms began [56]. A prevalence study demonstrated that as many as 25% of patients initially denied the use of cocaine in relation to their presentation of chest pain [3]. In a prospective study of patients presenting to the ED with cocaine-associated chest pain, 19% of patients presented later than 24 hours, with the chest pain beginning at a median time of 60 minutes after cocaine use and persisting for an average of 120 minutes. Reasons for delayed presentation are multifactorial [56].

Traditionally, the clinical characteristics of a patient's chest pain have been used by physicians to help determine a pretest probability that the

---

Box 1. Differential diagnosis of cocaine-associated chest pain

- Aortic dissection
- Endocarditis
- Musculoskeletal pain
- Myocardial ischemia and infarction
- Myocarditis
- Pericarditis
- Pneumomediastinum
- Pneumonia
- Pneumopericardium
- Pneumothorax
- Pulmonary embolus

---

patient's chest pain is ischemic in origin. This rule does not hold true for cocaine-associated chest pain. Neither the location, duration, quality, nor associated symptoms of the chest pain have been shown to be predictive of myocardial ischemia in this patient population [56].

The ECG, despite its shortcomings, is a time-honored tool that clinicians rely on heavily for evaluating patients presenting with chest pain. A cross-sectional study compared ECGs in patients with cocaine-associated chest pain against matched controls [57]. Benign early repolarization (BER) was found in 35% of the cocaine group and 30% of the controls. Normal readings or nonspecific were found in 46% of each group. The authors found no difference in the mean frequencies of ECG diagnoses between the two groups and concluded that normal variations (BER) account for many of the ECG changes observed in this patient population. This phenomenon has the potential to mislead the treating physician, who might mistake BER for an acute injury pattern. Hollander and colleagues [56] calculated a sensitivity of 35.7% and a specificity of 89.9% for the ECG in this clinical setting. In other words, the ECG possesses a high false-negative rate under these circumstances. Positive and negative likelihood ratios for the ECG would be 3.5 and 0.72, respectively.

Just as they use the ECG, clinicians use cardiac markers to make management and disposition decisions for patients with cocaine-associated chest pain. One can intuit that the creatine kinase (CK) and CK-MB levels might be elevated following cocaine use, secondary to agitation and subsequent skeletal muscle injury. Cardiac troponin I, by contrast, has no cross-reactivity with human skeletal muscle troponin I. Hollander and colleagues [58] tested the performance of cardiac markers in 97 patients with potential myocardial ischemia (20% with recent cocaine use). Myoglobin, CK-MB, and troponin I were drawn at the time of presentation and then serially every 8 to 12 hours. The specificity of myoglobin for AMI in patients without cocaine use was 82%, compared with only 50% in patients who had recently used cocaine. For CK-MB, the specificity was 88% (no cocaine) versus 75% (with cocaine), and for troponin I the specificity was 94% for both groups. The authors concluded that the specificity of troponin I was not affected by recent cocaine use. Kontos and colleagues [59] studied the usefulness of troponin I in patients with cocaine-associated chest pain. The study included 526 patients presenting to the ED with cocaine-associated chest pain, of which 246 patients were admitted. CK-MB criteria for AMI were found in 14% of the admitted patients, and for troponin I the figure was 16%. The authors concluded that troponin I has equivalent diagnostic accuracy to CK-MB in this patient population.

Myocardial perfusion imaging may provide the clinician with useful information in the assessment of the patient who has worrisome chest pain. Kontos and colleagues [60] used technetium-99m sestamibi scanning to study 216 low- and moderate-risk patients with cocaine-associated chest pain. All patients were injected with the isotope in the ED and then scanned within 60 to 90 minutes. No negative scan patients were found to have biochemical evidence of AMI. A total of five patients had positive scans, two of whom were found to have AMI. All patients with negative scans were followed for 90 days (8% were lost to follow-up), and no cardiac events occurred during this period. The authors concluded that early perfusion scanning could offer an alternative to inpatient evaluation.

Treatment

As with every sick or potentially sick patient, the clinician's initial focus should be on the patient's airway, breathing, and circulation (ABCs). Once these steps are completed, more goal-directed assessment and treatment may commence.

Only a few well-designed studies have compared the efficacy of the various treatment strategies for cocaine-associated chest pain. Recommendations for treatment are based on animal studies, observational series, case series, case reports, and small clinical trials. The American Heart Association (AHA), in its 2000 Guidelines for Cardiopulmonary Resuscitation and Emergency Cardiovascular Care, openly acknowledges that its recommendations related to the treatment options for cocaine-associated chest pain are based on a small number of studies [61].

The central nervous system plays a key role in many of the sympathomimetic manifestations of cocaine toxicity [62]. Clinical experience has confirmed that benzodiazepines blunt this response. Benzodiazepines have anxiolytic properties and hence may curb psychomotor agitation. Benzodiazepines also attenuate the rise in blood pressure and pulse secondary to cocaine. These effects could therefore result in a reduction of myocardial oxygen demand. The 2000 AHA guidelines recommend benzodiazepines as primary therapy [61].

On the premise that aspirin will impede thrombus formation, the 2000 AHA guidelines recommend aspirin as first-line therapy [61]. No clinical studies substantiate this premise, but it makes intuitive sense based on the pathophysiology involved (cocaine is thrombogenic), aspirin's safety profile and minimal cost, and the extensive investigations that have confirmed aspirin's efficacy in patients with coronary artery disease, myocardial ischemia, and myocardial infarction.

Nitrates are a mainstay of the treatment of myocardial ischemia, and they are believed to provide benefit in the setting of cocaine-associated myocardial ischemia as well. Hollander and colleagues [63] studied 246 patients with cocaine-associated chest pain. Of these, 83 patients were treated with nitroglycerin (NTG) at the discretion of the physician. NTG was found to be beneficial in nearly half the patients, and the only adverse outcome (hypotension) occurred in a patient with a right ventricular myocardial infarction. Two studies have compared nitroglycerin with benzodiazepines in this clinical setting. The first study, by Baumann and colleagues [64], enrolled 40 patients who had cocaine-associated chest pain and blindly randomized them to one of three treatment arms: sublingual NTG only, diazepam only, or sublingual NTG and diazepam. The investigators found no difference among the three treatment groups regarding change in vital signs or chest pain. They concluded that there is no clinical difference in response between agents and appears to be no additive effect. A second study by Honderick and colleagues [65] compared the use of lorazepam plus NTG with that of NTG alone in 27 patients with cocaine-associated acute coronary syndromes. The lorazepam-plus-NTG group experienced significantly greater pain relief at both 5 and 10 minutes. The authors concluded that the early use of lorazepam and NTG is both efficacious and safe in relieving cocaine-associated chest pain. The 2000 AHA guidelines view nitrates as first-line therapy [61].

As with aspirin, the efficacy of heparin in this patient population has not been studied [61]. Lewin and Hoffman [62] and Hahn and Hoffman [6] support the use of heparin based on the pathophysiology involved (thrombus formation). The risks of heparin, specifically bleeding, must be weighed against the potential for aortic dissection and intracranial hemorrhage in these patients.

Beta adrenergic blockade is standard treatment for patients with AMI. Traditionally, beta blockers have been avoided in the setting of cocaine-associated chest pain, based on the rationale that beta blockade would lead to the unopposed alpha adrenergic effects of cocaine. Clinically, this process could lead to an increase in blood pressure and a failure to control heart rate, with significant consequences. Labetalol might be an attractive alternative in this setting, but its beta blockade effects far outweigh its alpha blockade effects. No clinical ED studies have investigated this issue. One study evaluated intravenous labetalol in 15 patients undergoing cardiac catheterization who experimentally received IN cocaine [66]. The observed cocaine-induced coronary artery vasoconstriction was not diminished with labetalol. Other investigators call into question the strict avoidance of beta blockers in this setting [67]. The author of this editorial questions the traditional reasoning, arguing that the pathophysiology involved is probably more complex than the simple sympathomimetic model and that more selective beta blockers are now available. Others, too, have reported on the clinical safety of using beta antagonists in treating the cardiotoxic effects of cocaine [68].

Morphine is often used as a supplement in the setting of acute chest pain to help control the patient's discomfort. Saland and colleagues [69] studied 16 patients undergoing elective cardiac catheterization for evaluation of chest pain. Patients were randomized into two groups: cocaine/saline and cocaine/morphine. The findings showed that cocaine increased myocardial oxygen demand, and the subsequent administration of morphine did not further alter oxygen demand. At the same time, the administration of morphine following cocaine reversed the cocaine-induced arterial vasoconstriction. The investigators concluded that morphine was both safe and beneficial in this clinical setting.

Calcium channel blockade is not routinely advocated in the treatment of AMI. However, in the setting of cocaine-associated chest pain, some evidence indicates that calcium channel blockade may be of benefit. A study of 10 healthy volunteers demonstrated that verapamil relieved cocaine-induced vasospasm [70]. The 2000 AHA guidelines recommend calcium channel blockade as a second-line therapy [61]. Others do not endorse this concept and call for further clinical investigation [6].

Phentolamine, because it is a pure alpha antagonist, is theoretically an option in this clinical setting. A case report documented its efficacy in a patient unresponsive to traditional treatments for cocaine-associated chest pain who improved dramatically with its use [71].

Thrombolysis is an attractive treatment choice for cocaine-associated AMI because of the pathology of enhanced thrombogenesis noted with cocaine. However, several concerns must be kept in mind. First and foremost, the clinical benefit of thrombolysis in this setting is unclear (risk/benefit assessment). Vasospasm is thought to play a role in some patients. At catheterization, some of these patients are found not to have thrombus. Moreover, in this patient population, a high prevalence of BER is seen on ECG, leading to the possibility of false-positive interpretations meeting thrombolytic criteria. Overall, morbidity and mortality in this clinical setting are low. Unfortunately, there have been case reports of intracranial hemorrhage when thrombolysis is used in this patient population [72]. The most complete study that has attempted to address this clinical dilemma is a retrospective, cross-sectional study by Hollander and colleagues [73]. The primary endpoint of the study was the safety of thrombolytics in patients who had cocaine-associated AMI. Thrombolytics were given to 25 patients, who were then compared with 41 well-matched patients who met thrombolysis in myocardial infarction criteria but did not receive thrombolytics. No deaths occurred in either group, and there were no major complications (eg, intracranial hemorrhage, need for transfusion). Approximately two thirds of the patients were believed to have reperfused when given thrombolytics. No difference was found regarding peak cardiac marker levels or time to peak levels (indirect measures of efficacy). The authors advocate for adoption of a "cautious" policy for the use of thrombolytics in patients with cocaine-associated ST segment elevation. The 2000 AHA guidelines state that thrombolysis should not be considered unless there is evidence of evolving myocardial infarction that persists despite other medical therapy and timely percutaneous coronary intervention (PCI) is not accessible [61].

The 2000 AHA guidelines go on to suggest that PCI, when available, is the treatment of choice for ongoing ischemia. No studies have compared these two interventions in this patient population. Kontos and colleagues [47] reported on 90 patients who underwent coronary angiography within 5 weeks of an ED evaluation for cocaine-associated chest pain. They found that significant disease, defined as coronary artery, major branch, or bypass graft stenosis of greater than or equal to 50%, was present in 50% of patients. Significant disease was present in 77% of patients with AMI or elevated troponin levels, compared with 35% of patients without myonecrosis. These findings demonstrate that a high percentage of this patient population has underlying coronary artery disease, and thus lends credence to the argument that PCI should be the primary treatment for cocaine-associated AMI.

Several mechanisms have been suggested for the development of cocaine-associated dysrhythmias. These include increased ventricular irritability, lower ventricular arrhythmia threshold, prolonged QRS and Q–T intervals, similar to the effects of class 1 antiarrhythmics, and reduced vagal tone (Box 2). Most of the more lethal arrhythmias have been noted in the context of hemodynamic or metabolic derangements (ie, hypoxia, hypotension, seizure, AMI) and occur early in the course of the patient's presentation [56,74]. Because of cocaine's cardiac sodium channel blocking properties, sodium bicarbonate is suggested for the treatment of wide-complex tachycardias. Lidocaine, despite some concerns, has been used for cocaine-induced ventricular arrhythmias [6]. Class 1a (quinidine, procainamide, and disopyramide) should be avoided [75]. No literature reports the efficacy of amiodarone for cocaine-induced ventricular tachycardia or fibrillation.

Morbidity and mortality

Unsurprisingly, patients presenting with cocaine-associated chest pain may experience complications and death. Fortunately, their morbidity and mortality are strikingly low.

Box 2. Potential dysrhythmias secondary to cocaine

- Asystole
- Atrial fibrillation
- Bundle branch block
- Complete heart block
- Sinus bradycardia (early)
- Sinus tachycardia
- Supraventricular tachycardia
- Torsade de Pointes
- Ventricular tachycardia
- Ventricular fibrillation

Brody and colleagues [76] retrospectively summarized hospital visits for cocaine-related medical problems. This study consisted of a series of 233 consecutive visits to an urban ED. Most of the presenting complaints were cardiopulmonary in nature (56%), and the most common complaint was chest pain (40%). Acute mortality was less than 1%, with one of the ED deaths being preceded by a prehospital cardiac arrest and the other being a cardiac arrest in a patient with recent endocarditis. Hollander and colleagues [56] presented data from a prospective, cohort, multicenter study that evaluated 246 patients who had cocaine-associated chest pain. Approximately 90% of these patients reported insufflation or inhalation as the preferred route of use. The prevalence of myocardial infarction was 5.7%; congestive heart failure developed in four patients (1.6%), 10 patients sustained arrhythmias (4.0%), and two patients (0.8%) suffered a cardiac arrest—both in the prehospital setting. Once in the ED, no patients experienced a life-threatening complication. The authors were unable to identify any data from the history that could assist the physician in predicting or excluding myocardial ischemia or infarction. The clinical description of the pain and associated symptoms, along with cardiovascular risk factors, was not helpful.

A retrospective study by Weber and colleagues [74] evaluated 250 admitted patients who had cocaine-associated chest pain. The "rule-in" rate for AMI was 6%, and complications were uncommon. No complications developed more than 12 hours after ED presentation. A fourth study went one step further and reported on 130 patients with 136 episodes of AMI secondary to cocaine [77]. Mortality was 0% (confidence interval 0%–2%), with cardiovascular complications occurring in 36% of patients. Approximately 90% of these complications occurred within the first 12 hours (congestive heart failure in nine patients, arrhythmias in 55 patients), and all episodes of ventricular tachycardia and ventricular fibrillation occurred before hospital arrival. All patients who had complications were identified by one of the following: a 12-hour period of observation, an initial abnormal ECG, or an elevated CK-MB within the first 12 hours. From these data the authors make calculations and state that, for 1000 patients presenting to the ED with cocaine-associated chest pain, 1.6 patients might be expected to develop cardiovascular complications not identified by the above criteria. Notably, 52 of these patients went on to cardiac catheterization, and 67% were found to have at least single-vessel disease (more than 50% narrowing).

From this information, the clinician may draw several conclusions regarding the ED and hospital course for these patients. Approximately 6% of patients with cocaine-associated chest pain will ultimately be diagnosed with an AMI. Almost all anticipated complications will occur within the first 12 hours of presentation, with life-threatening arrhythmias being most prevalent in the prehospital setting, and the mortality for patients with cocaine-associated chest pain is low (less than 1%).

The previous section on differential diagnosis mentioned the possibility of an aortic dissection being present in the setting of cocaine-associated chest pain. Hsue and colleagues [55] report on a retrospective case series of 38 patients with acute aortic dissection. Fourteen patients (37%) had a dissection related to cocaine use, with a mean interval of 12 hours between cocaine use and the onset of symptoms (range 0–24 hours). The pattern of the dissection was type A in six patients and type B in eight patients. The majority (79%) of these 14 patients also had a history of hypertension. There were four deaths (29%).

Prognosis

Data are available regarding the prognosis of this patient population once discharged from the hospital. Hollander and colleagues [5] reported on 203 patients who were followed for a mean of 408 days after discharge for cocaine-associated chest pain. Mortality data were available for all 203 patients. The study endpoints consisted of 1-year mortality and the incidence of AMI. The survival rate was 97%. Six deaths occurred: three from HIV, one from end-stage renal disease, one from congestive heart failure, and one from sepsis. Two AMIs occurred, and both of these patients continued to use cocaine. Approximately 60% of the patients continued to use cocaine, and 75% of these patients experienced recurrent chest pain. No deaths or AMIs occurred in those patients claiming abstinence.

Disposition

At the crux of every ED patient encounter is the decision whether to admit the patient to the hospital or discharge the patient, usually to home. Several recent studies may help guide the clinician with disposition decisions in the patient with cocaine-associated chest pain. Kushman and colleagues

[78] from the Cincinnati Chest Pain Center retrospectively reported on 197 patients with cocaine-associated chest pain. Their evaluation protocol consisted of an initial ECG, continuous ST segment monitoring, and cardiac marker assays at 0, 3, 6, and 9 hours. Patients without evidence of myocardial necrosis or ischemia then underwent graded exercise testing. The investigators found that this provocative test was not positive in any patient for whom the initial evaluation protocol was negative. Weber and colleagues [79] prospectively evaluated 344 patients with cocaine-associated chest pain. Of this study population, 42 (12%) of the patients were admitted to the hospital, and 302 (88%) were evaluated in an ED chest pain observation unit. The initial ED evaluation protocol included provocative testing in all patients, but, because of the extremely low rate of positive tests (the number was not cited in the article), the protocol was altered, and stress testing before discharge ceased to be mandatory. Patients who had normal troponin I levels (0, 3, 6, and 9 hours), who were without new ischemic ECG changes, and who experienced no cardiovascular complications during the 9- to 12-hour period of observation were discharged home. During the 30-day follow-up period, four of the 256 patients for whom follow-up data were available had a nonfatal AMI. All these events occurred in patients who continued to use cocaine.

These studies lend strong support to the belief that if the initial and ongoing cardiac evaluation is unremarkable, the patient's symptoms resolve, and no other abnormalities are found, these patients may be safely discharged from the ED with appropriate follow-up arrangements. The studies also demonstrate that the patients at greatest risk are those who continue to use cocaine. Therefore, the physician should consider offering drug rehabilitation opportunities to these patients.

Summary

The pathophysiology of cocaine leading to myocardial ischemia is multifactorial. Given the paucity of well-designed clinical studies, treatment is directed toward the potential mechanisms involved in the development of myocardial ischemia. Fortunately, morbidity and mortality in this patient population are low, and the vast majority of patients will not suffer AMI or other cardiac complications. Long-term prognosis is excellent for those who abstain from continued cocaine use.

References

[1] 1999 National Household Survey on Drug Abuse: summary findings. Substance Abuse and Mental Health Services Administration. Available at: http://www.health.org/govstudy/bkd376. Accessed November 10, 2004.
[2] Leshner A. NIDA research report: cocaine abuse and addiction. National Institutes of Health. Available at: http://www.drugabuse.gov/ResearchReports/Cocaine/Cocaine.html. Accessed November 10, 2004.

[3] Hollander JE, Todd KH, Green G, et al. Chest pain associated with cocaine: an assessment of prevalence in suburban and urban emergency departments. Ann Emerg Med 1995;26(6): 671–6.

[4] Qureshi AI, Suri MF, Guterman LR, et al. Cocaine use and the likelihood of nonfatal myocardial infarction and stroke: data from the Third National Health and Nutrition Examination Survey. Circulation 2001;103(4):502–6.

[5] Hollander JE, Hoffman RS, Gennis P, et al. Cocaine-associated chest pain: one-year follow-up. Acad Emerg Med 1995;2(3):179–84.

[6] Hahn IH, Hoffman RS. Cocaine use and acute myocardial infarction. Emerg Med Clin North Am 2001;19(2):493–510.

[7] National Institute on Drug Abuse infofacts. Hospital visits. National Institutes of Health. Available at: http://www.nida.nih.gov/InfoFacts/hospital.html. Accessed November 10, 2004.

[8] Mouhaffel AH, Madu EC, Satmary WA, et al. Cardiovascular complications of cocaine. Chest 1995;107(5):1426–34.

[9] Benzaquen BS, Cohen V, Eisenberg MJ. Effects of cocaine on the coronary arteries. Am Heart J 2001;142(3):402–10.

[10] Kuhn FE, Johnson MN, Gillis RA, et al. Effect of cocaine on the coronary circulation and systemic hemodynamics in dogs. J Am Coll Cardiol 1990;16(6):1481–91.

[11] Hayes SN, Moyer TP, Morley D, et al. Intravenous cocaine causes epicardial coronary vasoconstriction in the intact dog. Am Heart J 1991;121(6 Pt 1):1639–48.

[12] Kuhn FE, Gillis RA, Virmani R, et al. Cocaine produces coronary artery vasoconstriction independent of an intact endothelium. Chest 1992;102(2):581–5.

[13] Egashira K, Pipers FS, Morgan JP. Effects of cocaine on epicardial coronary artery reactivity in miniature swine after endothelial injury and high cholesterol feeding. In vivo and in vitro analysis. J Clin Invest 1991;88(4):1307–14.

[14] Lange RA, Cigarroa RG, Flores ED, et al. Potentiation of cocaine-induced coronary vasoconstriction by beta-adrenergic blockade. Ann Intern Med 1990;112(12):897–903.

[15] Flores ED, Lange RA, Cigarroa RG, et al. Effect of cocaine on coronary artery dimensions in atherosclerotic coronary artery disease: enhanced vasoconstriction at sites of significant stenoses. J Am Coll Cardiol 1990;16(1):74–9.

[16] Moliterno DJ, Willard JE, Lange RA, et al. Coronary-artery vasoconstriction induced by cocaine, cigarette smoking, or both. N Engl J Med 1994;330(7):454–9.

[17] Majid PA, Cheirif JB, Rokey R, et al. Does cocaine cause coronary vasospasm in chronic cocaine abusers? A study of coronary and systemic hemodynamics. Clin Cardiol 1992;15(4): 253–8.

[18] Daniel WC, Lange RA, Landau C, et al. Effects of the intracoronary infusion of cocaine on coronary arterial dimensions and blood flow in humans. Am J Cardiol 1996; 78(3):288–91.

[19] Lange RA, Cigarroa RG, Yancy CW Jr, et al. Cocaine-induced coronary-artery vasoconstriction. N Engl J Med 1989;321(23):1557–62.

[20] Brogan WC III, Lange RA, Kim AS, et al. Alleviation of cocaine-induced coronary vasoconstriction by nitroglycerin. J Am Coll Cardiol 1991;18(2):581–6.

[21] Isner JM, Chokshi SK. Cardiac complications of cocaine abuse. Annu Rev Med 1991;42: 133–8.

[22] Perreault CL, Hague NL, Morgan KG, et al. Negative inotropic and relaxant effects of cocaine on myopathic human ventricular myocardium and epicardial coronary arteries in vitro. Cardiovasc Res 1993;27(2):262–8.

[23] Lange RA, Hillis LD, Pitts WR, et al. Cardiovascular complications of cocaine use. N Engl J Med 2001;345(5):351–8.

[24] Pitts WR, Vongpatanasin W, Cigarroa JE, et al. Effects of the intracoronary infusion of cocaine on left ventricular systolic and diastolic function in humans. Circulation 1998;97(13): 1270–3.

[25] Baumann BM, Perrone J, Hornig SE, et al. Cardiac and hemodynamic assessment of patients with cocaine-associated chest pain syndromes. J Toxicol Clin Toxicol 2000;38(3): 283–90.

[26] Kloner RA, Hale S, Alker K, et al. The effects of acute and chronic cocaine use on the heart. Circulation 1992;85(2):407–19.

[27] Perreault CL, Hague NL, Ransil BJ, et al. The effects of cocaine on intracellular Ca2+ handling and myofilament Ca2+ responsiveness of ferret ventricular myocardium. Br J Pharmacol 1990;101(3):679–85.

[28] Perreault CL, Morgan KG, Morgan JP. Effects of cocaine on intracellular calcium binding in cardiac and vascular smooth muscle. NIDA Res Monogr 1991;1(8):139–53.

[29] Woolf JH, Huang L, Ishiguro Y, et al. Negative inotropic effect of methylecgonidine, a major product of cocaine base pyrolysis, on ferret and human myocardium. J Cardiovasc Pharmacol 1997;30(3):352–9.

[30] Folts JD, Bonebrake FC. The effects of cigarette smoke and nicotine on platelet thrombus formation in stenosed dog coronary arteries: inhibition with phentolamine. Circulation 1982;65(3):465–70.

[31] Togna G, Tempesta E, Togna AR, et al. Platelet responsiveness and biosynthesis of thromboxane and prostacyclin in response to in vitro cocaine treatment. Haemostasis 1985; 15(2):100–7.

[32] Moliterno DJ, Lange RA, Gerard RD, et al. Influence of intranasal cocaine on plasma constituents associated with endogenous thrombosis and thrombolysis. Am J Med 1994; 96(6):492–6.

[33] Kugelmass AD, Oda A, Monahan K, et al. Activation of human platelets by cocaine. Circulation 1993;88(3):876–83.

[34] Goldfrank LR, Hoffman RS. The cardiovascular effects of cocaine. Ann Emerg Med 1991; 20(2):165–75.

[35] Nademanee K, Gorelick DA, Josephson MA, et al. Myocardial ischemia during cocaine withdrawal. Ann Intern Med 1989;111(11):876–80.

[36] Kolodgie FD, Virmani R, Cornhill JF, et al. Cocaine: an independent risk factor for aortic sudanophilia. A preliminary report. Atherosclerosis 1992;97(1):53–62.

[37] Kolodgie FD, Wilson PS, Mergner WJ, et al. Cocaine-induced increase in the permeability function of human vascular endothelial cell monolayers. Exp Mol Pathol 1999;66(2):109–22.

[38] Gan X, Zhang L, Berger O, et al. Cocaine enhances brain endothelial adhesion molecules and leukocyte migration. Clin Immunol 1999;91(1):68–76.

[39] Lai S, Lai H, Meng Q, et al. Effect of cocaine use on coronary calcium among black adults in Baltimore, Maryland. Am J Cardiol 2002;90(3):326–8.

[40] Karch SB, Billingham ME. Myocardial contraction bands revisited. Hum Pathol 1986;17(1): 9–13.

[41] Wiener RS, Lockhart JT, Schwartz RG. Dilated cardiomyopathy and cocaine abuse. Report of two cases. Am J Med 1986;81(4):699–701.

[42] Bertolet BD, Freund G, Martin CA, et al. Unrecognized left ventricular dysfunction in an apparently healthy cocaine abuse population. Clin Cardiol 1990;13(5):323–8.

[43] Chokshi SK, Moore R, Pandian NG, et al. Reversible cardiomyopathy associated with cocaine intoxication. Ann Intern Med 1989;111(12):1039–40.

[44] Mao JT, Zhu LX, Sharma S, et al. Cocaine inhibits human endothelial cell IL-8 production: the role of transforming growth factor–beta. Cell Immunol 1997;181(1):38–43.

[45] Besse S, Assayag P, Latour C, et al. Molecular characteristics of cocaine-induced cardiomyopathy in rats. Eur J Pharmacol 1997;338(2):123–9.

[46] Xiao Y, He J, Gilbert RD, et al. Cocaine induces apoptosis in fetal myocardial cells through a mitochondria-dependent pathway. J Pharmacol Exp Ther 2000;292(1):8–14.

[47] Kontos MC, Jesse RL, Tatum JL, et al. Coronary angiographic findings in patients with cocaine-associated chest pain. J Emerg Med 2003;24(1):9–13.

[48] Hollander JE, Hoffman RS. Cocaine-induced myocardial infarction: an analysis and review of the literature. J Emerg Med 1992;10(2):169–77.

[49] Mittleman MA, Mintzer D, Maclure M, et al. Triggering of myocardial infarction by cocaine. Circulation 1999;99(21):2737–41.

[50] Grant BF, Harford TC. Concurrent and simultaneous use of alcohol with cocaine: results of national survey. Drug Alcohol Depend 1990;25(1):97–104.

[51] Hearn WL, Flynn DD, Hime GW, et al. Cocaethylene: a unique cocaine metabolite displays high affinity for the dopamine transporter. J Neurochem 1991;56(2):698–701.

[52] Hearn WL, Rose S, Wagner J, et al. Cocaethylene is more potent than cocaine in mediating lethality. Pharmacol Biochem Behav 1991;39(2):531–3.

[53] Pirwitz MJ, Willard JE, Landau C, et al. Influence of cocaine, ethanol, or their combination on epicardial coronary arterial dimensions in humans. Arch Intern Med 1995;155(11): 1186–91.

[54] Nallamothu BK, Saint S, Kolias TJ, et al. Clinical problem-solving. Of nicks and time. N Engl J Med 2001;345(5):359–63.

[55] Hsue PY, Salinas CL, Bolger AF, et al. Acute aortic dissection related to crack cocaine. Circulation 2002;105(13):1592–5.

[56] Hollander JE, Hoffman RS, Gennis P, et al. Prospective multicenter evaluation of cocaine-associated chest pain. Cocaine Associated Chest Pain (COCHPA) Study Group. Acad Emerg Med 1994;1(4):330–9.

[57] Hollander JE, Lozano M, Fairweather P, et al. "Abnormal" electrocardiograms in patients with cocaine-associated chest pain are due to "normal" variants. J Emerg Med 1994;12(2): 199–205.

[58] Hollander JE, Levitt MA, Young GP, et al. Effect of recent cocaine use on the specificity of cardiac markers for diagnosis of acute myocardial infarction. Am Heart J 1998;135(2 Pt 1): 245–52.

[59] Kontos MC, Anderson FP, Ornato JP, et al. Utility of troponin I in patients with cocaine-associated chest pain. Acad Emerg Med 2002;9(10):1007–13.

[60] Kontos MC, Schmidt KL, Nicholson CS, et al. Myocardial perfusion imaging with technetium-99m sestamibi in patients with cocaine-associated chest pain. Ann Emerg Med 1999;33(6):639–45.

[61] Resuscitation AHA. Guidelines 2000 for cardiopulmonary resuscitation and emergency cardiovascular care. Part 8: Advanced challenges in resuscitation. Section 2: Toxicology in ECC. Circulation 2000;102(8):I223–8.

[62] Lewin NA, Hoffman RS. Cocaine. In: Goldfrank LR, Lewin NA, Flomenbaum NE, et al, editors. Goldfrank's toxicologic emergencies. 5th edition. Norwalk (CT): Appleton and Lange; 1994. p. 847–62.

[63] Hollander JE, Hoffman RS, Gennis P, et al. Nitroglycerin in the treatment of cocaine associated chest pain—clinical safety and efficacy. J Toxicol Clin Toxicol 1994;32(3):243–56.

[64] Baumann BM, Perrone J, Hornig SE, et al. Randomized, double-blind, placebo-controlled trial of diazepam, nitroglycerin, or both for treatment of patients with potential cocaine-associated acute coronary syndromes. Acad Emerg Med 2000;7(8):878–85.

[65] Honderick T, Williams D, Seaberg D, et al. A prospective, randomized, controlled trial of benzodiazepines and nitroglycerine or nitroglycerine alone in the treatment of cocaine-associated acute coronary syndromes. Am J Emerg Med 2003;21(1):39–42.

[66] Boehrer JD, Moliterno DJ, Willard JE, et al. Influence of labetalol on cocaine-induced coronary vasoconstriction in humans. Am J Med 1993;94(6):608–10.

[67] Leikin JB. Cocaine and beta-adrenergic blockers: a remarriage after a decade-long divorce? Crit Care Med 1999;27(4):688–9.

[68] Blaho K, Winbery S, Park L, et al. Cocaine use and acute coronary syndromes [comment]. Lancet 2001;358(9290):1368.

[69] Saland KE, Hillis LD, Lange RA, et al. Influence of morphine sulfate on cocaine-induced coronary vasoconstriction. Am J Cardiol 2002;90(7):810–1.

[70] Negus BH, Willard JE, Hillis LD, et al. Alleviation of cocaine-induced coronary vasoconstriction with intravenous verapamil. Am J Cardiol 1994;73(7):510–3.

[71] Hollander JE, Carter WA, Hoffman RS. Use of phentolamine for cocaine-induced myocardial ischemia. N Engl J Med 1992;327(5):361.

[72] LoVecchio F, Nelson L. Intraventricular bleeding after the use of thrombolytics in a cocaine user. Am J Emerg Med 1996;14(7):663–4 [see comment].

[73] Hollander JE, Burstein JL, Hoffman RS, et al. Cocaine-associated myocardial infarction. Clinical safety of thrombolytic therapy. Cocaine Associated Myocardial Infarction (CAMI) Study Group. Chest 1995;107(5):1237–41.

[74] Weber JE, Chudnofsky CR, Boczar M, et al. Cocaine-associated chest pain: how common is myocardial infarction? Acad Emerg Med 2000;7(8):873–7.

[75] Winecoff AP, Hariman RJ, Grawe JJ, et al. Reversal of the electrocardiographic effects of cocaine by lidocaine. Part 1. Comparison with sodium bicarbonate and quinidine. Pharmacotherapy 1994;14(6):698–703.

[76] Brody SL, Slovis CM, Wrenn KD. Cocaine-related medical problems: consecutive series of 233 patients. Am J Med 1990;88(4):325–31.

[77] Hollander JE, Hoffman RS, Burstein JL, et al. Cocaine-associated myocardial infarction. Mortality and complications. Cocaine-Associated Myocardial Infarction Study Group. Arch Intern Med 1995;155(10):1081–6.

[78] Kushman SO, Storrow AB, Liu T, et al. Cocaine-associated chest pain in a chest pain center. Am J Cardiol 2000;85(3):394–6, A310.

[79] Weber JE, Shofer FS, Larkin GL, et al. Validation of a brief observation period for patients with cocaine-associated chest pain. N Engl J Med 2003;348(6):510–7.

ELSEVIER
SAUNDERS

CLINICS IN
LABORATORY
MEDICINE

Clin Lab Med 26 (2006) 147–164

New Drugs of Abuse in North America

Rachel Haroz, MD[a],*,
Michael I. Greenberg, MD, MPh[b]

[a]Department of Emergency Medicine, Cooper Hospital University Medical Center,
Camden, NJ, USA
[b]Department of Emergency Medicine, Drexel University College of Medicine,
Medical College of Pennsylvania Hospital, Philadelphia, PA, USA

The term "drugs of abuse" usually brings to mind traditional street drugs, such as cocaine, heroin, marijuana, and methamphetamine. In recent years, these drugs have been joined by other abusable substances, such as the well-known "club drugs": ketamine, gamma hydroxybutyric acid, and Ecstasy. The drug scene, however, is constantly changing and evolving. As various law enforcement agencies pursue and dismantle distribution and production organizations of the usual drugs of abuse, dealers and users are turning to less known, more accessible, and often currently licit substances. The widespread growth of the Internet with its vast distribution of information has increased the accessibility of a host of substances and facilitated synthesis and production of various substances by individuals. This article discusses several new and emerging drugs of abuse, including new synthetic variations, plants, and pharmaceuticals diverted for abuse. It is not an all-inclusive list but rather an attempt to bring to light some lesser-known agents that appear to be growing in popularity.

Ecstasy-related compounds

In the 1990s, use of 3,4-methylenedioxy-N-methylamphetamine (MDMA, commonly known as Ecstasy) increased dramatically both in the United States and Europe [1]. At first, MDMA was associated almost exclusively with the rave and club drug scene. However, its use has continued to grow, and the consumer market has expanded. In addition, over the past several

---

Portions of this article were previously published in Holstege CP, Rusyniak DE: Medical Toxicology. 89:6, Med Clin North Am, 2005; with permission.

* Corresponding author. Department of Emergency Medicine, Cooper Hospital University Medical Center, One Cooper Plaza, Camden, NJ 08103.
E-mail address: rburshtein@aol.com (R. Haroz).

years, drugs have appeared on the market as so-called "legal sub-stitutes," touted as mimicking the "feel-good" and hallucinogenic effects of MDMA [2]. The production and sale of these Ecstasy-like drugs is intended to capitalize on the popularity of MDMA. Although these drugs may be sold individually, often they are purported actually to be Ecstasy tablets, and the consumers are unaware of the actual ingredients. This next generation of club drugs may be divided into three classes: tryptamines, phenylethylamines, and piperazines.

Tryptamines

Tryptamine compounds recently re-emerged on the drug scene. These compounds are actually synthetic hallucinogenic indolealkylamines and include N,N-alpha-methyltryptamine (AMT), 5-methoxy-N,N-alpha-methyl-tryptamine (5-MeO-AMT), N,N-dipropyltryptamine (DPT), N,N-dimethyl-tryptamine (DMT), 5-methoxy-N,N-diisopropyltryptamine (5-MeO-DIPT), and 5-methoxy-N,N-dimethyltryptamine (5-MeO-DMT), among others. These substances are structurally similar to psilocybin, psilocin, and bufotenine, all of which are classified as schedule I drugs under the Controlled Substance Act (Fig. 1). Psilocybin (4-phosphoryloxy-N,N-dimethyltrypta-mine) and its metabolite psilocin (4-OH N,N-dimethyltryptamine) are found in the genus of mushrooms known as *Psilocybe* and are also called "magic

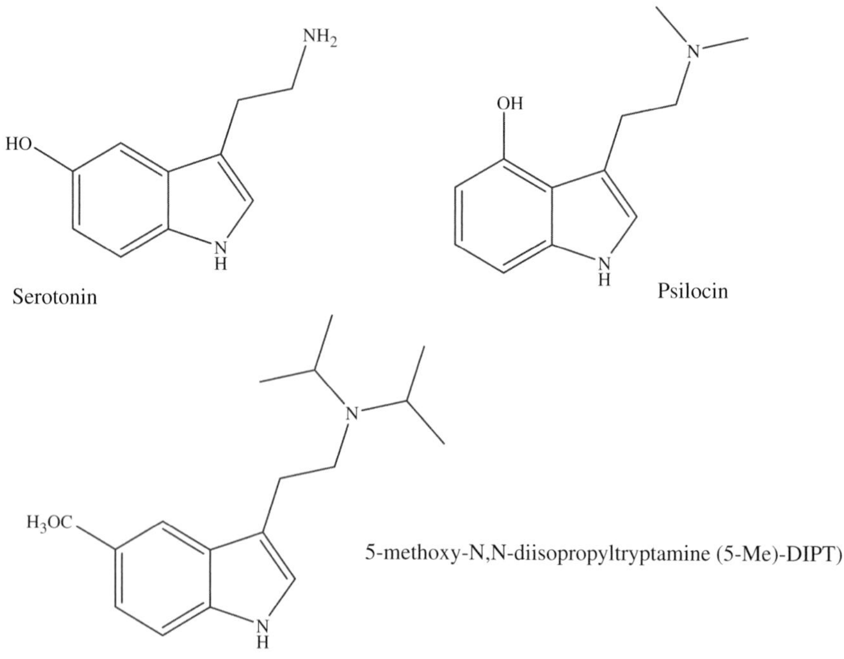

Serotonin

Psilocin

5-methoxy-N,N-diisopropyltryptamine (5-Me)-DIPT)

Fig. 1. Tryptamines.

mushrooms" because of their hallucinogenic properties. Bufotenine (5-OH dimethyltryptamine) is found in certain toads, including the *Bufo* species, and plants, such as *Anadenanthera* [2]. Tryptamine itself lacks significant stimulant and hallucinogenic properties. However, some of the derivatives of tryptamine contain indole ring structures and ethylamine substitutions that result in pharmacologic activity [2].

Use of DMT was first encountered in the United States in the 1960s, when it was known as a "businessman's lunch" because of the rapid onset of action when smoked (2 to 5 minutes) and short duration of action (20 minutes to 1 hour). DMT has long been used in South America for spiritual and medicinal purposes. This substance may be injected, inhaled, smoked, or even administered as an enema [3,4]. The most popular South American preparation containing DMT is known as "ayahuasca," a brewed tea made up of two plants: *Psychotria viridis* and *Banisteriopsis caapi*. *P viridis* contains DMT, whereas *B caapi* contains β-carboline compounds, including harmaline, harmine, and 1,2,3,4-tetrahydroharmine [4,5]. These β-carboline compounds possess sedative and hallucinogenic properties and may also act as monoamine oxidase inhibitors (MAOIs). Because MAO breaks down DMT, its inhibition allows DMT to be absorbed and become bioavailable orally. The β-carbolines also often cause nausea and vomiting [4]. Several plants found in the United States contain DMT as well as β-carbolines. These include *Peganum harmala* (Syrian rue) and *Passiflora incarnata* (passionflower) [4].

Historically, the illicit use of tryptamine compounds was infrequent. Except for DMT, these drugs were unscheduled until 2004, when the US Drug Enforcement Administration (DEA) placed 5-MeO-DIPT and AMT in the schedule I category. Use of these drugs has been increasing. For example, from 2001 through 2003, law enforcement officials reported the confiscation or use in 12 states of 5-MeO-DIPT (also known as "foxy" or "foxy methoxy") alone [6].

Although various routes of administration are possible for the hallucinogenic tryptamines, not all are active when ingested. Although 5-MeO-DIPT, AMT (known as "spirals"), and DPT are active when ingested, DMT and 5-MeO-DMT are ineffective when ingested owing to breakdown by MAOs and must be smoked or insufflated [6–9]. Coingestion of MAOIs, as mentioned earlier, may facilitate the oral bioavailability of these compounds.

Most of the tryptamines are available in capsule, tablet, or powder form; occasionally they are encountered as liquids. The liquid form may be impregnated on sugar cubes, candy, or blotter paper, as has been the case with 5-MeO-AMT [10]. A single oral dose of AMT is approximately 20 mg, a dose of 5-MeO-AMT is 2 to 4.5 mg, and a 5-MeO-DIPT dose is approximately 6 to 10 mg [3].

Although DMT has a rapid onset and a brief duration of action, orally ingested AMT has an onset of action as long as 4 hours and a duration of action of 12 to 24 hours, similar to 5-MeO-AMT [2,9,10]. 5-MeO-DIPT has an onset of action of 20 to 30 minutes, peaks at 1 to 1.5 hours, and lasts as long as 3 to 6 hours [2].

The mechanisms of action of tryptamines have not been fully elucidated. They may act similarly to the classical hallucinogens, such as LSD, namely as agonists at the 5HT2 and $5HT1_C$ receptors, causing an increase in serotonin. These compounds may be active at other serotonin receptors as well [11].

Users of tryptamines report a variety of acute effects, including empathy, euphoria, visual and auditory hallucinations, nausea, vomiting, diarrhea, and emotional distress. Clinical symptoms may include agitation, tachycardia, hypertension, diaphoresis, salivation, dystonia, mydriasis, tremors, confusion, and seizures [2,3,6,9]. Two case reports describe paralysis and catalepsy associated with 5-MeO-DIPT use [1,6,7]. Rhabdomyolysis has been described following the ingestion of DPT [8].

Treatment and management of tryptamine-intoxicated individuals is essentially supportive; there are no specific antidotes. Benzodiazepines have been used to treat the sympathomimetic symptoms and should be administered to an endpoint of peaceful sedation [9]. Routine urine drug screening will not be positive for amphetamines in the circumstance of tryptamine use.

Phenylethylamines

Amphetamine, methamphetamine, and the popular designer drugs MDMA ("Ecstasy," "Adam") and 3,4-methylenedioxy-N-ethylamphetamine (MDEA—"Eve," "love drug") are all derivatives of the phenylethylamine structure (Fig. 2). Newer designer analogues are based on the same structure with a variety of substitutions and include the so-called "2C" series: 4-bromo-2,5-dimethoxyphenethylamine (2C-B—Nexus, Bromo), 2, 5-dimethoxy-4-ethylthiophenethylamine (2C-T-2), and 2,5-dimethoxy-4-(n)-propylthiophenethylamine (2C-T-7—T7, Triptasy, Beautiful) are some examples. Other designer phenylethylamines include 4-methylthioamphetamine (4-MTA), 4-methyl-2,5-dimethoxyamphetamine (DOM), and 4-bromo-2,5-dimethoxyamphetamine (DOB); these are not discussed here. In all, approximately 200 designer phenylethylamine derivatives have been described [12].

A naturally occurring phenylethylamine is mescaline, found in peyote cacti along the Texas–Mexico border. Mescaline (β-3,4,5-trimethoxyphenethylamine) constitutes about 1.5% of the peyote and is well known for its hallucinogenic properties [4].

Although 2C-B emerged in the United States in the late 1970s, it became a schedule I drug only in 1995, followed by 2C-T-7. In Europe these drugs have only recently become illegal. Previously, they were sold in "smart shops," similar to health food stores, as supplements under various names [13].

Sulfur molecules are found in 2C-T-7 and 2C-T-2, whereas bromide is present in 2C-B, but they share the 2,5-dimethoxyphenethylamine structure

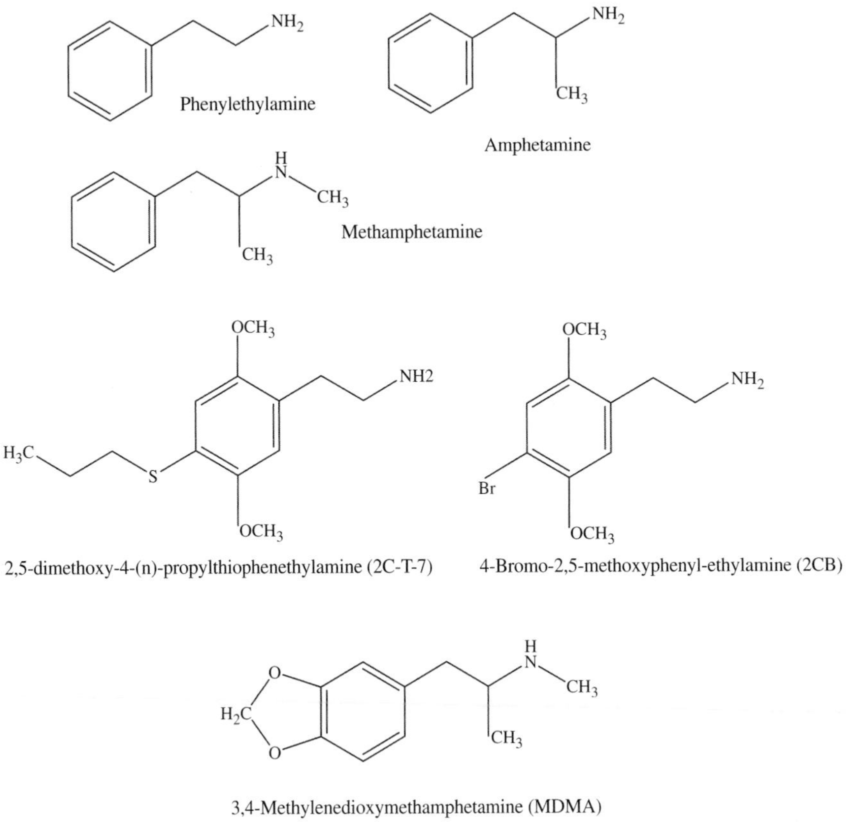

Phenylethylamine

Amphetamine

Methamphetamine

2,5-dimethoxy-4-(n)-propylthiophenethylamine (2C-T-7)

4-Bromo-2,5-methoxyphenyl-ethylamine (2CB)

3,4-Methylenedioxymethamphetamine (MDMA)

Fig. 2. Phenylethylamines.

that determines their activity. This structure enables them to bind to 5HT2 receptors and act as agonists [14]. As mentioned in the previous section, this binding to the 5HT2 and possibly other 5HT receptors, found in all the classic hallucinogens, conveys the hallucinogenic properties. The 2C series also has activity at the α_1-adrenergic receptors [15].

Dose ranges for the 2C series are approximately 10 to 30 mg, depending on the substance [14]. According to the DEA, 2C-B is active at about 0.1 to 0.2 mg/kg and lasts for 6 to 8 hours [16]. These new designer drugs are usually available in table or powder form, although occasionally they may be found as liquids or capsules. 2C-B has also been found adulterating sugar cubes [16]. The route of administration is usually oral, but there have been reports of insufflation, smoking, and rectal use, as well as intravenous and intramuscular administration [15]. Often these drugs are found in tablets sold as "Ecstasy" in various quantities [13].

Symptoms reported with 2C drug use are similar to those found with mescaline and MDMA use. These include hallucinations, euphoria, empathic and emotional responses, headaches, nausea, vomiting, anxiety, agitation, violent behavior, tachycardia, hypertension, respiratory depression, and seizures. Several fatalities have been reported with the use of 2C-T-7 [14,17]. Curtis and colleagues [17] describe a 20-year-old male who died after arriving in the emergency department in cardiac arrest. The patient allegedly had insufflated approximately 35 mg of 2C-T-7, began seizing 90 minutes later, and developed respiratory arrest en route to the emergency department. 2C-T-7 was later recovered from the urine at autopsy.

Management of phenylethylamine-intoxicated patients is primarily supportive and observational. Benzodiazepines may be used for the sympathomimetic symptoms. Gastrointestinal (GI) decontamination may be indicated, depending on the route of administration and time of ingestion. No specific antidotes are currently available. Routine drug urine analysis will generally not test positive [18].

Piperazines

Piperazine derivatives have recently emerged as potential drugs of abuse [19,20]. These derivatives are divided into two major groups: the benzylpiperazines, which include N-benzylpiperazine (BZP) and 1-(3,4-methylenedioxybenzyl)piperazine (MDBP), the methylene dioxy analogue, and the phenylpiperazines, which include 1-(3-chlorophenyl)piperazine (mCPP), 1-(4-methoxyphenyl)piperazine (MeOPP), and 1-(3-trifluorome-thylphenyl)piperazine (TFMPP) [21]. The most popular piperazines, BZP and TFMPP, are also known as "A2" and "Molly," respectively, and have been referred to collectively as "Legal E" or "Legal X" [22,23].

Piperazine compounds were originally used as antihelminthic agents in the 1950s. Although they are still used this way in animals, human use has been phased out. Nonetheless, Enactyl, an oral piperazine drug, is still available in Canada.

In the 1970s, N-benzyl-piperazine-picolinyl fumarate, whose active metabolite is 1-benzylpiperazine, was investigated as an antidepressant [20]. Animal studies at the time, however, demonstrated substantial side effects, including involuntary head movements, hyperactivity, and decreased reaction time. This evidence led to the hypothesis that piperazines, which share some structural features with amphetamines, shared physical effects as well. Further human pharmacodynamic studies confirmed the similarities in autonomic function and behavior. They also showed that former amphetamine addicts did not distinguish the effects of piperazines from those of dexamphetamine and found both favorable. The development of piperazines as antidepressants was therefore not pursued [20].

BZP and TFMPP were both emergently classified as schedule I drugs in 2002 in the United States. Since then, BZP has been permanently classified as schedule I, whereas the scheduling of TFMPP was lifted, leaving it currently unscheduled [24]. BZP doses range from 75 to 250 mg taken orally, with an approximate duration of action of 6 to 8 hours [20,25]. BZP is available as capsules containing 125 mg of BZP dihydrochloride, primarily in New Zealand, where it is legal. The other piperazines are available in semibulk quantities as a salt or free base. The tablets are often tan, yellow, and pink in color and may bear markings such as a fly, an "A," a butterfly, a heart, a bull's head, or spiders [19,26]. Piperazines may be found in combination with MDMA in tablets, unbeknownst to the user, or as a replacement for MDMA [19,27]. BZP and TFMPP have often been found as combination pills [23], typically with a BZP to TFMPP ratio of 2:1 [26].

The mechanism of action of BZP and TFMPP has been shown to be similar to that of MDMA: both drugs increase dopamine and serotonin levels. BZP increases levels of dopamine more than serotonin, accounting for an increased level of motor activity manifested as head bobbing, sniffing, and increased ambulation [23]. TFMPP acts as a partial agonist/antagonist at $5HT2_A$ receptors and a full agonist at other 5HT receptors and increases serotonin release [23]. However, TFMPP is roughly three times less potent than MDMA at similar concentrations. Interestingly, it was noted that together BZP and TFMPP produce a synergistic effect similar to MDMA. Furthermore, when BZP is used in combination with TFMPP at low doses, motor activity is decreased, making the experience more pleasurable [23]. This effect may explain the increased number of BZP/TFMPP combination pills that have been recovered. The BZP/TFMPP combination in high doses (10 mg/kg) reportedly causes seizures and ataxia in rats [23]. This effect has not been reported in humans.

Acute symptoms caused by piperazines reflect a combination of the stimulant and hallucinogenic properties, including euphoria, psychomotor agitation, increased energy, increased body temperature, increased heart rate and blood pressure, and hallucinations [19,21,25,27]. Stimulant effects are noted to resemble those caused by amphetamines, whereas the hallucinogenic properties tend to mirror the effects of MDMA [21]. Two deaths have been reported with BZP, although both involved coingestion of MDMA [20]. Balmelli and colleagues [26] report the death of a 23-year-old woman who developed massive brain edema and subsequent tonsillar herniation after ingesting BZP and MDMA. TFMPP and BZP are also known to be skin irritants, with inhalation leading to sore nasal passages and throats [28].

Management of piperazine-intoxicated individuals is supportive and requires adequate periods of observation. Although GI decontamination may be indicated in some cases, it should be remembered that antidotes are not currently available for these substances.

Khat

Plant-derived drugs of abuse are popular and often easy to obtain. Two lesser-known drugs that have increased in popularity are khat and *Salvia divinorum*. The former is illegal but has been increasingly available, whereas the latter is currently not an illegal substance.

Khat is derived from a shrub known as *Catha edulis Forssk*, Celastraceae, that is primarily cultivated in the Arabian Peninsula and East and Central Africa. It grows to roughly 3 to 4 m in height at altitudes of 1500 to 2000 m, mainly in arid regions. Distribution is in bundles of stalks with leaves, each weighing in the range of 500 g. The fresh leaves and stalks exist in different varieties of various quality. Young yellow leaves from the distal branches appear to be the most desirable [29]. The leaves from the lower branches are referred to as "qatal" and are less desirable (Fig. 3).

Khat, also called "Abyssinian tea," "chat," "qat," "miraa," and "African salad," is a cultural tradition in many African and Middle Eastern countries, and its use is widespread. As the numbers of immigrants to the United States from these countries have increased, the importation of khat has grown as well. According to a DEA drug intelligence brief, seizures of illegal khat rose from 800 kg in 1992 to 37.2 metric tons in 2002. In 1998, most of these seizures occurred at John F. Kennedy Airport in New York on flights via Great Britain [30]. Khat is usually wrapped in banana leaves or plastic bags and sprinkled with water to preserve moisture. It may arrive with passengers or be shipped as a "vegetable," such as molokheya, an Egyptian product [21].

The cultivation, exportation, and consumption of khat play an important economic role in many countries. In Yemen, for example, more than 33% of the gross national product is related to khat, and in Ethiopia it is the fourth largest export [29]. Although a khat cultivation operation was seized in 1998 in Salinas, California, khat production in the United States is not extensive at present; most khat is imported [30].

Khat leaves are usually chewed but may be smoked, sprinkled on food, or brewed into a tea. When chewed, khat is retained against the inner mucosa of the cheek so that the drug is intermittently released. Only the saliva mixed

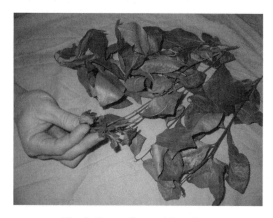

Fig. 3. Leaves from a khat plant.

with the plant juices is swallowed; the leaves are expectorated. In one study, only 10% of the original alkaloid content remained in the leaves after they were chewed for 1 hour. This study also demonstrated that the oral mucosa play a primary role in absorption [31].

Khat chewing is often a social pastime in Middle Eastern and African cultures, with use taking place in private homes in "khat rooms." Men tend to use khat more frequently than do women. During a khat use session, approximately 100 to 300 g are chewed, usually over a span of 3 to 4 hours [31].

Khat contains a variety of chemicals, including more than 40 glycosides, tannins, terpenoids, and alkaloids, as well as ascorbic acid, beta carotene, magnesium, and amino acids [5]. The central nervous system (CNS) effects of khat are due to two primary active substituents: cathine and cathinone. Cathine (norpseudoephedrine) is found in the dried leaves and stems and has mild stimulant activity. Cathinone (S-[-]-alpha-aminopropiophenone) is similar in chemical structure to amphetamine and appears to have a similar mechanism of action, increasing dopamine release and decreasing reuptake [5]. Cathinone is substantially more potent than cathine. This difference may be related to its higher lipid solubility, facilitating greater CNS entry [32]. Currently, cathine is a schedule IV substance, whereas cathinone is categorized as schedule I by the DEA.

Cathinone is found primarily in the fresh khat leaves and converts naturally to cathine within 48 hours as the leaves dry. Consequently, it is desirable to chew khat when it is fresh. Market value is directly related to cathinone content. A typical 100 g quantity of khat contains approximately 36 mg of cathinone. Younger leaves tend to have higher cathinone content [33]. A dried form of khat known as "graba" has recently been seized in the United States from Ethiopian and Somali nationals. Graba may contain higher concentrations of cathinone than regular dried khat and hence be more profitable to those who transport and sell it [34]. Methcathinone, referred to as "cat" or "Jeff," is a synthetic, more potent form of cathinone. Cat initially appeared in Russia but emerged in the United States Midwest in the 1990s; it is sold as a methamphetamine alternative [30].

Cathinone absorption is slow, and plasma levels peak at approximately 2 hours after use. The drug is metabolized in the liver to norephedrine, norpseudoephedrine, 3,6-dimethyl-2,5-diphenylpyrazine, and 1-phenyl-1, 2-propanedione [35].

Ingestion results in a variety of sympathomimetic effects manifested by increased cardiac chronotropy and inotropy; vasoconstriction, hyperthermia, increased oxygen consumption, hypertension, mydriasis, increased respiratory rate, extra systoles, insomnia, anorexia, and increased libido have all been described [36]. Brown teeth and a greenish tongue discoloration have been reported in frequent users [36]. Constipation is a common complication of khat use and is probably secondary to the high tannin content [5]. Decreased infant birth weight and decreased lactation in khat-using mothers have been described [32]. A recent article from Yemen reported that khat chewing might be related to an increased risk for acute myocardial infarction [37]. In addition, it is possible that individuals who chew khat may have an increased risk for oral malignancies, similar to the increased risk for individuals who chew tobacco [38].

The psychoactive effects associated with khat use include feelings of euphoria, excitation, clarity of thought, and cheerfulness. Users may also experience emotional lability and increased querulousness and anxiety [5,35]. Several case reports describe psychoses associated with khat use that manifested as disorientation, hallucinations, grandiose fantasies, and paranoia [35].

Users of khat do not generally present to the emergency department, because severe acute toxicity is rare and the sympathomimetic effects of the drug are not troublesome to the users. However, the treatment for acute khat intoxication when it presents does not differ from routine treatment for a sympathomimetic toxic syndrome of any cause. Rest, fluids, temperature control (in severely hyperthermic individuals), benzodiazepines for sedation, and supportive care usually suffice. GI decontamination may not be helpful, because absorption is usually by the oral mucosa. Although they are similar to amphetamines in chemical structure, cathinone and cathine may not be identified using routine urine drug testing [36].

Salvia

Salvia divinorum is a plant in the mint family used for medicinal and spiritual purposes by the Mazatec Indians in Oaxaca, Mexico. Today, Mexican youths often travel to the Sierra Mazateca region to purchase dried salvia and smoke it. Salvia is currently not classified as an illegal substance in the United States, Canada, or the United Kingdom; however, European nations such as Denmark, Italy, and Belgium have banned its use. Salvia became more popular in the United States several years ago and currently sells for $8.95 to $120 per ounce, depending on its potency, whereas the liquid extract runs $110 to $300 per ounce [39,40]. Salvia is also known as "La [or Maria] Pastora," "Yerba Maria," "Diviner's Mint [or Sage]," "Dalvia," and "The Shepherdess" [41]. The Mazatec Indians refer to it as "leaves of Mary, the Shepherdess" [42].

Salvia plants grow to a height of approximately 3 ft and have white flowers with characteristic purple calyces and large green leaves [43]. In the United States, salvia is grown primarily in Hawaii and California and imported from South and Central America. It is available from the Internet and from various "head shops" [39]. A number of active compounds have been isolated from the *Salvia divinorum* plant, including the neoclerodane diterpenoids, divinatorins (or salvinorins) A, B, and C. Divinatorin A is probably responsible for most of the hallucinogenic properties of salvia, although divinatorin C may have significant hallucinogenic potency as well

[44]. Although it possesses hallucinogenic properties, divinatorin A does not share structural similarities with classic hallucinogens, such as mescaline and LSD, nor does it exhibit any activity at 5HT2 receptors, known to be activated by these hallucinogens [45]. Divinatorin A appears to be a nonnitrogenous κ opioid receptor agonist [45]. These opioid receptors are known to have psychomimetic properties. Active agonists, however, are rare, and divinatorin A is hence unique [45].

Salvia may be used in various ways. Generally, fresh salvia leaves are chewed and swallowed. They may also be dried and smoked, similar to marijuana, or the leaves may be crushed and the juices extracted in liquid form for oral ingestion or inhalation. Alternatively, salvia may be brewed into a tea [39,42].

Salvia leaves generally contain between 0.89 and 3.7 mg/g of divinatorin A [42]. Two hundred to 500 mcg of divinatorin A extract may result in significant hallucinations lasting approximately 15 minutes when smoked and 1 hour when ingested. Ingestion tends to produce less intense symptoms than smoking [4]. Symptoms associated with salvia use are described by users as resembling those elicited by psilocybin, ketamine, and mescaline. These include out of body experiences, sensations of merging with inanimate objects, movement, body, and object distortion, uncontrolled laughter, synesthesia (eg, smelling colors, seeing sounds), and intense hallucinations [33,39]. The long-term effects of salvia use are unknown.

Management of salvia-intoxicated individuals has not been described but may be presumed to be largely supportive, similar to treatment of psilocybin and mescaline intoxication. It is not known whether naloxone, an opioid antagonist, has any effects on symptoms of salvia intoxication.

Dextromethorphan

Dextromethorphan (d-3-methoxy-N-methylmorphine) is the dextrorotatory isomer of levorphanol, a codeine analogue. Initially marketed in the 1960s as an antitussive agent, it is widely available today as a cough suppressant. Abuse of preparations containing dextromethorphan has been increasing in the United States, particularly among adolescents and young adults [46]. A recent survey of adolescents in New Mexico demonstrated that over-the-counter medications containing dextromethorphan were significantly more likely to be abused than those without [47]. Known as "robo," "red devil," or "dex," dextromethorphan is widely available in various over-the-counter cough and cold preparations. Popular preparations include Robitussin (Whitehall-Robins Healthcare, Madison, New Jersey; responsible for the slang "robotripping," "Robocop") and Coricidin HBP Cough and Cold tablets (Schering-Plough, Kenilworth, New Jersey; known on the streets as "CCC" or "Triple C") [48].

Despite its initial classification as an opioid, dextromethorphan was believed to lack abuse potential and addictive properties. However,

Romilar, a tablet form of dextromethorphan, was withdrawn in the 1960s because of widespread abuse. In 1992, Bern and Peck [49] documented 64 cases of dextromethorphan dependence, contradicting earlier studies.

Dextromethorphan is absorbed readily from the GI tract and undergoes polymorphic metabolism by the P540 cytochrome 2D6 isoenzyme. Although approximately 85% of the population metabolizes the drug quickly, roughly 5% to 10% of whites are poor metabolizers. The primary active metabolite formed is dextrorphan. Two other less active metabolites are D-methoxymorphinane and D-hydroxmorphinane [50].

Dextromethorphan is believed to act centrally at several sites. It appears to stimulate σ receptors in the medulla and thus to suppress cough impulses to the cough centers. However, dextromethorphan does not give rise to the typical opiate syndrome of respiratory depression, miosis, and decreased bowel sounds, nor does it have analgesic properties, because of its lack of activity at the κ, δ, and μ receptors. Dextromethorphan also increases release and blocks reuptake of serotonin, accounting for its serotonergic properties [46,50,51]. Both dextromethorphan and dextrorphan, similar to phencyclidine (PCP), bind and block N-methyl-D-aspartate receptors. However, dextrorphan has a much stronger affinity, similar to ketamine, and alone is believed to be responsible for the PCP-like effects. Hence, individuals who metabolize dextromethorphan to dextrorphan more efficiently experience more PCP-like symptoms. These individuals may be more prone to abuse of the drug than are slow metabolizers, who report more sedation and dysphoria [50].

The recommended dosage for therapeutic effects in adults is 15 to 30 mg three to four times a day. The onset of action is rapid (15 to 30 minutes), with the maximum serum level occurring at 2.5 hours. The duration of action ranges from 2 to 6 hours. Erowid, a popular Internet drug information site, lists a recreational dosage chart [48]. "Light intoxication" is listed as requiring 100 to 200 mg, whereas "heavy intoxication" may require as much as 1500 mg. A Coricidin Cough and Cold tablet contains 30 mg of dextromethorphan; hence "light intoxication" requires only five tablets, whereas for "heavy intoxication" approximately 50 may be required. A 12-ounce bottle of Robitussin contains approximately 710 mg of dextromethorphan, so two bottles would be sufficient for "heavy intoxication." The effects of dosages may vary, however, based on the metabolism of the individual. The psychologic effects of dextromethorphan use have been described by Wolfe and Caravati [46] and include euphoria, tactile, auditory, and visual hallucinations, paranoia, altered time perception, and disorientation. The authors also describe a withdrawal syndrome that features intense craving, dysphoria, and difficulty in sleeping.

Symptoms associated with dextromethorphan overdose are primarily CNS effects, such as lethargy, hyperexcitability, ataxia, slurred speech, tremors, fasciculations, rigidity, tachycardia, hyperreflexia, and hypertonia [46,47,50–55]. Other symptoms may include diaphoresis, hypertension, nystagmus and pupillary changes, and acute psychosis. Most patients exhibit normal or dilated pupils; however, pinpoint pupils have been described [46,47,50–55].

The treatment of the acute effects of dextromethorphan overdose is primarily supportive. Gut decontamination using activated charcoal may be helpful in patients who present early, because dextromethorphan should be efficiently adsorbed to charcoal. The use of naloxone in reversing symptoms of toxicity is controversial. Although several case reports have described successful use, others have described little or no effect [49,51,55].

The widespread availability of dextromethorphan in combination preparations containing multiple drugs leads to another potential problem: the inadvertent ingestion of other medications. The most common culprits are anticholinergic agents, such as chlorpheniramine maleate, found in Coricidin Cough and Cold, acetaminophen, and bromide, found in the dextromethorphan hydrobromide preparations. Anticholinergic symptoms may exacerbate the CNS symptoms of dextromethorphan and manifest with tachycardia, mydriasis, flushed skin, urinary retention, and mental status changes, including possible seizures and coma. Bromide toxicity from the bromine portion of the dextromethorphan compound is not well described and is presumed to occur only in chronic users. Symptoms associated with bromide toxicity include mental status changes, including slurred speech, psychosis, ataxia, and hallucinations; an acneiform rash and weight loss have been described as well. Serum bromide levels may not be readily available, but elevated bromine levels may be suspected when an elevated chloride level and a negative anion gap are present. Patients with severe bromide toxicity need prompt attention and may require dialysis [47,51,55].

Fentanyl patches and lollipops

Fentanyl (N-[1-phenethyl-4-piperidyl]propionanilide) is a synthetic opioid used for its high-potency analgesic properties and short duration of action. Fentanyl's potency is reportedly 80 times that of morphine [56]. Although usually administered in intravenous form in the hospital setting, fentanyl is also available in prescription form as a transdermal patch with continuous release (Duragesic; AZLA, Mountain View, California) and as a lollipop (Actiq; Cephalon, Salt Lake City, Utah).

Fentanyl is currently categorized as a schedule II drug by the US Food and Drug Administration. Both the licit and illicit use of fentanyl has dramatically increased over the past decade. According to the DEA, 0.5 million prescriptions in 1994 increased to more than 5.7 million in 2003 [57]. Abuse has increased as well, particularly of the patch and lollipop. Pharmaceutical diversion of fentanyl currently occurs through fraudulent prescriptions, illicit distribution, pharmacy theft, and nursing home and long-term care facility theft [57].

In intravenous form, fentanyl is generally administered as a dose of 50 to 100 mcg with rapid analgesia and sedation. It has a large volume of distribution (60 to 300 L), and 90% of the drug leaves the plasma in the first 5 minutes [56]. Transdermal fentanyl patches are currently available in 10 to 40 cm^2 sizes, designed to release between 25 mcg/h and 100 mcg/h based on surface area. The patch contains a polyester film outer layer, under which a fentanyl reservoir rests in a hydroxyethyl cellulose gel and alcohol mixture. Beneath the reservoir is a microporous ethylenevinyl copolymer membrane controlling the diffusion rate, followed by a silicone adhesive layer [58]. The fentanyl forms a depot in the keratinized layer of the skin and is absorbed continuously (Fig. 4). Serum fentanyl levels achieved with the patch equal those of continuous intravenous infusion [56]. The manufacturer recommends that the patches be replaced after 72 hours. At this point, the patches still contain substantial amounts of fentanyl (approximately 2800 mcg in a 10-mg patch), and the potential for abuse is obvious [58]. According to the DEA, patches may be sold on the street for as much as $100 per patch, depending on the dose and geographic location [57].

Fentanyl patches may be smoked or ingested, or the contents may be extracted and injected. One case report describes a patch that was steeped in hot water, similar to a tea bag [59]. Alternatively, multiple patches may be applied transdermally to increase absorption. A fatality was described when an individual placed patches on his thigh as well as transbuccally and arrived in the emergency department in respiratory arrest [60].

Some abusers reportedly smoke fentanyl patches by scraping the reservoir contents onto aluminum foil. The foil is then lit, and the smoke is inhaled with a pipe or pen casing [56,61]. Studies of nebulized fentanyl demonstrate that analgesia without respiratory depression may be achieved at low levels in the range of 100 to 300 mcg. Inhaling the heated, volatilized material from the patch, which contains large depots of fentanyl, may actually increase the bioavailability [58]. Patch ingestion has been reported

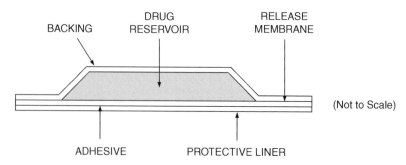

Fig. 4. Transdermal Fentanyl System diagram. (*From* Janssen Pharmaceutica, 1125 Trenton-Harbourton Road, Titusville, New Jersey 08560; with permission. Main phone number 609-730-2000; main fax number 609-730-2323. Janssen Pharmaceutica is a division of Johnson & Johnson.)

and has led to several fatalities [61,62]. GI absorption of fentanyl has not been well delineated and may vary depending on the condition of the patch and comorbidities of the individual.

Intravenous injection of the fentanyl involves extraction of the reservoir with subsequent bolus intravenous administration. Several fatalities have been described with this method of abuse [62,63]. Extraction of the reservoir is not a reliable dose predictor, and large amounts may be administered inadvertently. Intravenous injection of the fentanyl in the gel may also lead to other complications, such as abscesses, deep venous thrombosis, and superficial thrombophlebitis [63].

The fentanyl lollipop, Actiq, is currently used primarily for cancer break-through pain in patients tolerant of opioid therapy. Known as "perc-a-pops," these lozenges are being sold for approximately $20 a lollipop in the Philadelphia region, according to the DEA [64]. Absorption of the fentanyl is primarily transmucosal. Interestingly, to date, there have been no reports of fatalities from the abuse of fentanyl lollipops.

Patients presenting to the emergency department with adverse effects following fentanyl injection, patch ingestion, or inhalation are expected to exhibit symptoms of opioid intoxication, such as respiratory and CNS depression and miosis. Hypotension is less likely to occur, because of the lack of histamine release with fentanyl [65]. Treatment involves supportive care with special attention to airway maintenance. When ingestion of one or more fentanyl patches is suspected, GI decontamination using whole bowel irrigation may be indicated. Naloxone administration as an antidote may be necessary. The necessary doses of naloxone may be larger than those given for heroin and may need to be repeated or administered as an infusion.

Summary

Several new and emerging substances are being diverted for abuse. Most of these emerging abused substances do not cause traditional drug screens to turn positive. The health effects of these substances have not yet been fully elucidated. Health care providers should be aware of the existence of these new abused substances.

References

[1] Drug Enforcement Administration/Department of Justice. Intelligence brief. Ecstasy: rolling across Europe. August 2001.

[2] Drug Enforcement Administration/Department of Justice. DEA notice of intent to schedule alpha-methyltryptamine and 5-methoxy-N, N-diisopropyltryptamine. Fed Regist 2003;68(18).

[3] Drug Enforcement Agency. Drug intelligence brief. Trippin'on tryptamines. October 2003.

[4] Halpern JH. Hallucinogens and dissociative agents naturally growing in the United States. Pharmacol Ther 2004;102:131–8.

[5] Carlini EA. Plants and the central nervous system. Pharmacol Biochem Behav 2003;75: 501–12.

[6] Smolinske SC, Rastogi R, Schenkel S. Foxy methoxy: a new drug of abuse. Int J Med Toxicol 2004;7(1):3.

[7] Meatherall R, Sharma P. Foxy, a designer tryptamine hallucinogen. J Anal Toxicol 2003;27: 313–7.

[8] Dailey RM, Nelson LD, Scaglione JM. Tachycardia and rhabdomyolysis after intentional ingestion of N,N-dipropyltryptamine. J Toxicol Clin Toxicol 2003;41:742.

[9] Long H, Nelson LS, Hoffman RS. Alpha-methyltryptamine revisited via easy Internet access. Vet Hum Toxicol 2003;45(3):149.

[10] National Drug Intelligence Center. 5-MeO-AMT fast facts. 2004.

[11] Glennon RA. Classical hallucinogens: an introductory overview. NIDA Res Monogr 1994; 146:9–37.

[12] Christopherson AS. Amphetamine designer drugs—an overview and epidemiology. Toxicol Lett 2000;112:127–31.

[13] De Boer D, Gijzels MJ, Bosman IJ, et al. More data about the new psychoactive drug 2C-B. J Anal Toxicol 1999;23(3):227–8.

[14] De Boer D, Bosman I. A new trend in drugs-of-abuse: the 2C-series of phenethylamine designer drugs. Pharm World Sci 2004;26:110–3.

[15] European Monitoring Centre for Drugs and Drug Addiction. Report on the risk assessment of 2C-I, 2C-T-2, and 2C-T-7 in the framework of the joint action on new synthetic drugs. 2004.

[16] Drug Enforcement Administration/Department of Justice. Schedules of controlled substances: placement of 4-bromo-2,5-dimethoxyphenethylamine into schedule I. June 2, 1995.

[17] Curtis B, Harty L, Kemp P, et al. Preliminary investigation into identification and quantitation of 2,5 dimethoxy-N-propylthiophenethylamine also known as 2 C-T-7. Presented at the Fall Meeting of the Southwestern Association of Toxicologists. San Antonio (TX), November 1–3, 2001.

[18] US Department of Justice. Information bulletin. 2C-B (Nexus) reappears on the club drug scene. May 2001.

[19] De Boer D, Bosman IJ, Hidvegi E, et al. Piperazine-like compounds: a new group of designer drugs-of-abuse on the European market. Forensic Sci Int 2001;121:47–56.

[20] Wikstrom M, Holmgren P, Ahlner J. A2 (N-benzylpiperazine): a new drug of abuse in Sweden. J Anal Toxicol 2004;28(1):67–70.

[21] Maurer HH, Kraemer T, Springer D, et al. Chemistry, pharmacology, toxicology, and hepatic metabolism of designer drugs of the amphetamine (Ecstasy), piperazine, and pyrrolidinophenone types. Ther Drug Monit 2004;26(2):127–31.

[22] The vaults of EROWID. BZP. Available at: http://www.erowid.org/chemicals/bzp/bzp. shtml. Accessed December 2004.

[23] Bauman M, Clark RD, Budzynski AG, et al. N-substituted piperazines abused by humans mimic the molecular mechanism of 3,4-methylenedioxymethamphetamine (MDMA, or "Ecstasy"). Neuropsychopharmacology 2005;30(3):550–60.

[24] Drug Enforcement Administration (DEA), Department of Justice. Schedules of controlled substances; placement of 2,5-dimethoxy-4-(n)-propylthiophenethylamine and N-benzylpiperazine into Schedule I of the Controlled Substances Act. Final rule. Fed Regist 2004; 69(53):12794–7.

[25] Drug Enforcement Administration (DEA). Benzylpiperazine, trifluoromethylphenylpiperazine (BZP, TFMPP). Drugs and chemicals of concern. 2001.

[26] Balmelli C, Kupferschmidt H, Reutsch K, et al. Fatal brain oedema after ingestion of ecstasy and benzylpiperazine. Dtsch Med Wochenschr 2001;126:809–11.

[27] The Expert Advisory Committee on Drugs (EACD) advice to the Minister on: benzylpiperazine (BZP). April 2004.

[28] Drug Enforcement Administration/Department of Justice. Drug intelligence brief. BZP and TFMPP: chemicals used to mimic MDMA's effects. December 2001.
[29] Paris R. Abyssinian tea (Catha edulis Forssk, Celastraceae). United Nations Office on Drugs and Crime—Bulletin on Narcotics 1958;2:29–34.
[30] Drug Enforcement Administration/Department of Justice. Drug intelligence brief. Khat. June 2002.
[31] Toennes SW, Harder S, Schramm M, et al. Pharmacokinetics of cathinone, cathine, and norephedrine after chewing of khat leaves. Br J Clin Pharmacol 2003;56:125–30.
[32] Pantelis C, Hindler C, Taylor J. Use and abuse of khat (catha edulis): a review of the distribution, pharmacology, side effects and description of psychosis attributed to khat chewing. Psychol Med 1989;19(3):657–68.
[33] Sporkert F, Pragst F, Bachus R, et al. Determination of cathinone, cathine and norephedrine in hair of Yemenite khat chewers. Forensic Sci Int 2003;133:39–46.
[34] "Graba" (dried khat) seized in Kansas City. Intelligence brief. NDIC Narcotics Digest Weekly 2004;3(13):3.
[35] Spinella M. Psychopharmacology of herbal medicine. Cambridge (MA): MIT Press; 2001.
[36] Toennes SW, Kauert GF. Driving under the influence of khat—alkaloid concentrations and observations in forensic cases. Forensic Sci Int 2004;140:85–90.
[37] Al-Motarreb A, Al-Kebsi M, Al-Adhi B, et al. Khat chewing and acute myocardial infarction. Heart 2002;87:279–80.
[38] Kassie F, Darroudi F, Kundi M, et al. Khat (Catha edulis) consumption causes genotoxic effects in humans. Int J Cancer 2001;92:329–32.
[39] National Drug Intelligence Center. Department of Justice information bulletin. Salvia divinorum. April 2003.
[40] Leinwand D. Teens, and now DEA, are on trail of hallucinogenic herb. USA Today. June 22, 2003.
[41] The vaults of EROWID. Salvia divinorum. Available at: http://www.erowid.org/plants/salvia/salvia.shtml. Accessed December 2004.
[42] Giroud C, Felber F, Augsburger M, et al. Salvia divinorum: an hallucinogenic mint which might become a new recreational drug in Switzerland. Forensic Sci Int 2000;112:143–50.
[43] Drug Enforcement Administration. Salvia divinorum. Drugs and chemicals of concern. June 2004.
[44] Valdes LJ, Chang HM, Visger DC, et al. Salvinorin C, a new neoclerodane diterpene from a bioactive fraction of the hallucinogenic Mexican mint Salvia divinorum. Org Lett 2001; 3(24):3935–7.
[45] Roth BL, Baner K, Westkaemper R, et al. Salvinorin A: a potent naturally occurring nonnitrogenous κ opioid selective agonist. Proc Natl Acad Sci U S A 2002;99:11934–9.
[46] Wolfe T, Caravati E. Massive dextromethorphan ingestion and abuse. Am J Emerg Med 1995;13:174–5.
[47] Noonan W, Miller W, Feeney D. Dextromethorphan abuse among youth. Arch Fam Med 2000;9:790–3.
[48] The vaults of EROWID. DXM dosage. Available at: http://www.erowid.org/chemicals/dxm/dxm_dose.shtml. Accessed December 2004.
[49] Bern JL, Peck R. Dextromethorphan: an overview of safety issues. Drug Saf 1992;7: 190–9.
[50] Zawertailo L, Kaplan HL, Busto UE, et al. Psychotropic effects of dextromethorphan are altered by the CYP2D6 polymorphism: a pilot study. J Clin Psychopharmacol 1998;18: 332–7.
[51] Pender E, Parks B. Toxicity with dextromethorphan-containing preparations: a literature review and report of two additional cases. Pediatr Emerg Care 1991;7(3):163–5.
[52] Kirages T, Sule H, Mycyk M. Severe manifestations of coricidin intoxication. Am J Emerg Med 2003;21:473–5.
[53] Price L, Lebel J. Dextromethorphan-induced psychosis. Am J Psychiatry 2000;157(2):304.

[54] Shier J, Diaz J. Avoid unfavorable consequences: dextromethorphan can bring about a false positive phencyclidine urine drug screen. J Emerg Med 2000;18(3):379–83.

[55] Schneider S, Michelson EA, Boucek CD, et al. Dextromethorphan poisoning reversed by naloxone. Am J Emerg Med 1991;9:237–8.

[56] Poklis A. Fentanyl: a review for clinical and analytical toxicologists. J Toxicol Clin Toxicol 1995;33(5):439–48.

[57] Drug Enforcement Administration. Fentanyl. Drugs and chemicals of concern. DEA Diversion Program. October 2004.

[58] Marquardt KA, Tharratt SR. Inhalation abuse of fentanyl patch. J Toxicol Clin Toxicol 1994;32(1):75–9.

[59] Barrueto FJ. The fentanyl tea bag. Vet Hum Toxicol 2004;46(1):30–1.

[60] Kramer C, Tawney M. A fatal overdose of transdermally administered fentanyl. J Am Osteopath Assoc 1998;98(7):385–6.

[61] Purucker M, Swann W. Potential for duragesic patch abuse. Ann Emerg Med 2000;35(3): 314.

[62] Tharp AM, Winecker RE, Winston DC, et al. Fatal intravenous fentanyl abuse. Am J Forensic Med Pathol 2004;25(2):178–81.

[63] Reeves MD, Ginifer CJ. Fatal intravenous misuse of transdermal fentanyl. Med J Aust 2002; 177:552–3.

[64] Lollipop-shaped fentanyl products diverted in Eastern Pennsylvania. DEA microgram bulletin June 2004. Narcotics Digest Weekly 2004;3(20):1.

[65] Grossmann M, Abiose A, Tangphao O, et al. Morphine-induced venodilation in humans. Clin Pharmacol Ther 1996;60(5):554–60.

ELSEVIER
SAUNDERS

CLINICS IN
LABORATORY
MEDICINE

Clin Lab Med 26 (2006) 165–184

Hyperthermic Syndromes Induced by Toxins

Daniel E. Rusyniak, MD[a,b,c,]*, Jon E. Sprague, PhD[d,e]

[a]Division of Medical Toxicology, Department of Emergency Medicine,
Indiana University School of Medicine, Indianapolis, IN, USA
[b]Department of Neurology, Indiana University School of Medicine,
Indianapolis, IN, USA
[c]Department of Pharmacology and Toxicology,
Indiana University School of Medicine, Indianapolis, IN, USA
[d]Virginia College of Osteopathic Medicine, Blacksburg, VA, USA
[e]Department of Biomedical Sciences and Pathobiology, Virginia Polytechnic
Institute and State University, Blacksburg, VA, USA

Body temperature regulation is complex and requires a balance between heat production and dissipation. Hyperthermia occurs when metabolic heat production exceeds heat dissipation. Many exogenously administered xenobiotics are capable of altering the body's ability to maintain a constant temperature. For example, agents with anticholinergic activity may contribute to hyperthermia by eliminating sweating and evaporation [1]. Because both recognition and treatment vary with the cause of hyperthermia, it is important for clinicians to understand the various presentations and treatments of toxin-induced hyperthermic syndromes.

Body temperature regulation in warm-blooded (endothermic) animals is divided into obligatory and facultative thermogenesis. Metabolic processes required for normal basal function generate heat, which contributes to maintaining a constant body temperature in a process known as obligatory thermogenesis. Secondary to acute changes in environmental temperatures, however, humans and warm-blooded animals require an adaptive or facultative thermogenic process to adjust their body temperatures rapidly.

Portions of this article were previously published in Holstege CP, Rusyniak DE: Medical Toxicology. 89:6, Med Clin North Am, 2005; with permission.

* Corresponding author. Division of Medical Toxicology, Department of Emergency Medicine, Indiana University School of Medicine, 1050 Wishard Boulevard, Room 2200, Indianapolis, IN 46202.

E-mail address: drusynia@iupui.edu (D.E. Rusyniak).

This process is largely governed through hypothalamic regulation of the sympathetic nervous system [2] and mitochondrial oxidative phosphorylation, both of which may be adversely affected by a variety of toxins.

Normal thermogenesis

Adaptive thermogenesis refers to the body's ability rapidly to induce heat production through hypothalamic regulation of the sympathetic nervous system [2]. The preoptic nucleus of the anterior hypothalamus responds to core temperature changes and regulates the autonomic nervous system, inducing either cutaneous vasodilation, dissipating heat when body temperature is elevated, or vasoconstriction, conserving heat when the body is cold [3]. Similarly, through the activation of the autonomic nervous system, humans have the unique ability to sweat, dissipating heat by evaporative cooling. This process is affected by a patient's hydration status, ambient temperature, conditioning, and acclimation [4]. Increasing motor activity from either exercise or shivering also increases heat production, with shivering representing a unique feature of mammalian thermogenesis regulated by the coordinated interaction between the hypothalamus and motor neurons in the spinal cord [5].

Norepinephrine [6], dopamine [7], and serotonin [8] have all been suggested to play major roles in regulating hypothalamic control of body temperature. Drugs altering the hypothalamic levels of these neurotransmitters are therefore capable of altering body temperature regulation. Activation of the hypothalamic-pituitary-thyroid and the hypothalamic-pituitary-adrenal axes further assists in maintaining body temperature. Sympathetic nervous system activation contributes to effects on thermogenesis through cutaneous vasoconstriction and nonshivering thermogenesis [9]. Nonshivering thermogenesis occurs primarily by uncoupling of oxidative phosphorylation through the activity of a group of mitochondrial proteins known as uncoupling proteins (UCP).

Oxidative phosphorylation requires proteins in the mitochondrial inner membrane transport chain to shuttle electrons through a series of oxidation/reduction reactions that ultimately result in oxygen being converted to carbon dioxide, water, and protons being pumped from the cytosolic side of the inner membrane into the inner membrane space. This process creates an electrochemical gradient, with the inner membrane space being charged in comparison with the matrix. The potential energy of this gradient is then converted into adenosine triphosphate (ATP) through a protein known as ATP synthetase. To maintain ATP at a relatively constant level in cells, mitochondrial respiration is stoichiometrically coupled to and rate-limited by ATP synthesis or steady state levels of adenosine diphosphate (ADP) and ATP. This coupling is referred to simplistically as *respiratory control*. When any toxin or protein short circuits this system by facilitating the leak of protons across the inner membrane independent of ATP synthetase, this process results in the loss of potential energy being released as heat, a phenomenon known as uncoupling (Fig. 1) [10].

Uncoupling proteins, by providing a conduit for the passive flow of electrons across the inner membrane of the mitochondria, constitute a regulated source of heat production [11]. The stimulation of uncoupling protein-1 (UCP1) in brown adipose tissues represents the primary site of nonshivering thermogenesis in rodents [12]. Although adult humans have little brown fat, another uncoupling protein, UCP3, has been detected in abundance in human skeletal muscle [13]. Expression of UCP3 has been shown to increase threefold in rodent skeletal muscle exposed to 5°C for 24 hours, suggesting a thermoregulatory role for UCP3 in skeletal muscle mitochondria [14]. Norepinephrine and β_3-adrenoreceptor agonists are known to increase the activity of UCP-mediated thermogenesis in tissues containing UCP1 and UCP3 [15,16]. Thyroid hormones have a synergistic effect on norepinephrine-mediated mechanisms of thermogenesis [17,18], an interaction that appears to be mediated through α_1 and β_3 adrenergic receptors [19]. These findings suggest that drugs that affect thyroid hormone

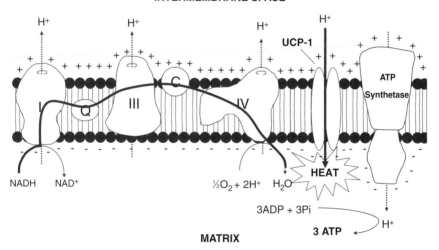

Fig. 1. Uncoupling. Process of uncoupling of oxidative phosphorylation. In normal oxidative phosphorylation, electrons donated by the tricyclic antidepressant cycle product NADH are shuttled along a series of proteins contained in the intermembrane space known as the electron transport chain. Through a series of oxidation reduction reactions within proteins I, II, III, and IV, protons are pumped against their concentration gradient into the intermembrane space. This process creates potential energy that under normal circumstances is converted to ATP through a unique protein known as ATP synthetase. Uncoupling occurs when potential energy of the intermembrane space is lost, either through the transport of protons through UCP or by chemicals that chaperone protons directly through the intermembrane space. Unable to provide useful work (ie, ATP), the potential energy is converted to heat. Pi, inorganic phosphate.

can affect thermogenesis. Chronically, thyroid hormones have also been shown to regulate the synthesis of UCPs [20], giving them both acute and chronic effects on temperature regulation.

Serotonin and sympathomimetic syndromes

Although many texts distinguish between the sympathomimetic syndrome and the serotonin syndrome, at times they are clinically indistinguishable. Because of their similar presentations and mechanisms of toxicity, the authors do not differentiate between the two syndromes. Acute intoxication with cocaine [21] and agents in the phenethylamine class (eg, amphetamine [22], methamphetamine [23], and 3,4–methylenedioxymethamphetamine [MDMA] [24]) may cause serotonin syndrome. Along with abuse, therapeutic usage of stimulants in combination with antidepressants has been reported to induce a serotonin syndrome [25,26].

With the plethora of serotonergically based antidepressant agents currently on the market and the increased popularity of the drug of abuse MDMA, there has been a marked increase in the number of case reports of and research conducted into serotonin syndrome. Although serotonin syndrome might appear to be a modern phenomenon, history is rich in cases. Numerous outbreaks of convulsive ergotism, from the contamination of grain with the fungus *Claviceps purpurea*, have been reported since the Middle Ages [27]. From one such outbreak it has been speculated that the Salem witch trials arose [28]. In the earliest medical case attributed to serotonin syndrome, reported in 1955, a patient experienced a recurrent drug reaction to the combination of meperidine and the monoamine oxidase inhibitor iproniazid [29]. In 1984, a possible case of serotonin syndrome would forever change the course of medical education in the United States. In that year, 18-year-old Libby Zion died of a presumed drug interaction between meperidine and phenelzine, a monoamine oxidase inhibitor [30]. Zion's father, an attorney and writer for the *New York Times*, used his influence to obtain a grand jury investigation into the conditions surrounding his daughter's death. The lasting ramifications of the jury's findings would include policies addressing resident supervision, resident duty hours, regulation of the use of restraints, and systems to prevent drug interactions [30].

Several good reviews on the clinical effects of serotonin syndrome have been conducted to date [26,31–34]. Although differences exist in the incidence of certain features seen in these reviews, the clinical findings are consistent. In most cases, patients present with the triad of altered mental status, autonomic instability, and abnormal neuromuscular activity. Altered mental status may manifest as coma, somnolence, confusion, agitation, and seizures, with some patients manifesting multiple symptoms in one presentation. Autonomic instability has been reported as fever, diaphoresis, tachycardia, hypertension or hypotension, and mydriasis. The neuromuscular derangements reported in serotonin syndrome include clonus, myoclonus, rigidity, and hyperreflexia; all are more commonly reported in the lower than the upper extremities. Although the literature contains published criteria for the diagnosis of serotonin syndrome [32,34], they tend to be either nonspecific or impractical for practicing physicians. Instead, the authors recommend the consideration of serotonin syndrome in any patient on serotonergic agents who presents with the triad of altered mental status, autonomic instability, and neuromuscular abnormalities.

Although most cases of serotonin syndrome are mild and self limited, severe and fatal cases have been reported [24,29]. Fatal intoxications usually produce a clinical picture characterized by diaphoresis, tachycardia, muscle rigidity, rhabdomyolysis, metabolic acidosis, seizures, hyperkalemia, coagulopathy, and marked hyperpyrexia, with temperatures as high as 43.9°C being reported [35]. In cases of serotonin syndrome from MDMA, mortality directly correlates with core body temperatures, with cases in which body temperature was greater than 41.5°C resulting in fatality two thirds of the time [36]. Although severe hyperthermia represents the most serious manifestation of serotonin syndrome, it is reported in only about a third of cases [37]. The onset of serotonin syndrome typically occurs within hours of medication initiation; however, as many as a quarter of patients may not present until more than 24 hours after taking their medication [37].

Numerous compounds have been associated with serotonin syndrome; several articles review these [26,31–34,37]. Essentially, any drug capable of increasing the concentration of serotonin in the central nervous system has the potential to cause this syndrome (Fig. 2). Although it is most common with a combination of drugs (ie, monoamine oxidase inhibitor and tricyclic antidepressants), serotonin syndrome has also been reported with single-agent therapy [38,39]. Although the serotonin reuptake inhibitors, tricyclic antidepressants, monoamine oxidase inhibitors, and many of the newer antidepressants are recognized by most physicians as having serotonergic activity, several commonly prescribed medications that can cause serotonin syndrome may not be as well recognized. Included in this group are dextromethorphan [40], meperidine [41], L-dopa [42], bromocriptine [42], tramadol [43], and lithium [44].

The mechanism of serotonin syndrome is complex and involves interaction between the environment, the central catecholamine release, the hypothalamic-pituitary-thyroid-adrenal axis, the sympathetic nervous system, and skeletal muscle (Fig. 3). The effect of ambient temperature on drugs that can cause serotonin syndrome has been well documented. In several animal studies, researchers have shown that elevating ambient temperature increases the body temperature and toxicity associated with MDMA [45] and methamphetamine [46,47], whereas lowering ambient temperature decreases these factors. This evidence supports the idea that MDMA and similar serotonergic agents cause a central deregulation of thermogenesis [48]. This idea is supported by the finding that deaths from cocaine are more frequent during months with elevated ambient temperatures [49], and it has important

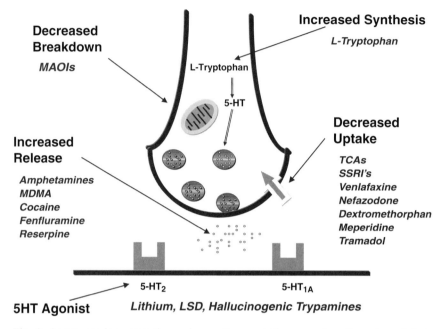

Fig. 2. Agents causing serotonin syndrome. Representative examples of agents and their various actions involving serotonin. Any agent capable of increasing serotonin concentrations in the synaptic cleft, increasing activity of or stimulating 5-HT2a receptors, or decreasing the activity of or inhibiting 5-HT1a receptors may, in theory, cause or contribute to hyperthermia from serotonin syndrome. MAOIs, monoamine oxidase inhibitors; SSRIs, serotonin selective reuptake inhibitors; TCAs, tricyclic antidepressants.

implications for users of recreational drugs such as MDMA in hot and crowded dance clubs.

Along with elevated ambient temperature, motor activity increases the toxicity of stimulants such as amphetamine and MDMA. Because motor activity can increase body temperature and exhaust supplies of ATP, it is not surprising that the combination of increased motor activity and stimulant use results in exaggerated toxicity [50,51]. This finding is particularly relevant to MDMA, which is typically taken at all-night dance parties. Recent work in the authors' laboratory using nuclear magnetic resonance has shown that MDMA decreases ATP in skeletal muscle of MDMA-treated anesthetized immobile rats, suggesting that MDMA impairs energy production in skeletal muscle [52]. When combined with the increased motor activity seen with MDMA, this impairment is a likely mechanism for the rhabdomyolysis seen in both humans [53] and experimental animals [54].

The hypothalamus is known to be a key thermoregulatory site in the central nervous system and is activated following MDMA treatment [55]. Thermoregulation within the hypothalamus has been suggested to be controlled by serotonin [7], dopamine [6], and norepinephrine [8]. Animal models of serotonin syndrome have likewise demonstrated acute elevations

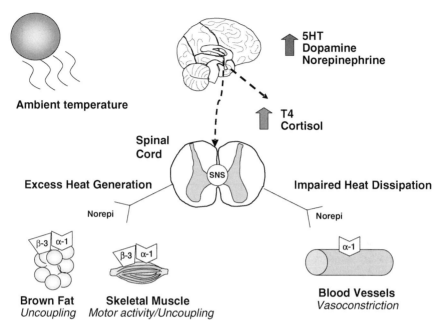

Fig. 3. Thermogenesis from serotonin syndrome. Serotonergic drugs increase central catecholamine release, activating the hypothalamus. The hypothalamus activates the pituitary/thyroid/adrenal glands to increase circulation levels of thyroid hormones and cortisol and the sympathetic nervous system to increase the peripheral release of norepinephrine. Norepinephrine activates α_1 and β_3 receptors on brown fat (rodents) and skeletal muscle (humans and rodents), causing uncoupling of oxidative phosphorylation and heat generation. Excess motor activity, which often accompanies serotonin syndrome, also increases heat generation. Elevated levels of norepinephrine cause vasoconstriction, impairing heat dissipation. Finally, ambient temperature plays an important role, with elevations resulting in higher body temperatures and increased morbidity and mortality. Norepi, norepinephrine; SNS, sympathetic nervous system.

in serotonin, norepinephrine, and dopamine in the anterior hypothalamus [56–58]. These findings correlate with elevated cerebrospinal fluid levels of these neurotransmitters in human cases of serotonin syndrome [59,60]. Direct and indirect stimulation of the hypothalamus by agents such as MDMA and methamphetamine activates the hypothalamic-pituitary-thyroid-adrenal axis, with subsequent thermogenesis and toxicity being dependent on the circulating levels of thyroid and adrenal hormones [61–64]. When activated neurons in the anterior hypothalamus stimulate the sympathetic nervous system, norepinephrine is released from nerve endings into the circulatory system. Significant elevations of norepinephrine have been shown by the authors' laboratory in rats treated with MDMA and have similarly been demonstrated in human users [65,66]. Acting through vascular α_1-adrenoreceptors (AR), norepinephrine release from MDMA in rats and cocaine in humans induces vasoconstriction and impaired heat dissipation [67,68]. In concert with the thyroid hormones, norepinephrine also binds to and activates α_1- and β_3-AR regulating the activity of thermogenic tissues, such as brown fat, through UCP [69]. Although the role of skeletal muscle UCPs in thermogenesis has been controversial, recent work suggests they may have an integral role in MDMA-induced hyperthermia [70]. Support for this notion comes from animal work showing that the combination of an α_1- and β_3-AR antagonist can prevent hyperthermia and mortality in a rat model of MDMA intoxication [62]. Similarly, mice lacking UCP3 express a blunted hyperthermic response to MDMA and are protected against its subsequent mortality [71]. In summary, serotonin syndrome appears to be a concerted action between central and peripheral catecholamine release, with resultant hypothalamic activation causing both impaired heat dissipation through vasoconstriction and excess heat generation through motor work and uncoupling (see Fig. 3).

Although mechanisms of serotonin syndrome are slowly beginning to come to light, the development of specific treatments has lagged behind. Part of the problem with developing treatments has been the incomplete understanding of which receptors are important for the generation and propagation of serotonin syndrome. In his original review article on the topic, Sternbach [32] made a case for the role of 5-hydroxytryptamine (5-HT1a) receptors in the development and treatment of serotonin syndrome. More recently, however, studies have placed an emphasis on 5-HT2a and D-1 receptors in mediating hyperthermia [72–74]. But these studies typically employ pretreatment models, which, although helpful in delineating mechanisms, offer little in the way of support for clinical treatments. Pretreatment models are particularly problematic with MDMA, because any drug that lowers core body temperature in rats, regardless of mechanism, is protective in MDMA intoxication. To date, the authors know of only two animal studies in which treatments employed after the establishment of MDMA-mediated hyperthermia showed a benefit. In one of these studies, the commonly used antipsychotics olanzapine and clozapine reduced MDMA hyperthermia and cutaneous vasoconstriction; in the other, carvedilol reduced MDMA hyperthermia and rhabdomyolysis [65,75]. Olanzapine and clozapine affect of variety of receptor systems, including 5-HT2a, 5-HT1a, D-1, D-2, and α_1 receptors, although which of these is responsible for its effects in MDMA hyperthermia is currently unknown. Carvedilol is an antagonist of $\beta_{1,2,3}$-AR, as well as α_1-AR. Hence it is a more attractive treatment choice for sympathomimetic and serotonin syndromes than other nonselective β-blockers, such as propranolol and nadolol. These lack affinity for α_1- or β_3-AR and so may enhance α_1-AR–mediated vasoconstriction and heat retention. In both of these studies, however, the agents were used at significantly larger doses than are commonly used in humans, and we lack any clinical reports or studies of their role in humans.

Given similarities in the clinical presentation of serotonin syndrome and malignant hyperthermia, it has become tempting to speculate and even assume that the molecular underpinnings of anesthesia- and MDMA-induced hyperthermic syndromes are the same. To date, however, both animal and human studies have shown mixed results, without convincing evidence of the usefulness of dantrolene in cases of serotonin syndrome [64,76–79].

The two most commonly reported beneficial drugs for serotonin syndrome are cyproheptadine and chlorpromazine [80–82]. Although both are reported to be beneficial, their utility is derived solely from case reports [82]. The purported benefits of these agents are thought to be mediated by their central serotonin antagonist properties. The recommended starting dose is 50 mg intramuscular (IM) for chlorpromazine and 4 to 16 mg of cyproheptadine orally. Other agents used in case reports include benzodiazepines, propranolol, and methysergide [82]. Of note is the theoretic benefit of benzodiazepines, which hyperpolarize neurons, reducing central mediated catecholamine release [83], and decrease hyperthermia from serotonin syndrome in rats [56]. Their anticonvulsant and anxiolytic properties, safety and availability, numerous routes of administration, potential titration to effect, and lack of contraindication in other causes of drug-induced hyperthermia make benzodiazepines a reasonable treatment choice in cases of sympathomimetic and serotonin syndromes.

Because hyperthermia represents one of the most serious complications of serotonin syndrome, it makes intuitive sense for physicians to seek actively to cool their patients. Few studies, however, have looked at the role of active cooling in serotonin syndrome. In one of these studies, dogs cooled through a femoral artery catheter after a lethal dose of amphetamine had dramatically increased survival times [84]. Although researchers have largely ignored this simple treatment step, teenagers and young adults have employed this method of treatment in the form of the chilled rooms available at rave parties, so-called "chill out" rooms. However, no research has been done on this topic in humans except in the setting of exertional and nonexertional heat stroke. In heat stroke, various means of external cooling, including cool water submersion and evaporative cooling with misting and fans, have shown rapid cooling of hyperthermic patients [85] and increased survival in animals [86]. Based on current knowledge, it appears prudent to recommend similar methods of cooling for patients with life-threatening hyperthermia from serotonin syndrome.

Neuroleptic malignant syndrome

Neuroleptic malignant syndrome (NMS) is a rare idiosyncratic reaction typically occurring in persons taking neuroleptics or after the sudden withdrawal of dopamine agonists. The prevalence of NMS is typically reported as between 0.02% and 2.44% for patients taking neuroleptics [87]. These numbers, however, were typically generated by retrospective reviews of the older, higher-potency neuroleptic agents. With the recent advent of the atypical antipsychotics, it was hoped that lower prevalence and severity of NMS would ensue, but a recent review of published cases casts doubt on this possibility [88].

NMS patients typically present with a clinical syndrome of hyperthermia, altered mental status, skeletal muscle rigidity, and autonomic dysfunction [89–93]. Hyperthermia is one of the most consistent features of NMS, with temperatures greater than 38°C being one of the key diagnostic features. Manifestations of altered mental status in NMS are variable, however, and include delirium, somnolence, coma, and mutism [93]. The muscle rigidity associated with NMS is typically described as "lead pipe," denoting a resistance to passive motion. Finally, autonomic dysfunction is typically seen, with tachycardia, hyper- or hypotension, and diaphoresis. Other symptoms seen in NMS include tremor, cogwheeling, dystonic reactions, and choreiform movements [92,94]. The clinical presentation of NMS may vary, and it can occur in the absence of some or all of the classic clinical features [89,90]. Although the sequential development of signs and symptoms is variable in patients with NMS, symptom progression has been suggested to proceed from mental status changes to muscle rigidity, autonomic instability, and hyperthermia [95]. Common laboratory abnormalities seen in NMS include leukocytosis, elevated creatine phosphokinase (CPK), and low serum iron [92,96].

With the increased use of atypical antipsychotics and serotonergic antidepressants, it may be difficult to differentiate between NMS and serotonin syndrome in patients presenting with fever, muscle rigidity, autonomic instability, and altered mental status on concomitant medications. The authors believe that the speed of onset of symptoms and the finding of hyperreflexia/clonus are the most distinguishing features between these two syndromes. Patients who have serotonin syndrome typically present acutely, within 24 hours of starting their medication, whereas patients who have NMS may present at any time in their drug course, with peak symptoms not occurring for days [93]. In patients who have serotonin syndrome, clonus, hyperreflexia, and myoclonus are commonly reported, whereas these symptoms are rarely reported in NMS [31].

Although NMS is most commonly reported with the use of high-potency neuroleptics, such as haloperidol, it does occur with the atypical neuroleptics (eg, risperidone, olanzapine) [88], as well as with nonneuroleptic drugs, including metaclopramide [97], prochlorperazine [98], and promethazine [99]; it may also result from the acute withdrawal of antiparkinsonian agents [100].

Difficulties in establishing an animal model for NMS have led to difficulties in understanding the cause [101]. Although NMS is believed to be due to central dopamine antagonism, particularly within the hypothalamus [102], the sympathetic nervous system also appears to play a critical role [103]. In patients with NMS, peripheral and cerebral spinal fluid catecholamines have been shown to be markedly elevated [104–106]. In particular, cerebral spinal fluid levels of norepinephrine during the acute phase of illness were two times greater than those of matched controls or during convalescence [104]. Similar findings have been reported for plasma concentrations of serotonin and epinephrine [107]. Although less is known about the cellular events leading to NMS, overlap between the clinical features and catecholamine levels of NMS and serotonin syndrome suggests similar mechanisms.

In NMS, as in all cases of drug-induced hyperthermia, the first step in managing the patient is the removal of the offending drug. The most commonly recommended drugs in the treatment of NMS are bromocriptine and dantrolene. The recommendations for the use of bromocriptine and dantrolene are based solely on case reports and retrospective reviews.

Bromocriptine is an orally administered dopamine agonist and has been used with reported success in treating NMS [108–110]. In one study, early discontinuation of bromocriptine resulted in recrudescence of NMS in two patients who responded to reinstitution of therapy [108]. Similarities between the clinical features of NMS and malignant hyperthermia have prompted many physicians to use dantrolene for patients with NMS, with some reported sucess [111]. A case-controlled analysis comparing dantrolene and dopamine agonists in treating NMS reported evidence for significant reduction in the mortality when dantrolene, bromocriptine, amantadine, and other dopamine agonists were used alone or in combination [112]. Other authors, however, have concluded the opposite and suggested that the use of dantrolene and bromocriptine may actually worsen the course of NMS over the use of supportive measures alone [113].

In patients with mild symptoms, drug withdrawal and supportive care are the mainstays of treatment. In patients with severe symptoms (ie, temperature greater than 40°C, coma, and severe rhabdomyolysis), the combined use of dantrolene and bromocriptine may be warranted [114,115]. The usual dose of bromocriptine to treat NMS ranges from 5 to 20 mg every 6 hours, with the most common side effects being hypotension, dyskinesia, and erythematous, tender lower extremities (erythromelalgia) [101,108]. Dantrolene should be administered intravenously at a dose ranging from 3 to 5 mg/kg divided three times a day. When patients are able to take oral medications, dantrolene may be given orally at a dose of 100 to 400 mg/d divided four times a day. The most serious side effect of dantrolene is liver toxicity; it should be avoided in patients with underlying liver disease. Treatment should be continued for 10 days beyond symptom resolution to prevent the recrudescence of NMS [115]. Benzodiazepines have also been used for the treatment of anxiety and catatonia associated with NMS [116,117] and may be effective single agents in mild cases [118]. Other agents that have been used in treatment include carbidopa/levodopa, L-dopa, carbamazepine, amantadine, and methylprednisolone [90]. More recently, a randomized clinical trial suggested some benefit in patients who have NMS and are treated with methylprednisolone [119]. For patients refractory to pharmacotherapy and supportive measures, electroconvulsive therapy

(ECT) may prove beneficial, but controlled studies comparing ECT, pharmacotherapy, and supportive care are lacking [101,115]. In those patients in whom NMS and serotonin syndrome cannot be differentiated, the authors recommend the use of benzodiazepines for treatment, because bromocriptine can potentially worsen serotonin syndrome and chlorpromazine could worsen NMS.

Because many patients are dependent on neuroleptic agents for the control of their mental illness, the question of when to reinstitute therapy is crucial. Although safe reinstitution of therapy with the same drug has been reported [120], reoccurrence has been reported as well [101]. Based on the unpredictable nature of the disease and the risk for recurrence, it is generally recommended to withhold therapy for at least 2 weeks after a case of NMS [120] and then reinstitute it, if possible with a lower-potency agent.

Malignant hyperthermia

Malignant hyperthermia (MH) was first described in 1960, when a 21-year-old Australian student requiring orthopedic surgery developed hyperthermia, hypotension, and cyanosis during anesthesia with halothane. A detailed family history revealed that 10 of his close relatives had died during or after anesthesia, clearly establishing a genetic link to his anesthesia reaction [121]. Before adequate screening and treatment for MH, the initial fatality rate of MH was approximately 70%, whereas today it is closer to 5% [122]. The prevalence of MH during general anesthesia varies from 1:15,000 in children to 1:50,000 in adults [123].

Clinical symptoms of MH are the consequences of uncontrolled calcium release in skeletal muscle and the subsequent uncoupling of oxidative phosphorylation and excess cellular metabolism. Exaggerated jaw rigidity after succinylcholine and excess carbon dioxide production are often the earliest signs [122]. As symptoms progress, skeletal muscle rigidity, tachycardia, and hyperthermia develop. As ATP depletion occurs, anaerobic metabolism with metabolic acidosis and lactate production occurs, followed ultimately by skeletal muscle breakdown with elevations in serum creatine kinase and hyperkalemic cardiac arrest. As with other causes of drug-related hyperthermia, consumptive coagulopathy, pulmonary edema, and cerebral edema can develop as late and potentially fatal complications [124].

Agents inciting MH include many inhalational volatile anesthetics (ether, halothane, enflurane, isoflurane, sevoflurane, desflurane) and depolarizing muscle relaxants such as succinylcholine and decamethonium [125]. Some patients have developed an MH reaction after undergoing previous general anesthesia with known triggering agents without problems. Although MH is typically associated with anesthetics, persons genetically susceptible to it may develop symptoms after excess exertion in warm environments [126,127].

MH occurs in persons with genetic defects at one of several receptors controlling the release of sarcoplasmic calcium in skeletal muscle [128]. When they are exposed to triggering agents, sudden increases in intracellular calcium result in a cascade of events, ultimately leading to the uncoupling of oxidative phosphorylation in the mitochondria with excess metabolic breakdown. The sympathetic nervous system plays an important role in mediating symptoms of MH such as significant elevations in circulating norepinephrine [129,130], and increased survival with therapeutic α-blockade has been demonstrated in animal models [131,132]. Nonetheless, norepinephrine does not appear to induce MH [133]. Activation of the hypothalamic-pituitary-adrenal axis is also believed to occur in MH, because pigs undergoing adrenalectomy appear more resistant to the lethal effects of a halothane challenge [132]. Elevated levels of serotonin have also been demonstrated in MH [134], with serotonergic drug agonists causing exaggerated responses in MH-susceptible pigs [135–137]. Serotonin antagonists, however, have not been shown to be effective in preventing MH in susceptible swine [138]. In summary, MH occurs secondary to unregulated calcium release with excess metabolic breakdown and uncoupling of oxidative phosphorylations, which likely contributes to the activation of the sympathetic nervous system and release of catecholamines.

Dantrolene sodium is an effective antidote for MH. Dantrolene causes complete and sustained relaxation of skeletal muscle contractures in vitro in MH-susceptible muscle and in vivo in both human and porcine MH [139]. Dantrolene inhibits intracellular calcium release in the myocyte by direct action on calcium release channels, with two separate binding sites proposed [140]. At low doses, dantrolene may actually release calcium, which could explain the recrudescence of symptoms in MH [140,141]. Side effects include muscle weakness, dizziness, and hepatic dysfunction [142]. Dosing of dantrolene is 1 to 3 mg/kg intravenously, repeated every 15 minutes as needed to a maximum dose of 10 mg/kg in the setting of acute MH. Recurrence is prevented by administration of dantrolene 1 mg/kg intravenously (or as much as 2 mg/kg orally) four times a day for 24 to 72 hours postoperatively. Those patients thought to have MH should be referred to an approved MH testing facility to arrange for genetic and muscle testing.

Summary

Toxin-induced hyperthermic syndromes are important to consider in the differential diagnosis of patients presenting with fever and muscle rigidity. If untreated, toxin-induced hyperthermia may result in fatal hyperthermia with multisystem organ failure. All of these syndromes have at their center the disruption of normal thermogenic mechanisms, resulting in the activation of the hypothalamus and sympathetic nervous systems. The result of this thermogenic dysregulation is excess heat generation combined with impaired heat dissipation. Although many similarities exist among the clinical presentations and pathophysiologies of toxin-induced hyperthermic syndromes, important differences exist among their triggers and treatments.

Serotonin syndrome typically occurs within hours of the addition of a new serotonergic agent or the abuse of stimulants such as MDMA or methamphetamine. Treatment involves discontinuing the offending agent and administering either a central serotonergic antagonist, such as cyproheptadine or chlorpromazine, a benzodiazepine, or a combination of the two. NMS typically occurs over hours to days in a patient taking a neuroleptic agent; its recommended treatment is generally the combination of a central dopamine agonist, bromocriptine or L-dopa, and dantrolene. In those patients in whom it is difficult to differentiate between serotonin and neuroleptic malignant syndromes, the physical examination may be helpful: clonus and hyperreflexia are more suggestive of serotonin syndrome, whereas lead-pipe rigidity is suggestive of NMS. In patients in whom serotonin syndrome and NMS cannot be differentiated, benzodiazepines represent the safest therapeutic option.

MH presents rapidly with jaw rigidity, hyperthermia, and hypercarbia. Although it almost always occurs in the setting of surgical anesthesia, cases have occurred in susceptible individuals during exertion. The treatment of MH involves the use of dantrolene. Future improvements in understanding the pathophysiology and clinical presentations of these syndromes will undoubtedly result in earlier recognition and better treatment strategies.

References

[1] Adubofour KO, Kajiwara GT, Goldberg CM, et al. Oxybutynin-induced heatstroke in an elderly patient. Ann Pharmacother 1996;30(2):144–7.
[2] Lowell BB, Spiegelman BM. Towards a molecular understanding of adaptive thermo-genesis. Nature 2000;404(6778):652–60.
[3] Charkoudian N. Skin blood flow in adult human thermoregulation: how it works, when it does not, and why. Mayo Clin Proc 2003;78(5):603–12.
[4] Nielsen B. Heat acclimation—mechanisms of adaptation to exercise in the heat. Int J Sports Med 1998;19(Suppl 2):S154–6.
[5] De Witte J, Sessler DI. Perioperative shivering: physiology and pharmacology. Anesthesiology 2002;96(2):467–84.
[6] Mallick BN, Jha SK, Islam F. Presence of alpha-1 adrenoreceptors on thermosensitive neurons in the medial preoptico-anterior hypothalamic area in rats. Neuropharmacology 2002;42(5):697–705.
[7] Cox B, Lee TF. Further evidence for a physiological role for hypothalamic dopamine in thermoregulation in the rat. J Physiol 1980;300:7–17.
[8] Rothwell NJ. CNS regulation of thermogenesis. Crit Rev Neurobiol 1994;8(1–2):1–10.
[9] Landsberg L, Saville ME, Young JB. Sympathoadrenal system and regulation of thermogenesis. Am J Physiol 1984;247(2 Pt 1):E181–9.
[10] Wallace KB, Starkov AA. Mitochondrial targets of drug toxicity. Annu Rev Pharmacol Toxicol 2000;40:353–88.

[11] Boss O, Muzzin P, Giacobino JP. The uncoupling proteins, a review. Eur J Endocrinol 1998;139(1):1–9.

[12] Nicholls DG, Locke RM. Thermogenic mechanisms in brown fat. Physiol Rev 1984;64(1): 1–64.

[13] Boss O, Samec S, Paoloni-Giacobino A, et al. Uncoupling protein-3: a new member of the mitochondrial carrier family with tissue-specific expression. FEBS Lett 1997;408(1): 39–42.

[14] Simonyan RA, Jimenez M, Ceddia RB, et al. Cold-induced changes in the energy coupling and the UCP3 level in rodent skeletal muscles. Biochim Biophys Acta 2001;1505(2–3): 271–9.

[15] Ribeiro MO, Lebrun FL, Christoffolete MA, et al. Evidence of UCP1-independent regulation of norepinephrine-induced thermogenesis in brown fat. Am J Physiol Endocrinol Metab 2000;279(2):E314–22.

[16] Gong DW, He Y, Karas M, et al. Uncoupling protein-3 is a mediator of thermogenesis regulated by thyroid hormone, beta 3-adrenergic agonists, and leptin. J Biol Chem 1997; 272(39):24129–32.

[17] Rubio A, Raasmaja A, Maia AL, et al. Effects of thyroid hormone on norepinephrine signaling in brown adipose tissue. I. Beta 1- and beta 2-adrenergic receptors and cyclic adenosine $3',5'$–monophosphate generation. Endocrinology 1995; 136(8):3267–76.

[18] Bianco AC, Carvalho SD, Carvalho CR, et al. Thyroxine $5'$-deiodination mediates norepinephrine-induced lipogenesis in dispersed brown adipocytes. Endocrinology 1998; 139(2):571–8.

[19] Silva JE. Thyroid hormone control of thermogenesis and energy balance. Thyroid 1995; 5(6):481–92.

[20] Reitman ML, He Y, Gong DW. Thyroid hormone and other regulators of uncoupling proteins. Int J Obes Relat Metab Disord 1999;23(Suppl 6):S56–9.

[21] Roberts JR, Quattrocchi E, Howland MA. Severe hyperthermia secondary to intravenous drug abuse. Am J Emerg Med 1984;2(4):373.

[22] Kendrick WC, Hull AR, Knochel JP. Rhabdomyolysis and shock after intravenous amphetamine administration. Ann Intern Med 1977;86(4):381–7.

[23] Ginsberg MD, Hertzman M, Schmidt-Nowara WW. Amphetamine intoxication with coagulopathy, hyperthermia, and reversible renal failure. A syndrome resembling heatstroke. Ann Intern Med 1970;73(1):81–5.

[24] Dar KJ, McBrien ME. MDMA induced hyperthermia: report of a fatality and review of current therapy. Intensive Care Med 1996;22(9):995–6.

[25] Prior FH, Isbister GK, Dawson AH, et al. Serotonin toxicity with therapeutic doses of dexamphetamine and venlafaxine. Med J Aust 2002;176(5):240–1.

[26] Bodner RA, Lynch T, Lewis L, et al. Serotonin syndrome. Neurology 1995;45(2):219–23.

[27] Eadie MJ. Convulsive ergotism: epidemics of the serotonin syndrome? Lancet Neurol 2003; 2(7):429–34.

[28] Caporael LR. Ergotism: the satan loosed in Salem? Science 1976;192(4234):21–6.

[29] Mitchell RS. Fatal toxic encephalitis occurring during iproniazid therapy in pulmonary tuberculosis. Ann Intern Med 1955;42:417–24.

[30] Asch DA, Parker RM. The Libby Zion case. One step forward or two steps backward? N Engl J Med 1988;318(12):771–5.

[31] Mills KC. Serotonin syndrome. A clinical update. Crit Care Clin 1997;13(4):763–83.

[32] Sternbach H. The serotonin syndrome. Am J Psychiatry 1991;148(6):705–13.

[33] Hilton SE, Maradit H, Moller HJ. Serotonin syndrome and drug combinations: focus on MAOI and RIMA. Eur Arch Psychiatry Clin Neurosci 1997;247(3):113–9.

[34] Radomski JW, Dursun SM, Reveley MA, et al. An exploratory approach to the serotonin syndrome: an update of clinical phenomenology and revised diagnostic criteria. Med Hypotheses 2000;55(3):218–24.

[35] Milroy CM, Clark JC, Forrest AR. Pathology of deaths associated with "ecstasy" and "eve" misuse. J Clin Pathol 1996;49(2):149–53.

[36] Gowing LR, Henry-Edwards SM, Irvine RJ, et al. The health effects of ecstasy: a literature review. Drug Alcohol Rev 2002;21(1):53–63.

[37] Mason PJ, Morris VA, Balcezak TJ. Serotonin syndrome. Presentation of 2 cases and review of the literature. Medicine 2000;79(4):201–9.

[38] Kolecki P. Isolated venlafaxine-induced serotonin syndrome. J Emerg Med 1997;15(4): 491–3.

[39] Lejoyeux M, Fineyre F, Ades J. The serotonin syndrome. Am J Psychiatry 1992;149(10): 1410–1.

[40] Skop BP, Finkelstein JA, Mareth TR, et al. The serotonin syndrome associated with paroxetine, an over-the-counter cold remedy, and vascular disease. Am J Emerg Med 1994; 12(6):642–4.

[41] Meyer D, Halfin V. Toxicity secondary to meperidine in patients on monoamine oxidase inhibitors: a case report and critical review. J Clin Psychopharmacol 1981;1(5):319–21.

[42] Sandyk R. L-dopa induced "serotonin syndrome" in a parkinsonian patient on bromocriptine. J Clin Psychopharmacol 1986;6(3):194–5.

[43] Mahlberg R, Kunz D, Sasse J, et al. Serotonin syndrome with tramadol and citalopram. Am J Psychiatry 2004;161(6):1129.

[44] Muly EC, McDonald W, Steffens D, et al. Serotonin syndrome produced by a combination of fluoxetine and lithium. Am J Psychiatry 1993;150(10):1565.

[45] Malberg JE, Seiden LS. Small changes in ambient temperature cause large changes in 3,4-methylenedioxymethamphetamine (MDMA)–induced serotonin neurotoxicity and core body temperature in the rat. J Neurosci 1998;18(13):5086–94.

[46] Ali SF, Newport GD, Holson RR, et al. Low environmental temperatures or pharmacologic agents that produce hypothermia decrease methamphetamine neurotoxicity in mice. Brain Res 1994;658(1–2):33–8.

[47] Miller DB, O'Callaghan JP. Elevated environmental temperature and methamphetamine neurotoxicity. Environ Res 2003;92(1):48–53.

[48] Gordon CJ, Watkinson WP, O'Callaghan JP, et al. Effects of 3,4-methylenedioxymethamphetamine on autonomic thermoregulatory responses of the rat. Pharmacol Biochem Behav 1991;38(2):339–44.

[49] Marzuk PM, Tardiff K, Leon AC, et al. Ambient temperature and mortality from unintentional cocaine overdose. JAMA 1998;279(22):1795–800.

[50] Duarte JA, Leao A, Magalhaes J, et al. Strenuous exercise aggravates MDMA-induced skeletal muscle damage in mice. Toxicology 2005;206(3):349–58.

[51] Harding M, Peterson DI. The effect of exercise and limitation of movement on amphetamine toxicity. J Pharmacol Exp Ther 1963;145:47–51.

[52] Rusyniak DE, Tandy SL, Hekmatyar SK, et al. The role of mitochondrial uncoupling in 3,4-methylenedioxymethamphetamine mediated skeletal muscle hyperthermia and rhabdomyolysis. J Pharmacol Exp Ther 2005;313(2):629–39.

[53] Henry JA, Jeffreys KJ, Dawling S. Toxicity and deaths from 3,4-methylenedioxymethamphetamine ("ecstasy"). Lancet 1992;340(8816):384–7.

[54] Sprague JE, Brutcher RE, Mills EM, et al. Attenuation of 3,4-methylenedioxymethamphetamine (MDMA, Ecstasy)–induced rhabdomyolysis with alpha1- plus beta3-adrenoreceptor antagonists. Br J Pharmacol 2004;142(4):667–70.

[55] Stephenson CP, Hunt GE, Topple AN, et al. The distribution of 3,4-methylenedioxymethamphetamine "Ecstasy"–induced c-fos expression in rat brain. Neuroscience 1999; 92(3):1011–23.

[56] Nisijima K, Shioda K, Yoshino T, et al. Diazepam and chlormethiazole attenuate the development of hyperthermia in an animal model of the serotonin syndrome. Neurochem Int 2003;43(2):155–64.

[57] Nisijima K, Yoshino T, Ishiguro T. Risperidone counteracts lethality in an animal model of the serotonin syndrome. Psychopharmacology (Berl) 2000;150(1):9–14.

[58] Shioda K, Nisijima K, Yoshino T, et al. Extracellular serotonin, dopamine and glutamate levels are elevated in the hypothalamus in a serotonin syndrome animal model induced by tranylcypromine and fluoxetine. Prog Neuropsychopharmacol Biol Psychiatry 2004;28(4): 633–40.

[59] Nisijima K, Nibuya M, Sugiyama H. Abnormal CSF monoamine metabolism in serotonin syndrome. J Clin Psychopharmacol 2003;23(5):528–31.

[60] Nisijima K. Abnormal monoamine metabolism in cerebrospinal fluid in a case of serotonin syndrome. J Clin Psychopharmacol 2000;20(1):107–8.

[61] Fernandez F, Aguerre S, Mormede P, et al. Influences of the corticotropic axis and sympathetic activity on neurochemical consequences of 3,4-methylenedioxymethamphet-amine (MDMA) administration in Fischer 344 rats. Eur J Neurosci 2002;16(4):607–18.

[62] Sprague JE, Banks ML, Cook VJ, et al. Hypothalamic-pituitary-thyroid axis and sympathetic nervous system involvement in hyperthermia induced by 3,4-methylenediox-ymethamphetamine (Ecstasy). J Pharmacol Exp Ther 2003;305(1):159–66.

[63] Sprague JE, Mallett NM, Rusyniak DE, et al. UCP3 and thyroid hormone involvement in methamphetamine-induced hyperthermia. Biochem Pharmacol 2004; 68(7):1339–43.

[64] Makisumi T, Yoshida K, Watanabe T, et al. Sympatho-adrenal involvement in methamphetamine-induced hyperthermia through skeletal muscle hypermetabolism. Eur J Pharmacol 1998;363(2–3):107–12.

[65] Sprague JE, Moze P, Caden D, et al. Carvedilol reverses hyperthermia and attenuates rhabdomyolysis induced by 3,4-methylenedioxymethamphetamine (MDMA, Ecstasy) in an animal model. Crit Care Med 2005;33(6):1311–6.

[66] Stuerenburg HJ, Petersen K, Baumer T, et al. Plasma concentrations of 5-HT, 5-HIAA, norepinephrine, epinephrine and dopamine in ecstasy users. Neuro Endocrinol Lett 2002; 23(3):259–61.

[67] Pedersen NP, Blessing WW. Cutaneous vasoconstriction contributes to hyperthermia induced by 3,4-methylenedioxymethamphetamine (ecstasy) in conscious rabbits. J Neuro-sci 2001;21(21):8648–54.

[68] Crandall CG, Vongpatanasin W, Victor RG. Mechanism of cocaine-induced hyperthermia in humans. Ann Intern Med 2002;136(11):785–91.

[69] Zhao J, Cannon B, Nedergaard J. Alpha1-adrenergic stimulation potentiates the thermogenic action of beta3-adrenoreceptor–generated cAMP in brown fat cells. J Biol Chem 1997;272(52):32847–56.

[70] Mills EM, Rusyniak DE, Sprague JE. The role of the sympathetic nervous system and uncoupling proteins in the thermogenesis induced by 3,4-methylenedioxymethamphet-amine. J Mol Med 2004;82(12):787–99.

[71] Mills EM, Banks ML, Sprague JE, et al. Uncoupling the agony from ecstasy. Nature 2003; 426:403–4.

[72] Nisijima K, Yoshino T, Yui K, et al. Potent serotonin (5-HT)(2A) receptor antagonists completely prevent the development of hyperthermia in an animal model of the 5-HT syndrome. Brain Res 2001;890(1):23–31.

[73] Mechan AO, Esteban B, O'Shea E, et al. The pharmacology of the acute hyperthermic response that follows administration of 3,4-methylenedioxymethamphetamine (MDMA, "ecstasy") to rats. Br J Pharmacol 2002;135(1):170–80.

[74] Van Oekelen D, Megens A, Meert T, et al. Role of 5-HT(2) receptors in the tryptamine-induced 5-HT syndrome in rats. Behav Pharmacol 2002;13(4):313–8.

[75] Blessing WW, Seaman B, Pedersen NP, et al. Clozapine reverses hyperthermia and sympathetically mediated cutaneous vasoconstriction induced by 3,4-methylenedioxyme-thamphetamine (ecstasy) in rabbits and rats. J Neurosci 2003;23(15):6385–91.

[76] Rusyniak DE, Banks ML, Mills EM, et al. Dantrolene use in 3,4-methylenedioxymetham-phetamine (ecstasy)–mediated hyperthermia. Anesthesiology 2004;101(1):263 [author reply: 264].

[77] Singarajah C, Lavies NG. An overdose of ecstasy. A role for dantrolene. Anaesthesia 1992; 47(8):686–7.

[78] Watson JD, Ferguson C, Hinds CJ, et al. Exertional heat stroke induced by amphetamine analogues. Does dantrolene have a place? Anaesthesia 1993;48(12):1057–60.

[79] Webb C, Williams V. Ecstasy intoxication: appreciation of complications and the role of dantrolene. Anaesthesia 1993;48(6):542–3.

[80] Graudins A, Stearman A, Chan B. Treatment of the serotonin syndrome with cyproheptadine. J Emerg Med 1998;16(4):615–9.

[81] Lappin RI, Auchincloss EL. Treatment of the serotonin syndrome with cyproheptadine. N Engl J Med 1994;331(15):1021–2.

[82] Gillman PK. The serotonin syndrome and its treatment. J Psychopharmacol 1999;13(1): 100–9.

[83] Vogel WH, Miller J, DeTurck KH, et al. Effects of psychoactive drugs on plasma catecholamines during stress in rats. Neuropharmacology 1984;23(9):1105–8.

[84] Zalis EG, Lundberg GD, Kaplan G, et al. The effect of extracorporeal cooling on amphetamine toxicity. Arch Int Pharmacodyn Ther 1966;159(1):189–95.

[85] Hadad E, Rav-Acha M, Heled Y, et al. Heat stroke: a review of cooling methods. Sports Med 2004;34(8):501–11.

[86] Chou YT, Lai ST, Lee CC, et al. Hypothermia attenuates circulatory shock and cerebral ischemia in experimental heatstroke. Shock 2003;19(4):388–93.

[87] Khan M, Farver D. Recognition, assessment and management of neuroleptic malignant syndrome. S D J Med 2000;53(9):395–400.

[88] Ananth J, Parameswaran S, Gunatilake S, et al. Neuroleptic malignant syndrome and atypical antipsychotic drugs. J Clin Psychiatry 2004;65(4):464–70.

[89] Balzan MV. The neuroleptic malignant syndrome: a logical approach to the patient with temperature and rigidity. Postgrad Med J 1998;74(868):72–6.

[90] Carbone JR. The neuroleptic malignant and serotonin syndromes. Emerg Med Clin North Am 2000;18:317–25.

[91] Caroff SN, Mann SC. Neuroleptic malignant syndrome. Med Clin North Am 1993;77(1): 185–202.

[92] Nierenberg D, Disch M, Manheimer E, et al. Facilitating prompt diagnosis and treatment of the neuroleptic malignant syndrome. Clin Pharmacol Ther 1991;50(5 Pt 1): 580–6.

[93] Rosebush P, Stewart T. A prospective analysis of 24 episodes of neuroleptic malignant syndrome. Am J Psychiatry 1989;146(6):717–25.

[94] Oppenheim G. Mutism and hyperthermia in a patient treated with neuroleptics. Med J Aust 1973;2(5):228–9.

[95] Velamoor VR, Norman RMG, Caroff SN, et al. Progression of symptoms in neuroleptic malignant syndrome. J Nerv Ment Dis 1994;182:168–73.

[96] Rosebush PI, Mazurek MF. Serum iron and neuroleptic malignant syndrome. Lancet 1991; 338(8760):149–51.

[97] Friedman LS, Weinrauch LA, D'Elia JA. Metoclopramide-induced neuroleptic malignant syndrome. Arch Intern Med 1987;147(8):1495–7.

[98] Pesola GR, Quinto C. Prochlorperazine-induced neuroleptic malignant syndrome. J Emerg Med 1996;14(6):727–9.

[99] Chan-Tack KM. Neuroleptic malignant syndrome due to promethazine. South Med J 1999; 92(10):1017–8.

[100] Rainer C, Scheinost NA, Lefeber EJ. Neuroleptic malignant syndrome. When levodopa withdrawal is the cause. Postgrad Med 1991;89(5):175–8, 180.

[101] Olmsted TR. Neuroleptic malignant syndrome: guidelines for treatment and reinstitution of neuroleptics. South Med J 1988;81(7):888–91.

[102] Henderson VW, Wooten GF. Neuroleptic malignant syndrome: a pathogenetic role for dopamine receptor blockade? Neurology 1981;31(2):132–7.

[103] Gurrera RJ. Sympathoadrenal hyperactivity and the etiology of neuroleptic malignant syndrome. Am J Psychiatry 1999;156(2):169–80.

[104] Nisijima K, Oyafuso K, Shimada T, et al. Cerebrospinal fluid monoamine metabolism in a case of neuroleptic malignant syndrome improved by electroconvulsive therapy. Biol Psychiatry 1996;39(5):383–4.

[105] Feibel JH, Schiffer RB. Sympathoadrenomedullary hyperactivity in the neuroleptic malignant syndrome: a case report. Am J Psychiatry 1981;138(8):1115–6.

[106] Gurrera RJ, Romero JA. Sympathoadrenomedullary activity in the neuroleptic malignant syndrome. Biol Psychiatry 1992;32(4):334–43.

[107] Spivak B, Maline DI, Vered Y, et al. Prospective evaluation of circulatory levels of catecholamines and serotonin in neuroleptic malignant syndrome. Acta Psychiatr Scand 2000;102(3):226–30.

[108] Dhib-Jalbut S, Hesselbrock R, Mouradian MM, et al. Bromocriptine treatment of neuroleptic malignant syndrome. J Clin Psychiatry 1987;48(2):69–73.

[109] Janati A, Webb RT. Successful treatment of neuroleptic malignant syndrome with bromocriptine. South Med J 1986;79(12):1567–71.

[110] Verhoeven WM, Elderson A, Westenberg HG. Neuroleptic malignant syndrome: successful treatment with bromocriptine. Biol Psychiatry 1985;20(6):680–4.

[111] Bismuth C, de Rohan-Chabot P, Goulon M, et al. Dantrolene—a new therapeutic approach to the neuroleptic malignant syndrome. Acta Neurol Scand Suppl 1984;100:193–8.

[112] Sakkas P, Davis JM, Janicak PG, et al. Drug treatment of the neuroleptic malignant syndrome. Psychopharmacol Bull 1991;27(3):381–4.

[113] Rosebush PI, Stewart T, Mazurek MF. The treatment of neuroleptic malignant syndrome. Are dantrolene and bromocriptine useful adjuncts to supportive care? Br J Psychiatry 1991; 159:709–12.

[114] Schvehla TJ, Herjanic M. Neuroleptic malignant syndrome, bromocriptine, and anticholinergic drugs. J Clin Psychiatry 1988;49(7):283–4.

[115] Velamoor VR, Swamy GN, Parmar RS, et al. Management of suspected neuroleptic malignant syndrome. Can J Psychiatry 1995;40(9):545–50.

[116] Lew TY, Tollefson G. Chlorpromazine-induced neuroleptic malignant syndrome and its response to diazepam. Biol Psychiatry 1983;18(12):1441–6.

[117] Miyaoka H, Shishikura K, Otsubo T, et al. Diazepam-responsive neuroleptic malignant syndrome: a diagnostic subtype? Am J Psychiatry 1997;154(6):882.

[118] Kontaxakis VP, Christodoulou GN, Markidis MP, et al. Treatment of a mild form of neuroleptic malignant syndrome with oral diazepam. Acta Psychiatr Scand 1988;78(3):396–8.

[119] Sato Y, Asoh T, Metoki N, et al. Efficacy of methylprednisolone pulse therapy on neuroleptic malignant syndrome in Parkinson's disease. J Neurol Neurosurg Psychiatry 2003;74(5):574–6.

[120] Rosebush PI, Stewart TD, Gelenberg AJ. Twenty neuroleptic rechallenges after neuroleptic malignant syndrome in 15 patients. J Clin Psychiatry 1989;50(8):295–8.

[121] Denborough MA, Lovell RRH. Anaesthetic deaths in a family. Lancet 1960;2:45.

[122] Denborough M. Malignant hyperthermia. Lancet 1998;9134(352):1131–6.

[123] Loke J, MacLennan DH. Malignant hyperthermia and central core disease: disorders of Ca2+ release channels. Am J Med 1998;104(5):470–86.

[124] Hopkins PM. Malignant hyperthermia: advances in clinical management and diagnosis. Br J Anaesth 2000;85(1):118–28.

[125] Naguib M, Magboul MM. Adverse effects of neuromuscular blockers and their antagonists. Drug Saf 1998;18(2):99–116.

[126] Tobin JR, Jason DR, Challa VR, et al. Malignant hyperthermia and apparent heat stroke. JAMA 2001;286(2):168–9.

[127] Wappler F, Fiege M, Steinfath M, et al. Evidence for susceptibility to malignant hyperthermia in patients with exercise-induced rhabdomyolysis. Anesthesiology 2001; 94(1):95–100.

[128] Kaus SJ, Rockoff MA. Malignant hyperthermia. Pediatr Clin North Am 1994;41(1): 221–37.

[129] Haggendal J, Jonsson L, Carlsten J. The role of sympathetic activity in initiating malignant hyperthermia. Acta Anaesthesiol Scand 1990;34(8):677–82.

[130] Williams CH, Dozier SE, Buzello W, et al. Plasma levels of norepinephrine and epinephrine during malignant hyperthermia in susceptible pigs. J Chromatogr 1985;344:71–80.

[131] Lister D, Hall GM, Lucke JN. Porcine malignant hyperthermia. III. Adrenergic blockade. Br J Anaesth 1976;48(9):831–8.

[132] Lucke JN, Denny H, Hall GM, et al. Porcine malignant hyperthermia. VI. The effects of bilateral adrenalectomy and pretreatment with bretylium on the halothane-induced response. Br J Anaesth 1978;50(3):241–6.

[133] Maccani RM, Wedel DJ, Hofer RE. Norepinephrine does not potentiate porcine malignant hyperthermia. Anesth Analg 1996;82(4):790–5.

[134] Gerdes C, Richter A, Annies R, et al. Increase of serotonin in plasma during onset of halothane-induced malignant hyperthermia in pigs. Eur J Pharmacol 1992;220(1):91–4.

[135] Loscher W, Witte U, Fredow G, et al. Pharmacodynamic effects of serotonin (5-HT) receptor ligands in pigs: stimulation of 5-HT2 receptors induces malignant hyperthermia. Naunyn Schmiedebergs Arch Pharmacol 1990;341(6):483–93.

[136] Fiege M, Wappler F, Weisshorn R, et al. Induction of malignant hyperthermia in susceptible swine by 3,4-methylenedioxymethamphetamine ("ecstasy"). Anesthesiology 2003;99(5):1132–6.

[137] Gerbershagen MU, Wappler F, Fiege M, et al. Effects of a 5HT(2) receptor agonist on anaesthetized pigs susceptible to malignant hyperthermia. Br J Anaesth 2003;91(2):281–4.

[138] Loscher W, Gerdes C, Richter A. Lack of prophylactic or therapeutic efficacy of 5-HT2A receptor antagonists in halothane-induced porcine malignant hyperthermia. Naunyn Schmiedebergs Arch Pharmacol 1994;350(4):365–74.

[139] Ward A, Chaffman MO, Sorkin EM. Dantrolene. A review of its pharmacodynamic and pharmacokinetic properties and therapeutic use in malignant hyperthermia, the neuroleptic malignant syndrome and an update of its use in muscle spasticity. Drugs 1986;32(2):130–68.

[140] Nelson TE, Lin M, Sapata-Sudo G, et al. Dantrolene sodium can increase or attenuate activity of skeletal muscle ryanodine receptor calcium release channel: clinical implications. Anesthesiology 1996;84(6):1368–79.

[141] Jurkat-Rott K, McCarthy T, Lehmann-Horn F. Genetics and pathogenesis of malignant hyperthermia. Muscle Nerve 2000;23(1):4–17.

[142] Wedel DJ, Quinlan JG, Iaizzo PA. Clinical effects of intravenously administered dantrolene. Mayo Clin Proc 1995;70(3):241–6.

ELSEVIER
SAUNDERS

Clin Lab Med 26 (2006) 185–209

CLINICS IN
LABORATORY
MEDICINE

Chemically Induced Seizures

Brandon Wills, DO, MS[a,b,*],
Timothy Erickson, MD, FACEP, FACMT, FAACT[c]

[a]*University of Washington, Seattle, WA, USA*
[b]*Department of Emergency Medicine, Madigan Army Medical Center, Tacoma, WA, USA*
[c]*Department of Emergency Medicine, University of Illinois, Chicago, IL, USA*

Generalized seizure activity may be a presenting symptom of poisoning or a preterminal manifestation of serious toxicity. Seizures may result from a large number of drugs and toxins, such as isoniazid (INH), carbon monoxide, theophylline, cyclic antidepressants, and salicylates. Additionally, withdrawal states, such as from ethanol and sedative hypnotic agents, may induce refractory seizure activity.

In this article the authors review the pathophysiology of drug- and toxin-associated seizures (DTS), discuss the differential diagnosis, and provide a logical approach to management of DTS. Their aim is to discuss those specific agents for which seizure activity is a primary sequela in therapeutic use, exposure, or overdose.

Epidemiology

It is difficult to estimate the true incidence of DTS, because the literature shows a paucity of epidemiologic data. The Toxic Exposure Surveillance System [1] is an annually updated database documenting outcomes for all poisonings reported to regional poison centers throughout the United States, but it does not record data for seizures in its own category. A prospective study of status epilepticus (SE) by Delorenzo and colleagues [2] reported that, of 204 SE events, ethanol-related seizures were responsible for 13%, whereas drug overdose was responsible for less than 5%, with case/fatality rates of approximately 20% and 25%, respectively. A retrospective review of

---

Portions of this article were previously published in Holstege CP, Rusyniak DE: Medical Toxicology. 89:6, Med Clin North Am, 2005; with permission.

* Corresponding author. Madigan Army Medical Center, Department of Emergency Medicine, MCHJ-EM, Tacoma, WA 98431.

E-mail address: bkwills@gmail.com (B. Wills).

California Poison Control System data from 1993 reported that the most common DTS were cyclic antidepressants (29%), stimulants (29%), antihistamines (7%), theophylline (5%), and isoniazid (5%) [3]. The same authors reviewed poison center data from 2003 and found that the leading causes for drug-induced seizures had evolved to the following agents: bupropion (23%), diphenhydramine (8.3%), cyclic antidepressants (7.7%), tramadol (7.5%), amphetamines (6.9%), INH (5.9%), and venlafaxine (5.9%) [4]. In this series, 68% had only one seizure, 27% had two or more seizures, and only 3.6% had SE. The definition of SE is in evolution; however, some believe that it should be defined as either continuous seizures for more than 5 minutes or two or more seizures without a lucid interval [5,6].

Pathophysiology

Nerve signals in the central nervous system (CNS) are generally transmitted by neurotransmitters. Neurotransmitter binding results in either nerve signal propagation or termination. Neurotransmitter receptors located at the postsynaptic nerve terminal mediate opening or closing of ion channels. Receptors may be directly linked to an ion channel or modulate ion channels by stimulation of a second messenger (ie, cyclic adenosine monophosphate or cAMP). Nerve signal propagation occurs when the resting membrane potential rises to the threshold potential that triggers an action potential. Generally, excitation occurs with influx of sodium ions or a decrease in either chloride conduction or potassium efflux. Inhibition results from a decrease in sodium influx or an increase in either chloride influx or potassium efflux.

All seizure activity is a result of chaotic electrical discharge in the CNS. With tremendous advances in neurobiochemistry, a variety of neurochemical linked pathways have been implicated in the genesis of seizures. Seizure and epilepsy research frequently uses a kindling model to study the effects of proconvulsant agents. *Kindling* is a paradigm in which CNS stimulation from a xenobiotic or electrical stimulus results in epileptiform activity. Kindling also refers to sensitization of neuronal tissue by the addition of a drug or electrical stimulus that renders it susceptible to subsequent seizure activity [7]. Certainly, not all pathways for the genesis of seizures have been elucidated. The following are descriptions of specific neurochemical pathways known to induce seizures.

Gamma-aminobutyric acid

Gamma-aminobutyric acid (GABA) is the main inhibitory neurotransmitter of the CNS. When stimulated, GABA receptors modulate chloride ion flux, inhibiting membrane depolarization [8]. Conversely, GABA antagonists or functional depletion of GABA increases membrane depolarization and may result in seizures [9]. GABA agonists (direct or indirect) therefore play a vital role in seizure termination [6]. Loss of GABA-mediated inhibition results in seizures, as occurs in withdrawal from ethanol, sedative hypnotics, gamma-hydroxybutyrate, and baclofen [10].

Glutamate

The excitatory amino acid glutamate binds one of four glutamate receptors, allowing the influx of sodium, calcium, or both and causing neuron depolarization. Excessive neuronal excitation by glutamate by means of N-methyl-D-aspartate (NMDA), alpha-amino-3-hydroxy-5-methyl-4-isoxazolepropionic acid (AMPA), or kainate receptors may result in seizures [11,12].

Glycine

Glycine is another excitatory neurotransmitter that binds to NMDA receptors, causing sodium influx in the CNS. Postsynaptic glycine receptors modulate chloride influx. Postsynaptic glycine antagonists, such as strychnine, cause seizure-like myoclonic activity, but this occurs with an intact mental status that is not a true seizure [13].

Sodium channel blockade

Because depolarizations generated in the nerve body are propagated down the axon through the opening of sodium channels, local anesthetics slow neuronal transmission by virtue of sodium channel blockade. This phenomenon has led to the use of lidocaine as a possible treatment for SE [14]. Conversely, in overdose, it is known to produce seizures by an unknown mechanism. Other pharmaceuticals that block sodium channels, such as carbamazepine, may be anticonvulsant in therapeutic doses and yet produce seizures in overdose. It has been suggested that the local anesthetic effects of cocaine may potentiate seizures [15]. Concomitant administration of cocaine and lidocaine has additive effects on seizure incidence in an animal model [16].

Norepinephrine

Autonomic overstimulation may occur as a direct or indirect effect of drugs. Ethanol withdrawal, despite having multifactorial effects, results in marked sympathetic outflow. Ethanol withdrawal results in increased norepinephrine release and may lead to seizures [17].

Acetylcholine

Cholinergic overstimulation may result in seizures [8]. This effect may be seen with exposure to cholinesterase inhibitors, such as carbamates and organophosphate pesticides, or nerve agents [18].

Adenosine

Adenosine-1 (A_1) receptors are found in the CNS [19]. Experimentally, agonists of A_1 receptors inhibit glutamate release, causing an anticonvulsant effect, whereas A_1 antagonists markedly increase spontaneous seizure activity [20]. This mechanism may be a contributing factor in theophylline toxicity.

Histamine

Histamine may have anticonvulsive properties mediated by the central H_1 receptor [21]. Administration of toxic doses of antihistamines in animal models results in generalized seizures and is attenuated by the addition of the histamine precursor—histidine [21,22].

Metabolic disturbances

Disturbances in electrolyte or glucose homeostasis may result in seizures; these may include hyponatremia, hypernatremia, hypomagnesemia, hypocalcemia, hypoglycemia, and hyperglycemia [23].

Differential diagnosis and clinical presentation

Differentiation of DTS from epilepsy is challenging. Without any history of a predisposing cause or overdose, few "screening" tests will help to narrow the differential diagnosis. If a seizure patient is suspected of having a drug or toxin as the cause, the clinician must attempt to use all potential historians (family, paramedics, bystanders, coworkers, pharmacy, primary care physician) to provide clues to the possible causative agent. Box 1 contains a list of agents implicated in DTS. On a more lighthearted note, the mnemonic "Otis Campbell" (the town drunk from the Andy Griffith television show) has been used as a teaching tool to recall common causes of DTS (Box 2).

Specific clinical presentations may assist in narrowing the differential diagnosis. A sympathomimetic toxidrome preceding seizure activity may involve cocaine, amphetamines, or drug withdrawal. Patients with a history of foraging for wild plants or mushrooms may have inadvertently ingested water hemlock (ie, *Cicuta douglassi*) or false morel mushrooms (eg, *Gyromitra*). Patients with a psychiatric history may have overdosed from their own psychiatric medications, which could include such agents as antidepressants (ie, cyclic antidepressants, bupropion, and venlafaxine), lithium, or carbamazepine. A history of recent positive purified protein derivative (PPD) skin test or cavitary lesion on chest radiograph may be a clue to INH exposure. A presentation of seizures with an associated widened QRS interval on electrocardiogram may be a clue to cyclic antidepressants, propoxyphene, venlafaxine, diphenhydramine, or other agents (Box 3).

Patients may present with myoclonic activity with or without mental status alteration mimicking seizures. Possible seizure mimics include strychnine [13] and serotonin syndrome [24]. Opioid analgesic overdose traditionally presents with the toxidrome of mental status depression, respiratory depression, and miosis. In addition to the classic toxidrome, the opioids meperidine, tramadol, and propoxyphene may precipitate seizures [25–28]. Additionally, these opioids may produce mydriasis rather than miosis. Severe hypokalemia may be a clue to methylxanthine toxicity.

Discussion of selected agents

Drugs of abuse

A past review of 49 cases of seizures related to recreational drug use between 1975 and 1987 found that 65% were related to cocaine, 22% to amphetamines, 14% to heroin, and 8% to 1-phenylcyclohexyl-piperidine (PCP) [29]. With the emergence of new d esigner drugs of abuse, seizures induced by different agents, such as 3,4-methylenedioxymethamphetamine (MDMA) and gamma hydroxybutyric acid (GHB) are being reported.

Stimulants

Cocaine and the amphetamines increase the release of norepinephrine [30] and serotonin [31]. Hallucinogenic amphetamines (eg, MDMA) may have greater serotonergic effects [31]. Seizures from MDMA may be a result of direct drug effect or may be secondary to hyponatremia. MDMA-induced hyponatremia may be due to a central effect or marked consumption of water at "rave" parties [32]. Cocaine and drugs within the amphetamine family all can produce a sympathomimetic toxidrome and have been associated with seizures [31–33]. Seizures from cocaine intoxication may be mediated by its effects on serotonin receptors [34]. Cocaine body stuffing and packing can result in delayed-onset toxicity and seizures [35]. Treatment should be focused on supportive measures, including intravenous fluids and evaporative cooling for hyperthermia [31]. Liberal doses of benzodiazepines should be considered first-line therapy for the treatment of both the autonomic signs and seizure activity [30,31].

Gamma hydroxybutyric acid

GHB and its precursors (gamma-butyrolactone and 1,4-butanediol) produce a variety of CNS effects, most commonly mental status depression and coma [36]. From its early use as an induction agent for anesthesia, GHB has been noted to cause myoclonic jerking in humans and has been associated with seizures in animal models [36–38].

Abrupt cessation of GHB following chronic abuse has been associated with a profound withdrawal syndrome that includes many features similar

Box 1. Pharmaceuticals and toxins associated with seizures

Analgesics
  Meperidine
  Propoxyphene
  Tramadol
  Salicylates

Anticonvulsants
  Carbamazepine
  Phenytoin

Cellular asphyxiants
  Carbon monoxide
  Cyanide
  Hydrogen sulfide
  Azides

Drugs of abuse
  Cocaine
  Amphetamines
  Phencyclidine
  Gamma-hydroxybutyric acid

Envenomations
  Scorpion
  Elapid

Heavy metals
  Arsenic
  Lead
  Thallium

Plants, herbs, and natural products
  Water hemlock
  Gyromitra esculenta mushroom
  Ephedra
  Nicotine

Psychiatric medications
  Bupropion
  Cyclic antidepressants
  Lithium
  Olanzapine
  Selective serotonin reuptake inhibitors
  Venlafaxine

Rodenticides
Bromethalin
Zinc phosphide

Withdrawal
Ethanol
Sedative-hypnotic
Baclofen

Miscellaneous
Boric acid
Camphor
Diphenhydramine
Fluoride
Isoniazid
Iron
Lidocaine and local anesthetics
Methylxanthines (theophylline, caffeine)
Organochlorine pesticides (dichlorodiphenyltrichloroethane
[DDT], Lindane)
Organophosphates and carbamates
Thujone
Quinine

to ethanol and sedative withdrawal [39,40]. Despite similarities, including sympathomimetic syndrome, tremor, and visual hallucinations, seizures have not been reported [39,41] and were not observed in an animal model of GHB withdrawal [42].

1-Phenylcyclohexyl-piperidine (phencyclidine, PCP)
    PCP and its derivative ketamine are NMDA antagonists that produce a myriad of physical and behavioral effects [32]. Substantial alterations in behavior may include agitation, bizarre actions, hallucinations, and violence [43,44]. Other features of PCP intoxication include nystagmus, hypertension, hyperthermia, rhabdomyolysis, and seizures [44]. One review of 1000 cases of PCP intoxication reported generalized seizures in approximately 3% [44]. However, seizures were not reported in a poison center review of 28 cases of ketamine abuse [45]. Despite being structurally similar to PCP, ketamine may actually have antiepileptic properties and is used by some clinicians for intractable seizures. One animal model of SE using high-dose ketamine [46] and one pediatric case series of nonconvulsive SE [47] demonstrated effective seizure termination with ketamine.

Box 2. Agents that cause seizures

OTIS CAMPBELL[a]
Organophosphates
Tricyclic antidepressants
Isoniazid, insulin
Sympathomimetics
Camphor, cocaine
Amphetamines, anticholinergics
Methylxanthines (theophylline, caffeine)
Phencyclidine (PCP)
Benzodiazepine withdrawal, botanicals (water hemlock)
Ethanol withdrawal
Lithium, lidocaine
Lead, lindane

---

[a] The "town drunk" on *The Andy Griffith Show.*

Withdrawal

Ethanol
   Ethanol withdrawal resembles the sympathomimetic toxidrome and is manifested by agitation, tachycardia, hypertension, hyperthermia, and

---

Box 3. Drugs potentially causing both wide QRS interval and seizures

Amantadine
Bupropion
Carbamazepine
Citalopram
Cocaine
Cyclic antidepressants
Diphenhydramine
Disopyramide
Hydroxychloroquine
Procainamide
Propoxyphene
Quinidine
Quinine
Thioridazine
Venlafaxine

---

seizures [48]. In describing the temporal course of ethanol withdrawal, Victor and Adams [49] found that seizures often preceded autonomic overactivity. Treatment for severe withdrawal and delirium tremens is generally targeted at the autonomic signs, which are often difficult to control. Withdrawal seizures that typically precede autonomic signs and delirium tend not to be protracted. Benzodiazepines are first-line agents to control both withdrawal seizures and autonomic hyperactivity; high doses may be required. Cumulative doses of 2640 mg of diazepam and 2850 mg of midazolam were reported in severe withdrawal cases [50,51]. Intravenous phenobarbital and propofol have been used successfully to treat refractory ethanol withdrawal [52–54].

Sedative hypnotics/flumazenil

Withdrawal from sedative hypnotic medications resembles ethanol withdrawal. Key differences are that withdrawal from sedatives may be delayed or prolonged depending on the pharmacokinetics of the agent [55]. Similarly, the benzodiazepine antagonist flumazenil may induce seizures in selected patient populations. A paper analyzing 43 cases of seizures associated with flumazenil administration found that 47% were due to reversal of benzodiazepines given to control a drug-induced seizure (42% of this group coingested a cyclic antidepressant), 16% were due to reversal of a benzodiazepine given to control a seizure disorder, 12% were due to reversal of a benzodiazepine suppressing non–drug-induced seizures, 7% were due to reversal of chronic benzodiazepine dependence, 5% were due to reversal of benzodiazepines given for procedural sedation, and 14% had no apparent relationship [56]. Based on these data, one author suggests narrowing the potential indications for flumazenil to iatrogenic overdose, pediatric ingestion, or paradoxical response to benzodiazepines [57].

Baclofen

Baclofen is a $GABA_B$ agonist and is used for muscle spasticity [58]. Withdrawal has been noted from both intrathecal pump failure and discontinuation of oral therapy [58–61]. The clinical presentation of baclofen withdrawal is similar to that of ethanol and sedative withdrawal, including autonomic sympathomimetic signs, hallucinations, and seizures. Treatment includes benzodiazepines and the readministration of oral baclofen. However, in those patients experiencing intrathecal pump failure, it is difficult to obtain adequate cerebrospinal fluid concentrations with oral baclofen [58,59]. Dantrolene is reported to reduce muscle spasticity and hyperthermia from refractory baclofen withdrawal due to pump removal [62].

Psychiatric medications

Cyclic antidepressants

Cyclic antidepressants (TCA) have a variety of pharmacologic effects that give rise to several features in overdose. The psychopharmacologic action of

TCA is the inhibition of the reuptake of serotonin and norepinephrine [63]. In addition, TCA are antagonists of histamine (H_1), muscarinic, and alpha (α_1) receptors [63]. In overdose, TCA can produce anticholinergic toxidrome, hypotension, QRS interval prolongation, ventricular arrhythmias, and seizures (see Box 3) [63]. The presence of seizures increases mortality from TCA overdose [64].

Much investigation has been performed to identify surrogate markers for those patients who are at risk for seizures, arrhythmias, and death in TCA overdose. Some authors have suggested that level of consciousness predicts outcome [65,66], whereas others have predicted outcome by investigating TCA serum levels and electrocardiographic markers. In a recent meta-analysis, Bailey and colleagues [67] evaluated the performance of TCA levels and ECG for predicting seizures, arrhythmias, and death. They found the sensitivity and specificity for predicting seizures using QRS were 0.69 and 0.69, respectively, compared with 0.75 and 0.72 using TCA level [67]. Given that the pooled sensitivities and specificities had large confidence intervals and that it is difficult to obtain rapid quantitative TCA levels, the ECG remains a helpful tool to stratify patients at risk. Treatment of severe TCA overdose should include aggressive resuscitation and supportive care, benzodiazepines for seizures, and sodium bicarbonate loading for cardiac toxicity [63]. Beneficial effects of sodium bicarbonate may be due to both elevation of pH and increase in the sodium gradient [68]. Although some authors have suggested a role for phenytoin in cyclic overdoses, animal studies suggest it is helpful neither for seizures nor for ventricular arrythmias [63,69].

Antidepressants: other

The newer classes of antidepressants are thought to be generally safer than TCA in overdose. However, all selective serotonin reuptake inhibitors (SSRI) may be associated with seizures in overdose [70,71]. Among the SSRI, citalopram may have a higher occurrence of seizures in overdose, with a 6% prevalence in one series [72]. Data on other antidepressants that have substantial toxicity in large overdose are emerging.

Bupropion. Bupropion is a unique antidepressant and smoking cessation aid. Its mechanism is not fully understood, but it is thought to inhibit reuptake of dopamine, norepinephrine, and serotonin [73]. Despite being structurally dissimilar to TCA, bupropion has similarities to them in overdose. Of 2424 intentional bupropion exposures, seizures were noted in 15%, compared with less than 1% for unintentional exposures [74]. Conduction delay noted on ECG has been reported in bupropion overdose [74–77] but occurs in only 2% to 3% of symptomatic overdoses (see Box 3) [74,75]. The observed conduction delay does not appear to lead to ventricular arrythmias [75] or to respond to sodium bicarbonate therapy [77].

Venlafaxine. Like bupropion, venlafaxine is a unique class: an inhibitor of norepinephrine and serotonin and, to a lesser extent, dopamine reuptake

[73]. Cardiotoxicity has been reported, including tachycardia, widened QRS, and arrythmias (see Box 3) [78,79]. Two reviews found that venlafaxine had only modest effect on the QRS compared with TCA [72,80]. Seizures, however, are common with venlafaxine, occurring between 8% and 14% in two case series [72,80].

Other psychiatric medications

Antipsychotic agents. The first-generation antipsychotic agents (eg, chlorpromazine) may lower the seizure threshold. Of the "novel" antipsychotic agents, clozapine and olanzapine have been associated with seizures [81,82]. In general, novel antipsychotic agents antagonize serotonin, dopamine, muscarinic, H_1, and α_1 receptors [73]. There is little experience with this class of antipsychotics in overdose. Two case reports of patients with history of seizure disorder and one of a patient without such a history have documented seizures temporally related to the addition of olanzapine [83–85].

Lithium. Lithium continues to be a challenging overdose to manage. Last year there were 5296 exposures and 13 deaths reported to United States poison centers [1]. Despite lithium's having been used for over a century [86], little is known about its pharmacologic mechanism, although it likely has effects on neuronal ion transport and inhibition of reuptake of norepinephrine and serotonin [73]. Features of intoxication include vomiting, tremor and myoclonus, ataxia, mental status changes, and seizures [86,87]. Toxicity may result in persistent neurologic sequelae and usually involves cerebellar dysfunction, including ataxia and dysarthria [88]. No antidotal therapy for lithium intoxication exists, and treatment has hence focused on supportive measures, intravenous hydration and anticonvulsants, gastrointestinal decontamination, and enhanced elimination by means of hemodialysis. Lithium does not significantly adsorb to activated charcoal [86]. Whole bowel irrigation using polyethylene glycol solution may be effective if instituted soon after overdose of a sustained-release preparation [89]. The use of the cation exchange resin polystyrene sulfonate (SPS) has been investigated as a potential modality of reducing lithium concentration. In both animal models [90,91] and humans [92,93], SPS treatment shortened elimination half life and area under the plasma concentration-time curve. However, the use of SPS in lithium intoxication is not universally recommended and carries a theoretic risk for hypokalemia [86]. Controversy exists regarding both the effectiveness of and indications for the use of hemodialysis, especially in chronic intoxication [94]. The decision to institute hemodialysis is complex and should be based on interpretation of serum levels in the context of timing of the overdose (usually 8 to 12 hours postingestion), acute versus chronic intoxication, renal function, and clinical symptomatology [86,94].

Opioids

Propoxyphene
Overdose of propoxyphene results in a clinical presentation similar to that of TCA, including mental status depression, cardiotoxicity, and seizures [95]. Cardiotoxicity may manifest as bradycardia, tachycardia, hypotension, and QRS interval prolongation (see Box 3) [28,95]. In one series of propoxyphene overdoses, seizures were observed in 10% of patients, whereas 48% developed hypotension and approximately 20% exhibited widened QRS [28]. Propoxyphene-induced cardiotoxicity, like that induced by TCA, may be due to myocardial fast sodium channel blockade and is responsive to sodium bicarbonate therapy [96,97].

Tramadol
Tramadol is an analgesic with weak mu-opioid receptor agonist and inhibits serotonin and norepinephrine reuptake [98]. Tramadol has been reported to cause seizures in therapeutic use [99] and overdose [100]. Seizure risk appears to be higher with chronic dosing [99]; however, one case control study cosponsored by McNeil Pharmaceuticals found no increased seizure risk compared with other analgesics [101]. One review of 87 tramadol-only overdoses found the incidence of seizures to be 8% [27]. Naloxone reversed sedation in four of eight patients, with one report of seizure following its use [27].

Meperidine
Meperidine is metabolized by N-demethylation to normeperidine or hydrolysis to meperidinic acid, both of which are renally excreted [26]. Accumulation of normeperidine, either following administration of large doses of meperidine or in persons with renal insufficiency, may lead to myoclonic activity and seizures [25,26].

Natural agents

Water hemlock
Water hemlock (*Cicuta douglasii*), commonly referred to as wild carrot, is profoundly toxic. This plant contains cicutoxin, a neurotoxin that causes seizures [102]. Intractable seizures and death have been reported from even a few bites of the root [102,103]. Other than traditional care, there is no specific antidotal therapy.

Mushrooms
The cytotoxic mushroom *Gyromitra esculenta,* or "false morel," is frequently mistaken for the edible true morel or *Morchella* sp. These mushrooms contain gyromitrins, a family of hydrazines that are metabolized to monomethylhydrazine, which is structurally related to INH and some types of rocket fuel [104]. The pathophysiology of hydrazines is discussed in the INH

section. Ingestion may result in delayed gastrointestinal symptoms, seizures, and hepatic and renal toxicity [105]. Severe intoxications are rare in the United States and occur more frequently in Eastern Europe [1,104].

Ephedra

In December 2003, the US Food and Drug Administration banned an herbal supplement for the first time. Sale of the supplement ephedra (Ma Huang) was banned because of large numbers of reported adverse effects [106]. Haller and Benowitz [107] reviewed adverse events that were either possibly or probably related to the consumption of ephedra and found that seizures occurred in 7% of the events. Other herbal supplements reported to cause seizures include black cohosh, bearberry, kava kava, yohimbe, monkshood, pennyroyal, and guarana [108].

Anticonvulsant overdose

"Paradoxical seizures" from anticonvulsant overdose are uncommon; however, among the anticonvulsants, carbamazepine and phenytoin toxicity appear to induce this clinical phenomenon [109,110]. Valproic acid toxicity produces significant mental status depression and coma, cerebral edema, and hypotension, but seizures are generally not observed [109,111,112].

Heavy metals

Acute exposure to lead, arsenic, and thallium may result in severe toxicity and neurologic manifestations. Each of these metals may be found in a wide array of industries, but lead exposure from the environment is still common [113]. Thallium and arsenic share the distinction of being used for homicidal poisoning [113]. In acute overdose these metals share many similarities in clinical presentation. Symptoms may include severe gastrointestinal symptoms and neurologic manifestations, including confusion, delirium, encephalopathy, and seizures [113,114]. In addition to supportive measures, decontamination with whole bowel irrigation may be helpful when radiopaque material is seen in the gastrointestinal tract [89]. For severe acute toxicity, chelation therapy with dimercaprol (British Anti Lewisite, BAL) for arsenic, BAL/ethylenediaminetetraacetic acid (EDTA) for lead, or Prussian blue for thallium should be instituted [113,115].

Miscellaneous agents

Isoniazid

Like the *Gyromitra* mushroom species discussed above, INH is metabolized to hydrazines. In overdose, these cause a functional pyridoxine (vitamin B6) deficiency by inhibition of pyridoxine phosphokinase, the enzyme that converts pyridoxine to active B6 [116,117]. Activated B6 is required by glutamic acid decarboxylase to convert glutamic acid to GABA.

Decreased levels of GABA are believed to lead to seizures. Severe lactic acidosis may develop as a result of seizure activity. INH also inactivates nicotinamide adenine dinucleotide (NAD) and interferes with NAD synthesis. Decrease in functional NAD inhibits the conversion of lactate to pyruvate, resulting in more profound lactic acidosis [117]. Acute INH overdose is associated with a triad consisting of seizures refractory to conventional therapy, severe metabolic acidosis, and coma [117]. Initial manifestations may include nausea, vomiting, ataxia, tachycardia, mydriasis, and CNS depression, which could mimic an anticholinergic toxidrome [116]. One retrospective chart review evaluated 52 cases of INH overdose and reported associated complications [118]. Seizures were found in 100% of patients, CNS depression in 53%, vomiting in 45%, leukocytosis in 75%, metabolic acidosis in 29%, elevated hepatic enzymes in 21%, and elevated creatine phosphokinase (CPK) in 60% [118].

Activated charcoal readily absorbs INH. When given concomitantly with INH, activated charcoal will diminish toxicity [119]; however, patients often present several hours after ingestion. One study of healthy volunteers found that administration of activated charcoal 1 hour after INH dose resulted in a 20% decrease in area under the plasma concentration-time curve, which was not statistically significant [120]. Benzodiazepines should be first-line agents for seizures [116]. Seizures may be refractory to benzodiazepines, however, because these require the presence of GABA for their anticonvulsant activity. If benzodiazepines are unsuccessful, barbiturates should be used. As soon as INH overdose is suspected or confirmed by history, intravenous (IV) pyridoxine should be administered [116]. Pyridoxine will terminate seizures, possibly reverse coma [121], and improve lactic acidosis. The dose for an unknown ingestion is 5 g IV. When the amount of INH ingested is known, pyridoxine should be given in a dose of 1 g IV for each gram of INH ingested [116,117]. A hospital's supply of IV pyridoxine may be insufficient to treat a significant INH overdose. One study found that approximately 50% of pediatric institutions had less than 5 g of IV pyridoxine available [122].

Methylxanthines

Methylxanthines antagonize adenosine receptors and increase cAMP through inhibition of phosphodiesterase and beta-adrenergic activity [123,124]. Seizures are a frequent sequela of theophylline toxicity and do not appear to be solely due to its effects at the adenosine receptor [123]. Other causes may include depletion of pyridoxine [125] and inhibition of GABA [126]. A large retrospective review of 399 cases of theophylline toxicity (122 cases from overdose) found that the most common clinical effects of theophylline toxicity included nausea and vomiting (79%), tachycardia (75%), hypokalemia (28%), and seizures (27%) [124]. Seizures are less likely to occur with serum levels of less than 60 mg/dL [124], but they have been reported with therapeutic or mildly elevated levels [127].

First-line therapy for seizures should include benzodiazepines or barbiturates. Additionally, because theophylline may affect pyridoxine levels, a rationale may exist for the use of pyridoxine as adjunctive therapy [125]. Phenytoin is not recommended for theophylline-induced seizures. In animal models, phenytoin was not effective treatment [128] and actually lowered seizure threshold in one study [129]. Short-acting beta blockers may also be helpful for the hemodynamic effects of theophylline, even in the face of hypotension [124]. Additional treatment of severe theophylline toxicity should include enhancing its elimination with multidose activated charcoal and hemodialysis [124,130].

Diphenhydramine

Diphenhydramine is an antihistamine (H_1) with anticholinergic and sedating properties [73]. Overdose may produce significant anticholinergic symptoms, QRS prolongation, and seizures [131,132]. One series of 136 diphenhydramine overdoses reported seizures in less than 5% of cases [132].

Local anesthetics

The local anesthetics are associated with cardiotoxicity and neurologic symptoms in overdose. Ropivacaine and bupivacaine probably possess greater cardiotoxicity than lidocaine [133]. Overdose and seizures have been reported from oral administration of viscous lidocaine [134], from large subcutaneous infiltration [135], from IV overdose [136], and in association with the use of bupivacaine for Bier blocks [137,138]. Treatment of local anesthetic toxicity is supportive and includes benzodiazepines for seizures. Phenytoin lowered seizure threshold and increased mortality in an animal model [139]. Another animal study found that propofol was as effective as midazolam for lidocaine-induced seizures [140]. Propofol is an attractive agent for additional study, given that lipid emulsion is a promising experimental treatment for lidocaine-induced cardiotoxicity [141,142].

Organochlorine pesticides

Organochlorine pesticides encompass a diverse group of compounds with various effects on the CNS. Acute toxicities of dichlorodiphenyltrichloroethane (DDT) and hexachlorocyclohexane (Lindane) include seizures [143,144]. Lindane is a commonly used scabicide and pediculicide. It is thought to antagonize $GABA_A$ receptors at the picrotoxin binding site [114]. Neurotoxicity, including uncontrolled psychomotor activity and seizures, has been reported from both topical application [145] and oral ingestion [144]. As a result, Lindane is no longer recommended in children or as a first-line scabicide in adults. Cholestyramine may be an effective agent for gastrointestinal decontamination of Lindane [146]. Treatment of seizures should employ benzodiazepines or barbiturates [144].

Terpenes

Toxicity from terpene hydrocarbons, namely camphor and thujone, may result in seizures [147,148]. Thujone is a constituent of the essential oil of wormwood and is contained in the illicit beverage absinthe [149]. Camphor was previously found in mothballs and is currently used in many over-the-counter rubefacient products [150]. Last year more than 10,000 camphor exposures were reported to United States poison centers, with only 10 major outcomes reported [151]. Mental status depression and seizures are frequently seen even with small ingestions [148,152]. Treatment should focus on airway protection and termination of seizures with benzodiazepines or barbiturates. A rationale may exist for nasogastric aspiration of liquid ingestions for patients presenting early after exposure, but there is no published experience with this approach. Enhanced elimination of camphor with lipid dialysis has been reported but is unlikely to be available [153].

Treatment of drug- and toxin-associated seizures

A rational approach to consider for every patient presenting with a potential toxicologic condition includes attention to airway, breathing, and circulation, focused history and physical examination, rapid glucose determination and ancillary diagnostic testing, gastrointestinal decontamination, enhanced elimination, and specific or antidotal therapy.

When the clinician is faced with a patient seizing from an uncertain cause, the history is of paramount importance, because few drugs or toxins will be easily diagnosed by laboratory testing. When indicated, specific laboratory testing based on history and clinical presentation may be helpful to narrow the differential diagnosis. Distinguishing characteristics of many drug- and toxin-associated seizures are discussed in the earlier section on differential diagnosis and clinical presentation. When managing suspected toxin-induced seizures, it is imperative not to overlook coexisting head injuries, spinal injuries, rhabdomyolysis, infection, or hyperthermia.

By virtue of administering large doses of sedative agents or the presence of refractory seizures, endotracheal intubation may be required for airway protection and ventilation. Neuromuscular blockade will likely be necessary to facilitate intubation. Succinylcholine, despite having favorable kinetics, has drawbacks in regard to increasing potassium and possibly intracranial pressure. Shorter-acting, nondepolarizing agents, such as rocuronium, are preferred [6]. Long-acting neuromuscular blocking agents should be avoided; if they are used, electroencephalographic monitoring should be performed [154].

A large body of literature deals with the treatment of SE. It is difficult to determine whether these treatment strategies will be equally efficacious for DTS. No trials have investigated an optimal anticonvulsant or treatment algorithm for DTS. In general, benzodiazepines followed by barbiturates are the first- and second-line therapies for DTS unless a specific antidote is available. Lorazepam appears to be the preferred agent for SE [6,155]; however, diazepam and midazolam are also appropriate.

Although phenytoin is the second-line agent indicated in the treatment of most causes of seizures, it is usually not efficacious in the management of drug-induced seizures. Phenytoin is not effective for TCA or ethanol withdrawal seizures [63,156,157] and may worsen seizures from theophylline, local anesthetics, and Lindane [128,129,139,144]. IV phenytoin has also been associated with arrhythmias and hypotension, probably owing to the rate of infusion [158].

IV administration of valproic acid is a new strategy for SE [159,160], but its role in DTS remains to be evaluated. Reports of hemodynamic compromise in pediatric patients exist [161,162], but other studies have reported no hemodynamic effects even with large doses [160]; valproic acid did not alter blood pressure in a group already on vasopressors for hypotension [163]. IV dosing for various anticonvulsants is listed in Table 1.

Much controversy exists in the area of gastrointestinal decontamination; no one modality is universally recommended. Patients presenting with seizures or with the anticipation of seizures introduce additional potential for morbidity, especially in regard to airway protection and aspiration. Patients being considered for gastrointestinal decontamination procedures should either be alert with intact protective airway reflexes or have their airway secured by cuffed endotracheal intubation if obtunded. In general, it is not recommended to intubate patients solely for the purpose of performing gastrointestinal decontamination procedures; the decision should be based on the clinical status of the patient.

Table 1
Intravenous anticonvulsant dosing

Anticonvulsant	Loading dose (mg/kg)	Comments
Benzodiazepines		
Diazepam	Titrate up to 0.15 mg/kg	Onset: 1–5 min
Lorazepam	Titrate up to 0.1 mg/kg	Onset: 5 min
Midazolam	Titrate up to 0.2 mg/kg	Onset: 1–5 min
Other agents		
Phenobarbital	15–20 mg/kg	Loading infusion rate: 50–75 mg/min
Phenytoin[a]	15–20 mg/kg	Loading infusion rate: 50 mg/min
Propofol	3–5 mg/kg	Maintenance infusion: 30–100 mcg/kg/min
Valproic acid	15–25 mg/kg	Loading infusion rate: 20–50 mg/min (up to 6 mg/kg/min)
Pyridoxine		Pyridoxine dose should equal estimated INH dose
		If amount is unknown, 5 g should be administered

With all sedatives, larger doses may be needed to control-status seizures, and endotracheal intubation may be required for airway protection and ventilation.

[a] Phenytoin is generally not expected to be helpful for drug and toxin-induced seizures and may cause harm (see text for details) [129].

Table 2
Agents that may require specific therapy in addition to common therapy

Therapy	Agent
Atropine/pralidoxime	Organophosphate insecticides and nerve agents
BAL/EDTA	Lead and arsenic
Prussian blue	Thallium
Dextrose	Insulin, sulfonylurea, or other hypoglycemic agent
Hemodialysis	Lithium, theophylline, salicylates
Hyperbaric oxygen	Carbon monoxide
Octreotide	Sulfonylurea
Pyridoxine	INH, *Gyrometria* mushrooms, hydrazines, theophylline

Activated charcoal may be considered at a dose of 1 g/kg for agents that are known to adsorb to it. The airway must be intact to reduce the likelihood of aspiration. Whole bowel irrigation may be considered for body stuffers, body packers, heavy metals, or large ingestions of sustained-release preparations. It cannot be recommended for patients who are actively seizing, who have hemodynamic instability, or who have an ileus. Multidose activated charcoal may be useful for enhancing the elimination of methylxanthines or carbamazepine [130]. Hemodialysis is useful for enhancing the elimination of lithium, methylxanthines, and salicylates. Directed or antidotal therapy is discussed in individual drug or toxin headings and is summarized in Table 2.

Summary

Drug- and toxin-associated seizures may result from exposure to a wide variety of agents. Obtaining a comprehensive history behind the exposure is generally more helpful than diagnostic testing. Most DTS may be managed with supportive care, including benzodiazepines, except in the case of agents that require a specific intervention or antidote.

References

[1] American Association of Poison Control Centers. Toxic Exposure Surveillance System. Available at: http://www.aapcc.org. Accessed November 2004.
[2] DeLorenzo RJ, Hauser WA, Towne AR, et al. A prospective, population-based epidemiologic study of status epilepticus in Richmond, Virginia. Neurology 1996;46(4): 1029–35.
[3] Olson KR, Kearney TE, Dyer JE, et al. Seizures associated with poisoning and drug overdose. Am J Emerg Med 1994;12(3):392–5.
[4] Thundiyil JGKT, Olson KR. Evolving epidemiology of drug-induced seizures reported to a poison control center system. J Toxicol Clin Toxicol 2004;42(5):730.
[5] Lowenstein DH, Bleck T, Macdonald RL. It's time to revise the definition of status epilepticus. Epilepsia 1999;40(1):120–2.
[6] Marik PE, Varon J. The management of status epilepticus. Chest 2004;126(2):582–91.

[7] Loscher W. Pharmacology of glutamate receptor antagonists in the kindling model of epilepsy. Prog Neurobiol 1998;54(6):721–41.

[8] Fountain NB, Lothman EW. Pathophysiology of status epilepticus. J Clin Neurophysiol 1995;12(4):326–42.

[9] Cohen PG. The metabolic basis for the genesis of seizures: the role of the potassium-ammonia axis. Med Hypotheses 1984;13(3):311–6.

[10] Dyer JE, Roth B, Hyma BA. Gamma-hydroxybutyrate withdrawal syndrome. Ann Emerg Med 2001;37(2):147–53.

[11] Morimoto K, Fahnestock M, Racine RJ. Kindling and status epilepticus models of epilepsy: rewiring the brain. Prog Neurobiol 2004;73(1):1–60.

[12] Teitelbaum JS, Zatorre RJ, Carpenter S, et al. Neurologic sequelae of domoic acid intoxication due to the ingestion of contaminated mussels. N Engl J Med 1990;322(25): 1781–7.

[13] Shadnia S, Moiensadat M, Abdollahi M. A case of acute strychnine poisoning. Vet Hum Toxicol 2004;46(2):76–9.

[14] Walker IA, Slovis CM. Lidocaine in the treatment of status epilepticus. Acad Emerg Med 1997;4(9):918–22.

[15] Marley RJ, Witkin JM, Goldberg SR. A pharmacogenetic evaluation of the role of local anesthetic actions in the cocaine kindling process. Brain Res 1991;562(2):251–7.

[16] Derlet RW, Albertson TE, Tharratt RS. Lidocaine potentiation of cocaine toxicity. Ann Emerg Med 1991;20(2):135–8.

[17] Linnoila M, Mefford I, Nutt D, et al. NIH conference. Alcohol withdrawal and noradrenergic function. Ann Intern Med 1987;107(6):875–89.

[18] Tuovinen K. Organophosphate-induced convulsions and prevention of neuropathological damages. Toxicology 2004;196(1–2):31–9.

[19] Fredholm BB, IJzerman AP, Jacobson KA, et al. International Union of Pharmacology. XXV. Nomenclature and classification of adenosine receptors. Pharmacol Rev 2001;53(4): 527–52.

[20] Etherington LA, Frenguelli BG. Endogenous adenosine modulates epileptiform activity in rat hippocampus in a receptor subtype–dependent manner. Eur J Neurosci 2004;19(9): 2539–50.

[21] Yokoyama H, Sato M, Iinuma K, et al. Centrally acting histamine H1 antagonists promote the development of amygdala kindling in rats. Neurosci Lett 1996;217(2–3):194–6.

[22] Kamei C, Ohuchi M, Sugimoto Y, et al. Mechanism responsible for epileptogenic activity by first-generation H1-antagonists in rats. Brain Res 2000;887(1):183–6.

[23] Delanty N, Vaughan CJ, French JA. Medical causes of seizures. Lancet 1998;352(9125): 383–90.

[24] Carbone JR. The neuroleptic malignant and serotonin syndromes. Emerg Med Clin North Am 2000;18(2):317–25, x.

[25] Knight B, Thomson N, Perry G. Seizures due to norpethidine toxicity. Aust N Z J Med 2000;30(4):513.

[26] Armstrong PJ, Bersten A. Normeperidine toxicity. Anesth Analg 1986;65(5):536–8.

[27] Spiller HA, Gorman SE, Villalobos D, et al. Prospective multicenter evaluation of tramadol exposure. J Toxicol Clin Toxicol 1997;35(4):361–4.

[28] Sloth Madsen P, Strom J, Reiz S, et al. Acute propoxyphene self-poisoning in 222 consecutive patients. Acta Anaesthesiol Scand 1984;28(6):661–5.

[29] Alldredge BK, Lowenstein DH, Simon RP. Seizures associated with recreational drug abuse. Neurology 1989;39(8):1037–9.

[30] Spivey WH, Euerle B. Neurologic complications of cocaine abuse. Ann Emerg Med 1990; 19(12):1422–8.

[31] Graeme KA. New drugs of abuse. Emerg Med Clin North Am 2000;18(4):625–36.

[32] Freese TE, Miotto K, Reback CJ. The effects and consequences of selected club drugs. J Subst Abuse Treat 2002;23(2):151–6.

[33] Koppel BS, Samkoff L, Daras M. Relation of cocaine use to seizures and epilepsy. Epilepsia 1996;37(9):875–8.

[34] O'Dell LE, Kreifeldt MJ, George FR, et al. The role of serotonin(2) receptors in mediating cocaine-induced convulsions. Pharmacol Biochem Behav 2000;65(4):677–81.

[35] Yao ICMS, O'Koren K, Guffey MA, et al. Delayed onset of seizure in a body stuffer. J Toxicol Clin Toxicol 2003;41(5):650.

[36] Mason PE, Kerns WP II. Gamma hydroxybutyric acid (GHB) intoxication. Acad Emerg Med 2002;9(7):730–9.

[37] Hu RQ, Cortez MA, Man HY, et al. Gamma-hydroxybutyric acid–induced absence seizures in GluR2 null mutant mice. Brain Res 2001;897(1–2):27–35.

[38] Hu RQ, Cortez MA, Man HY, et al. Alteration of GLUR2 expression in the rat brain following absence seizures induced by gamma-hydroxybutyric acid. Epilepsy Res 2001; 44(1):41–51.

[39] Craig K, Gomez HF, McManus JL, et al. Severe gamma-hydroxybutyrate withdrawal: a case report and literature review. J Emerg Med 2000;18(1):65–70.

[40] Mycyk MB, Wilemon C, Aks SE. Two cases of withdrawal from 1,4-Butanediol use. Ann Emerg Med 2001;38(3):345–6.

[41] McDonough M, Kennedy N, Glasper A, et al. Clinical features and management of gamma-hydroxybutyrate (GHB) withdrawal: a review. Drug Alcohol Depend 2004;75(1): 3–9.

[42] Bania TC, Ashar T, Press G, et al. Gamma-hydroxybutyric acid tolerance and withdrawal in a rat model. Acad Emerg Med 2003;10(7):697–704.

[43] Barton CH, Sterling ML, Vaziri ND. Phencyclidine intoxication: clinical experience in 27 cases confirmed by urine assay. Ann Emerg Med 1981;10(5):243–6.

[44] McCarron MM, Schulze BW, Thompson GA, et al. Acute phencyclidine intoxication: incidence of clinical findings in 1,000 cases. Ann Emerg Med 1981;10(5):237–42.

[45] Vieira L, Weiner A. Ketamine abusers presenting to the emergency department: a case series. J Toxicol Clin Toxicol 1998;36(5):505.

[46] Borris DJ, Bertram EH, Kapur J. Ketamine controls prolonged status epilepticus. Epilepsy Res 2000;42(2–3):117–22.

[47] Mewasingh LD, Sekhara T, Aeby A, et al. Oral ketamine in paediatric non-convulsive status epilepticus. Seizure 2003;12(7):483–9.

[48] Isbell HFH, Wikler A, Belleville RE, et al. An experimental study of the etiology of "rum fits" and delirium tremens. Q J Stud Alcohol 1955;16:1–33.

[49] Victor M, Adams RD. The effect of alcohol on the nervous system. Res Publ Assoc Res Nerv Ment Dis 1953;32:526–73.

[50] Nolop KB, Natow A. Unprecedented sedative requirements during delirium tremens. Crit Care Med 1985;13(4):246–7.

[51] Lineaweaver WC, Anderson K, Hing DN. Massive doses of midazolam infusion for delirium tremens without respiratory depression. Crit Care Med 1988;16(3):294–5.

[52] Coomes TR, Smith SW. Successful use of propofol in refractory delirium tremens. Ann Emerg Med 1997;30(6):825–8.

[53] McCowan C, Marik P. Refractory delirium tremens treated with propofol: a case series. Crit Care Med 2000;28(6):1781–4.

[54] Young GP, Rores C, Murphy C, et al. Intravenous phenobarbital for alcohol withdrawal and convulsions. Ann Emerg Med 1987;16(8):847–50.

[55] Petursson H. The benzodiazepine withdrawal syndrome. Addiction 1994;89(11):1455–9.

[56] Spivey WH. Flumazenil and seizures: analysis of 43 cases. Clin Ther 1992;14(2):292–305.

[57] Seger DL. Flumazenil—treatment or toxin. J Toxicol Clin Toxicol 2004;42(2):209–16.

[58] Greenberg MI, Hendrickson RG. Baclofen withdrawal following removal of an intrathecal baclofen pump despite oral baclofen replacement. J Toxicol Clin Toxicol 2003;41(1):83–5.

[59] Green LB, Nelson VS. Death after acute withdrawal of intrathecal baclofen: case report and literature review. Arch Phys Med Rehabil 1999;80(12):1600–4.

[60] Peng CT, Ger J, Yang CC, et al. Prolonged severe withdrawal symptoms after acute-on-chronic baclofen overdose. J Toxicol Clin Toxicol 1998;36(4):359–63.

[61] Kofler M, Arturo Leis A. Prolonged seizure activity after baclofen withdrawal. Neurology 1992;42(3 Pt 1):697–8.

[62] Khorasani A, Peruzzi WT. Dantrolene treatment for abrupt intrathecal baclofen withdrawal. Anesth Analg 1995;80(5):1054–6.

[63] Pimentel L, Trommer L. Cyclic antidepressant overdoses. A review. Emerg Med Clin North Am 1994;12(2):533–47.

[64] Frommer DA, Kulig KW, Marx JA, et al. Tricyclic antidepressant overdose. A review. JAMA 1987;257(4):521–6.

[65] Hulten BA, Adams R, Askenasi R, et al. Predicting severity of tricyclic antidepressant overdose. J Toxicol Clin Toxicol 1992;30(2):161–70.

[66] Emerman CL, Connors AF Jr, Burma GM. Level of consciousness as a predictor of complications following tricyclic overdose. Ann Emerg Med 1987;16(3):326–30.

[67] Bailey B, Buckley NA, Amre DKA. Meta-analysis of prognostic indicators to predict seizures, arrhythmias or death after tricyclic antidepressant overdose. J Toxicol Clin Toxicol 2004;42(6):877–88.

[68] McCabe JL, Cobaugh DJ, Menegazzi JJ, et al. Experimental tricyclic antidepressant toxicity: a randomized, controlled comparison of hypertonic saline solution, sodium bicarbonate, and hyperventilation. Ann Emerg Med 1998;32(3 Pt 1):329–33.

[69] Callaham M, Schumaker H, Pentel P. Phenytoin prophylaxis of cardiotoxicity in experimental amitriptyline poisoning. J Pharmacol Exp Ther 1988;245(1):216–20.

[70] Isbister GK, Bowe SJ, Dawson A, et al. Relative toxicity of selective serotonin reuptake inhibitors (SSRIs) in overdose. J Toxicol Clin Toxicol 2004;42(3):277–85.

[71] Raju GV, Kumar TC, Khanna S. Seizures associated with sertraline. Can J Psychiatry 2000; 45(5):491.

[72] Kelly CA, Dhaun N, Laing WJ, et al. Comparative toxicity of citalopram and the newer antidepressants after overdose. J Toxicol Clin Toxicol 2004;42(1):67–71.

[73] Fuller MA. Drug information handbook for psychiatry. 3rd edition. Husdon (OH): Lexi-Comp; 2002.

[74] Belson MG, Kelley TR. Bupropion exposures: clinical manifestations and medical outcome. J Emerg Med 2002;23(3):223–30.

[75] Druteika D, Zed PJ. Cardiotoxicity following bupropion overdose. Ann Pharmacother 2002;36(11):1791–5.

[76] Paris PA, Saucier JR. ECG conduction delays associated with massive bupropion overdose. J Toxicol Clin Toxicol 1998;36(6):595–8.

[77] Wills BKM, Aks S. QRS prolongation associated with bupropion ingestion. J Toxicol Clin Toxicol 2004;42(5):724.

[78] Blythe D, Hackett LP. Cardiovascular and neurological toxicity of venlafaxine. Hum Exp Toxicol 1999;18(5):309–13.

[79] Cumpston KCM, Pallasch E. Massive venlafaxine overdose resulting in arrhythmogenic death. J Toxicol Clin Toxicol 2003;41(5):659.

[80] Whyte IM, Dawson AH, Buckley NA. Relative toxicity of venlafaxine and selective serotonin reuptake inhibitors in overdose compared to tricyclic antidepressants. QJM 2003; 96(5):369–74.

[81] Hedges D, Jeppson K, Whitehead P. Antipsychotic medication and seizures: a review. Drugs Today (Barc) 2003;39(7):551–7.

[82] Lee KC, Finley PR, Alldredge BK. Risk of seizures associated with psychotropic medications: emphasis on new drugs and new findings. Expert Opin Drug Saf 2003;2(3): 233–47.

[83] Lee JW, Crismon ML, Dorson PG. Seizure associated with olanzapine. Ann Pharmacother 1999;33(5):554–6.

[84] Woolley J, Smith S. Lowered seizure threshold on olanzapine. Br J Psychiatry 2001;178(1): 85–6.

[85] Wyderski RJ, Starrett WG, Abou-Saif A. Fatal status epilepticus associated with olanzapine therapy. Ann Pharmacother 1999;33(7–8):787–9.

[86] Timmer RT, Sands JM. Lithium intoxication. J Am Soc Nephrol 1999;10(3):666–74.

[87] Amdisen A. Clinical features and management of lithium poisoning. Med Toxicol Adverse Drug Exp 1988;3(1):18–32.

[88] Kores B, Lader MH. Irreversible lithium neurotoxicity: an overview. Clin Neuropharmacol 1997;20(4):283–99.

[89] Position paper. Whole bowel irrigation. J Toxicol Clin Toxicol 2004;42(6):843–54.

[90] Linakis JG, Savitt DL, Wu TY, et al. Use of sodium polystyrene sulfonate for reduction of plasma lithium concentrations after chronic lithium dosing in mice. J Toxicol Clin Toxicol 1998;36(4):309–13.

[91] Linakis JG, Eisenberg MS, Lacouture PG, et al. Multiple-dose sodium polystyrene sulfonate in lithium intoxication: an animal model. Pharmacol Toxicol 1992;70(1): 38–40.

[92] Roberge RJ, Martin TG, Schneider SM. Use of sodium polystyrene sulfonate in a lithium overdose. Ann Emerg Med 1993;22(12):1911–5.

[93] Gehrke JC, Watling SM, Gehrke CW, et al. In-vivo binding of lithium using the cation exchange resin sodium polystyrene sulfonate. Am J Emerg Med 1996;14(1):37–8.

[94] Jaeger A, Sauder P, Kopferschmitt J, et al. When should dialysis be performed in lithium poisoning? A kinetic study in 14 cases of lithium poisoning. J Toxicol Clin Toxicol 1993; 31(3):429–47.

[95] Lawson AA, Northridge DB. Dextropropoxyphene overdose. Epidemiology, clinical presentation and management. Med Toxicol Adverse Drug Exp 1987;2(6):430–44.

[96] Stork CM, Redd JT, Fine K, et al. Propoxyphene-induced wide QRS complex dysrhythmia responsive to sodium bicarbonate—a case report. J Toxicol Clin Toxicol 1995;33(2): 179–83.

[97] Whitcomb DC, Gilliam FR III, Starmer CF, et al. Marked QRS complex abnormalities and sodium channel blockade by propoxyphene reversed with lidocaine. J Clin Invest 1989; 84(5):1629–36.

[98] Potschka H, Friderichs E, Loscher W. Anticonvulsant and proconvulsant effects of tramadol, its enantiomers and its M1 metabolite in the rat kindling model of epilepsy. Br J Pharmacol 2000;131(2):203–12.

[99] Gardner JS, Blough D, Drinkard CR, et al. Tramadol and seizures: a surveillance study in a managed care population. Pharmacotherapy 2000;20(12):1423–31.

[100] Tobias JD. Seizure after overdose of tramadol. South Med J 1997;90(8):826–7.

[101] Gasse C, Derby L, Vasilakis-Scaramozza C, et al. Incidence of first-time idiopathic seizures in users of tramadol. Pharmacotherapy 2000;20(6):629–34.

[102] From the Centers for Disease Control and Prevention. Water hemlock poisoning—Maine, 1992. JAMA 1994;271(19):1475.

[103] Heath KB. A fatal case of apparent water hemlock poisoning. Vet Hum Toxicol 2001;43(1): 35–6.

[104] Michelot D, Toth B. Poisoning by Gyromitra esculenta—a review. J Appl Toxicol 1991; 11(4):235–43.

[105] Karlson-Stiber C, Persson H. Cytotoxic fungi—an overview. Toxicon 2003;42(4):339–49.

[106] US Food and Drug Administration. Consumer alert for ephedrine alkaloids. Available at: http://www.fda.gov. Accessed November 2004.

[107] Haller CA, Benowitz NL. Adverse cardiovascular and central nervous system events associated with dietary supplements containing ephedra alkaloids. N Engl J Med 2000; 343(25):1833–8.

[108] Tyagi A, Delanty N. Herbal remedies, dietary supplements, and seizures. Epilepsia 2003; 44(2):228–35.

[109] Perucca E, Gram L, Avanzini G, et al. Antiepileptic drugs as a cause of worsening seizures. Epilepsia 1998;39(1):5–17.

[110] Spiller HA, Carlisle RD. Status epilepticus after massive carbamazepine overdose. J Toxicol Clin Toxicol 2002;40(1):81–90.

[111] Sztajnkrycer MD. Valproic acid toxicity: overview and management. J Toxicol Clin Toxicol 2002;40(6):789–801.

[112] Singh SM, McCormick BB, Mustata S, et al. Extracorporeal management of valproic acid overdose: a large regional experience. J Nephrol 2004;17(1):43–9.

[113] Sullivan J, Krieger G. Clinical environmental health and toxic exposures. 2nd edition. Philadelphia: Lippincott Williams & Wilkins; 2001.

[114] Toxicologic profiles ATSDR. Available at: http://www.atsdr.cdc.gov/toxprofiles. Accessed November 2004.

[115] Hoffman RS. Thallium toxicity and the role of Prussian blue in therapy. Toxicol Rev 2003; 22(1):29–40.

[116] Alvarez FG, Guntupalli KK. Isoniazid overdose: four case reports and review of the literature. Intensive Care Med 1995;21(8):641–4.

[117] Boyer E. Goldfrank's toxicologic emergencies. 7th edition. New York: McGraw-Hill; 2002.

[118] Panganiban LR, Makalinao IR, Corte-Maramba NP. Rhabdomyolysis in isoniazid poisoning. J Toxicol Clin Toxicol 2001;39(2):143–51.

[119] Siefkin AD, Albertson TE, Corbett MG. Isoniazid overdose: pharmacokinetics and effects of oral charcoal in treatment. Hum Toxicol 1987;6(6):497–501.

[120] Scolding N, Ward MJ, Hutchings A, et al. Charcoal and isoniazid pharmacokinetics. Hum Toxicol 1986;5(4):285–6.

[121] Brent J, Vo N, Kulig K, et al. Reversal of prolonged isoniazid-induced coma by pyridoxine. Arch Intern Med 1990;150(8):1751–3.

[122] Santucci KA, Shah BR, Linakis JG. Acute isoniazid exposures and antidote availability. Pediatr Emerg Care 1999;15(2):99–101.

[123] Hornfeldt CS, Larson AA. Adenosine receptors are not involved in theophylline-induced seizures. J Toxicol Clin Toxicol 1994;32(3):257–65.

[124] Paloucek FP, Rodvold KA. Evaluation of theophylline overdoses and toxicities. Ann Emerg Med 1988;17(2):135–44.

[125] Glenn GM, Krober MS, Kelly P, et al. Pyridoxine as therapy in theophylline-induced seizures. Vet Hum Toxicol 1995;37(4):342–5.

[126] Sugimoto T, Sugimoto M, Uchida I, et al. Inhibitory effect of theophylline on recombinant GABA(A) receptor. Neuroreport 2001;12(3):489–93.

[127] Bahls FH, Ma KK, Bird TD. Theophylline-associated seizures with "therapeutic" or low toxic serum concentrations: risk factors for serious outcome in adults. Neurology 1991; 41(8):1309–12.

[128] Hoffman A, Pinto E, Gilhar D. Effect of pretreatment with anticonvulsants on theophylline-induced seizures in the rat. J Crit Care 1993;8(4):198–202.

[129] Blake KV, Massey KL, Hendeles L, et al. Relative efficacy of phenytoin and phenobarbital for the prevention of theophylline-induced seizures in mice. Ann Emerg Med 1988;17(10): 1024–8.

[130] Position statement and practice guidelines on the use of multi-dose activated charcoal in the treatment of acute poisoning. American Academy of Clinical Toxicology; European Association of Poisons Centres and Clinical Toxicologists. J Toxicol Clin Toxicol 1999; 37(6):731–51.

[131] Goetz CM, Lopez G, Dean BS, et al. Accidental childhood death from diphenhydramine overdosage. Am J Emerg Med 1990;8(4):321–2.

[132] Koppel C, Ibe K, Tenczer J. Clinical symptomatology of diphenhydramine overdose: an evaluation of 136 cases in 1982 to 1985. J Toxicol Clin Toxicol 1987;25(1–2):53–70.

[133] Feldman HS, Arthur GR, Covino BG. Comparative systemic toxicity of convulsant and supraconvulsant doses of intravenous ropivacaine, bupivacaine, and lidocaine in the conscious dog. Anesth Analg 1989;69(6):794–801.

[134] Smith M, Wolfram W, Rose R. Toxicity-seizures in an infant caused by (or related to) oral viscous lidocaine use. J Emerg Med 1992;10(5):587–90.

[135] Ryan CA, Robertson M, Coe JY. Seizures due to lidocaine toxicity in a child during cardiac catheterization. Pediatr Cardiol 1993;14(2):116–8.

[136] Jonville AP, Barbier P, Blond MH, et al. Accidental lidocaine overdosage in an infant. J Toxicol Clin Toxicol 1990;28(1):101–6.

[137] Rosenberg PH, Kalso EA, Tuominen MK, et al. Acute bupivacaine toxicity as a result of venous leakage under the tourniquet cuff during a Bier block. Anesthesiology 1983;58(1): 95–8.

[138] Arai T, Kuzume K. Bupivicaine toxicity and Bier blocks. Anesthesiology 1983;59(5):481.

[139] Sawaki K, Ohno K, Miyamoto K, et al. Effects of anticonvulsants on local anaesthetic-induced neurotoxicity in rats. Pharmacol Toxicol 2000;86(2):59–62.

[140] Momota Y, Artru AA, Powers KM, et al. Posttreatment with propofol terminates lidocaine-induced epileptiform electroencephalogram activity in rabbits: effects on cerebrospinal fluid dynamics. Anesth Analg 1998;87(4):900–6.

[141] Weinberg G, Ripper R, Feinstein DL, et al. Lipid emulsion infusion rescues dogs from bupivacaine-induced cardiac toxicity. Reg Anesth Pain Med 2003;28(3):198–202.

[142] Weinberg GL, VadeBoncoeur T, Ramaraju GA, et al. Pretreatment or resuscitation with a lipid infusion shifts the dose-response to bupivacaine-induced asystole in rats. Anesthesiology 1998;88(4):1071–5.

[143] Ozucelik DN, Karcioglu O, Topacoglu H, et al. Toxicity following unintentional DDT ingestion. J Toxicol Clin Toxicol 2004;42(3):299–303.

[144] Aks SE, Krantz A, Hryhrczuk DO, et al. Acute accidental lindane ingestion in toddlers. Ann Emerg Med 1995;26(5):647–51.

[145] Fischer TF. Lindane toxicity in a 24-year-old woman. Ann Emerg Med 1994;24(5):972–4.

[146] Kassner JT, Maher TJ, Hull KM, et al. Cholestyramine as an adsorbent in acute lindane poisoning: a murine model. Ann Emerg Med 1993;22(9):1392–7.

[147] Burkhard PR, Burkhardt K, Haenggeli CA, et al. Plant-induced seizures: reappearance of an old problem. J Neurol 1999;246(8):667–70.

[148] Phelan WJ III. Camphor poisoning: over-the-counter dangers. Pediatrics 1976;57(3): 428–31.

[149] Strang J, Arnold WN, Peters T. Absinthe: what's your poison? Though absinthe is intriguing, it is alcohol in general we should worry about. BMJ 1999;319(7225):1590–2.

[150] Micromedex Healthcare Series. Poisindex. Available at: http://www.micromedex.com. Accessed November 2004.

[151] Watson WA, Litovitz TL, Klein-Schwartz W, et al. 2003 annual report of the American Association of Poison Control Centers Toxic Exposure Surveillance System. Am J Emerg Med 2004;22(5):335–404.

[152] Trestrail JH III, Spartz ME. Camphorated and castor oil confusion and its toxic results. Clin Toxicol 1977;11(2):151–8.

[153] Ginn HE, Anderson KE, Mercier RK, et al. Camphor intoxication treated by lipid dialysis. JAMA 1968;203(3):230–1.

[154] ACEP Clinical Policies Committee. Clinical Policies Subcommittee on Seizures. Clinical policy: critical issues in the evaluation and management of adult patients presenting to the emergency department with seizures. Ann Emerg Med 2004;43(5):605–25.

[155] Alldredge BK, Gelb AM, Isaacs SM, et al. A comparison of lorazepam, diazepam, and placebo for the treatment of out-of-hospital status epilepticus. N Engl J Med 2001;345(9): 631–7.

[156] Alldredge BK, Lowenstein DH, Simon RP. Placebo-controlled trial of intravenous diphenylhydantoin for short-term treatment of alcohol withdrawal seizures. Am J Med 1989;87(6):645–8.

[157] Chance JF. Emergency department treatment of alcohol withdrawal seizures with phenytoin. Ann Emerg Med 1991;20(5):520–2.

[158] Earnest MP, Marx JA, Drury LR. Complications of intravenous phenytoin for acute treatment of seizures. Recommendations for usage. JAMA 1983;249(6):762–5.

[159] Hodges BM, Mazur JE. Intravenous valproate in status epilepticus. Ann Pharmacother 2001;35(11):1465–70.

[160] Yu KT, Mills S, Thompson N, et al. Safety and efficacy of intravenous valproate in pediatric status epilepticus and acute repetitive seizures. Epilepsia 2003;44(5):724–6.

[161] Kumar P, Vallis CJ, Hall CM. Intravenous valproate associated with circulatory collapse. Ann Pharmacother 2003;37(12):1797–9.

[162] White JR, Santos CS. Intravenous valproate associated with significant hypotension in the treatment of status epilepticus. J Child Neurol 1999;14(12):822–3.

[163] Sinha S, Naritoku DK. Intravenous valproate is well tolerated in unstable patients with status epilepticus. Neurology 2000;55(5):722–4.

CLINICS IN
LABORATORY
MEDICINE

Clin Lab Med 26 (2006) 211–226

Brown Recluse Spider Envenomation

R. Brent Furbee, MD, FACMT*, Louise W. Kao, MD, Danyal Ibrahim, MD

Department of Emergency Medicine, Indiana University School of Medicine, Room AG373, 1701 North Senate Boulevard, Indianapolis, IN 46206, USA

Willis Caveness [1] is credited with the first account of toxicity from *Loxosceles reclusa* in 1872 involving a Tennessee man with fever following an insect bite. It was not until 1929 that Schmaus [2] described skin injury associated with the bite. In 1957, Atkins and colleagues [3] proposed that the bite of *L reclusa* caused skin necrosis similar to that of its South American relative *L laeta.* "...[I]t is not unduly presumptive tentatively to assign to *L reclusus* the same relationship with cutaneous arachnoidism [*sic*] in Missouri that *L laeta* bears to that condition in South America" [3]. From the beginning, the diagnosis of brown recluse spider bite was based on supposition much more than fact.

The spider

Of the genus *Loxosceles, L reclusa,* commonly known as the brown recluse spider (BRS), is one of nearly 50 related species endemic to the Unites States and 100 species throughout the world. It first was described in 1940 by Gersch [4]. Other species, such as *L laeta, L gaucho,* and *L intermedia,* long have been reported to cause cutaneous and systemic injury in South America. In the United States, *L reclusa* is found in the south from western Florida to the eastern third of Texas and ranges as far north as northern Illinois and southern Iowa (Fig. 1). Southern California and southwest Arizona are home to *L deserta.* Several less known species reside from southwest Texas to the southern half of Arizona, and *L rufescens* is found along the Gulf of Mexico [5].

Brown recluse, also known as fiddleback spiders, are noted for the violin-shaped marking on the cephalothorax (Fig. 2), though some immature spiders

---

* Corresponding author.
E-mail address: bfurbee@clarian.org (R.B. Furbee).

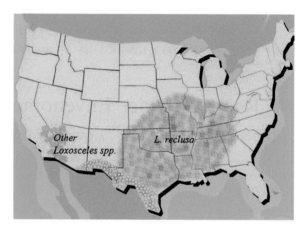

Fig. 1. Reported distribution of *L spp.* in the United States.

may not display that hallmark [5]. Their color ranges from yellow-brown to gray-brown. The adult's leg span is approximately 5 cm with body length of 6 to 11 mm. A helpful identifying feature is the presence of six eyes arranged in three pairs (dyads) as opposed to the more common eight eyes found in most spiders. Although not limited to *L spp.*, the number of eyes can be viewed under a microscope to aid in identification (Fig. 3). Legs are long in comparison to body length and have spiked hairs.

BRS may be found indoors or out. They prefer undisturbed areas, such as boxes or furniture in garages or basements. They are nocturnal and avoid areas of human and other animal activity. BRSs generally are nonaggressive and prefer dead prey [6]. Bites typically are defensive and usually occur when the spider is trapped against clothing or bedding. Contrary to popular belief, *Loxosceles* species do not predate human beings. In fact, Vetter and Barger [7] reported on a house infested with *L reclusa*, identifying more than

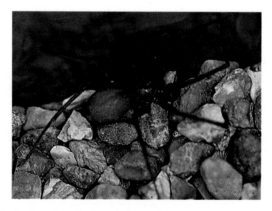

Fig. 2. *L reclusa* displays violin marking on the cephalothorax.

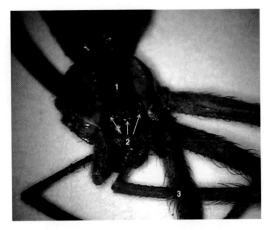

Fig. 3. *L reclusa* displays classic violin markings on the cephalothorax (*1*), three pairs of eyes (*2*), and hairy legs (*3*). Note several legs are missing.

2000 spiders in a 6-month period without a single known human bite during that time.

The bite

The necrotizing bite of the BRS has been studied intensively. Loxoscelism, necrotic arachnidism, or gangrenocutaneous arachnidism has been used to describe the clinical effects of BRS envenomation and includes the necrotizing lesion and systemic effects, such as fever, chills, rash, joint pains, and hemolysis [8].

Cutaneous effects from confirmed bites usually are found under clothing and on the thigh, lateral torso, or upper arm. Confirmed bites are defined as bites associated with a captured or recovered spider found in close proximity to the bite and correctly identified by a qualified person. They are uncommon on the neck and rare on the hands, feet, or face [9]. Erythema, burning pain, pruritus, and swelling may develop within a few hours of the bite. Less commonly, a hemorrhagic vesicle may develop several hours to days later. If necrosis develops it typically is central, well defined, and surrounded by mixed erythema and vasoconstriction. Similar lesions, however, are associated with many other causes. The vast majority of confirmed bites require no treatment and resolve without incident. Based on confirmed envenomations, the need for surgical intervention seems to be uncommon.

Rees and colleagues [10] reported 17 confirmed bites; a generalized macular rash occurred in 29%. Fig. 4 demonstrates the skin lesions described by Rees. In this case, a 14-year-old girl awoke with pain, redness, and swelling in her left axilla. She found a spider in her bed. Using a colposcope, the spider was identified as an *L reclusa* (see Fig. 3). She developed a generalized

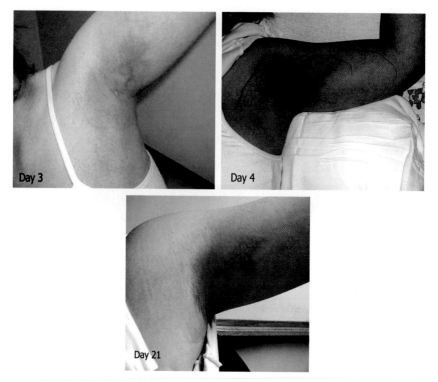

Fig. 4. Bite wound at days 3, 4, and 21 postinfliction.

maculopapular rash that completely resolved 3 weeks after the initial envenomation without any evidence of soft tissue necrosis.

Hemolysis has been associated with numerous case reports of *L reclusa*
bites [9,11–24]. Although most of these occurred with unconfirmed bites,
some reports with confirmed envenomation have demonstrated that brown
recluse venom can cause red cell destruction. In confirmed cases of hemolysis reported by Anderson and colleagues [9] transient renal failure also has
occurred.

Fatalities

Few deaths have been reported following *L reclusa* bites [19,21,22,24–27].
The clinical picture is that of rapid cardiovascular collapse with fever and
massive hemolysis. Although onset from time of bite is impossible to determine, the reported course ranged from about 18 hours [22,26] to nine days
[21]. Autopsy findings include skin lesions with thrombosis of dermal and
subcutaneous vessels. Coagulopathy frequently was apparent. Pulmonary
edema and renal tubular damage also were reported. Most victims were children and wound or blood cultures were not reported. Although some

fatality reports are suggestive of a spider bite, none were confirmed. Toxic Exposure Surveillance System data show eight fatalities attributed to *L reclusa* in the period from 1983 to 2004. In all of these cases the spider was presumed to cause the illness and subsequent death without confirmation, however [28–34]. In reported fatalities, patients presented with signs of hemolysis, including jaundice and dark urine; a retrospective diagnosis of spider bite was made when a skin lesion was identified.

Differential diagnosis

Numerous articles have concluded the skin lesions attributed to BRS bites in fact may be attributable to other causes. These articles warn that the diagnosis of BRS envenomation is purely speculative without a definite witnessing of the spider and subsequent identification of a BRS. In the case of such bites the diagnosis is said to be clinical or presumptive when in fact it is simple conjecture. Box 1 shows a listing of possible causes that should be ruled out before making the diagnosis of BRS bite in the absence of a spider [3,5,8,35–41].

Human reports

A review of multiple case reports of *L spp.* envenomations in the United States reflects the relative percentage of confirmed bites. Confirmed bites required a spider present at the bite site and identified as a brown recluse by an arachnologist, health care provider, or other person trained in such identification (Table 1).

Of 908 cases, only 7.9% were confirmed according to the definition above. Though impossible to analyze reliably, confirmed bites appear to require surgery less often, with only 4% undergoing surgery compared with 12.9% of unconfirmed cases treated surgically.

Animal studies of envenomation

Animal studies of loxoscelism have focused on several areas:

- Identification of venom and its mechanism of action
- Clinical effects of venom
- Diagnostic testing for true BRS bites
- Treatment of envenomation

Experimentally, BRS venom has been obtained by way of electrostimulation and expression from the live spider or by way of dissection of the venom sacs. Venom used in studies may be crude or purified. Unfortunately, many factors, such as gastric or salivary contamination and purification

Box 1. Causes to be ruled out before diagnosis of BRS bite

Angioedema
Ant bite or sting
Bacterial infection (staphylococcal, streptococcal)
Bedsores
Bee sting
Bromoderma use
Burns
Cutaneous anthrax
Cellulitis
Coumadin use
Diabetic ulcer
Drug injections
Ergot alkaloids
Erysipelas
Erythema multiforme
Erythema nodosum
Extravasation of chemotherapeutic agents
Factitious injection
Fat herniation with infarction
Flea bite
Focal vasculitis
Foreign body
Frostbite
Gonococcal hemorrhagic lesion
Heparin use
Herpes simplex infection
Hypersensitivity angiitis
Keratin-mediated response to a fungus
Lyme disease
Lymphoid papulosis
Malignancy causing arterial obstruction
Mosquito bite
Mycobacterial infection
Necrotizing fasciitis
Other arthropods
Periarteritis nodosa
Poison ivy
Poison oak
Purpura fulminans
Pyoderma gangrenosum
Reduviidae spp. bite
Scleroderma

Scorpion sting
Sporotrichosis
Stasis ulcers
Steven-Johnson syndrome
Thromboembolism
Tick bite
Toxic epidermal necrolysis
Trauma

method, lead to difficulty in developing a homogeneous product. In addition, studies often only use a portion of the venom obtained (such as a specific protein fraction). Many investigators test the venom (or protein fractions) obtained by mixing specific concentrations and testing animals for the development of a specific size of lesion before deciding on a dose to administer for the research project. Attempting to quantify the protein content of crude venom by comparison to a bovine standard is also used. In addition, there is significant interspecies variation in response to BRS venom, with rabbits being about 300 times more susceptible than rats [74].

Identification of venom and its mechanism of action

Loxosceles venom has been shown to contain several enzymes, including alkaline phosphatase, 5′ ribonucleotide phosphohydrolase, esterase, protease, and hyaluronidase. Hyaluronidase may be responsible for the spread of lesions. The most important enzyme causing loxoscelism seems to be sphingomyelinase D [75–77]. Sphingomyelinase D degrades sphingomyelin on cellular membranes resulting in lysis and cell death and also causes the release of prostaglandins, activates the complement cascade, stimulates platelet aggregation, and enhances neutrophil chemotaxis [78]. The dermonecrotic portion of venom that contains sphingomyelinase D is found to adhere to platelets suggesting a possible mechanism for BRS-induced coagulopathy [77]. Sphingomyelinase toxins from Loxosceles spiders have been shown to induce complement-dependent hemolysis of erythrocytes by way of activation of membrane-bound metalloproteinase [79–81]. The rate of sphingomyelin hydrolysis has been found to be related directly to temperature and to require the presence of divalent calcium. The rate of sphingomyelin hydrolysis is greater in crude venom than in purified fraction containing sphingomyelinase, suggesting a synergistic effect with other venom enzymes [82].

BRS venom adsorbs to cell membranes [10] and hemolyzes human erythrocytes in vitro [83]. Venom does not hemolyze washed erythrocytes in the absence of serum, however, thereby implicating serum factors in the pathophysiology of BRS envenomation [84]. Likewise the addition of complement

Table 1
Case reports of brown recluse spider envenomation

Reference	No. of patients	Unconfirmed	Spider present	Confirmed	Surgery
Arnold [42]	5	5	0	0	3
Berger [43]	2	0	2	2	0
Bey et al [44]	1	0	1	1	0
Borkan et al [45]	34	33	1	1	0
Broughton [46]	1	0	1	1	0
Chu and Rush [11]	1	0	1	1	0
Clowers [47]	39	39	0	0	?
Delozier et al [48]	31	20	?	11	6
Dillaha et al [12]	16	16	3	0	1
Edwards et al [49]	1	0	0	0	1
Eichner [13]	2	2	1	0	1
Goto [50]	1	0	1	1	?
Gross et al [51]	1	0	1	1	0
Hampton Taylor and Olive [52]	1	0	1	1	0
Hansen and Russell [53]	1	0	0	0	0
Hardman et al [54]	1	0	0	0	0
Hillis et al [55]	1	1	0	0	0
Hollabaugh [56]	18	18	0	0	18
Hoover [57]	1	1	0	0	1
Ingber et al [58]	35	35	0	0	5
King and Rees [59]	1	0	1	1	0
Leung [60]	1	1	1	0	0
Masters [61]	1	0	1	1	1
Maynor and Abt [38]	14	14	0	0	1
Murray and Segar [17]	1	1	0	0	0
Rees et al [62]	31	31	?	0	15
Rees et al [10]	17	0	17	17	0
Rees et al [63]	3	2	1	1	3
Ruelle et al [64]	1	1	0	0	0
Sauer [65]	1	1	0	0	0
Schenone and Prats [66]	40	21	25	19	3
Schuman and Caldwell [67]	478	478	0	0	43
Silcox and Miller [20]	1	1	1	0	0
Svendsen [68]	6	6	0	0	0
Taylor and Denny [21]	1	1	0	0	0
Vorse and Seccareccio [105]	1	1	0	0	0
Wasserman and Mydler [23]	5	5	0	0	0
Wesley et al [69]	1	1	0	0	1
Wille and Morrow [70]	1	1	0	0	0
Williams and Khare [24]	2	2	0	0	1
Wright et al [71]	110	98	22	13	3
Yiannais and Winkelman [72]	1	0	0	0	1
Young [73]	1	1	0	0	0
Totals	908	836	82	72	107
Percent of cases		92%	9%	7.9%	11.8%

inhibitors and ethylenediaminetetraacetic acid decreases hemolysis [85–87]. C-reactive protein has been implicated as a cofactor also, possibly by complement activation [84]. Along with complement activation, platelet aggregation occurs in a calcium-dependent fashion [78] requiring serum amyloid P [88]. Hemolysis is not seen with venom-exposed erythrocytes bathed in neonatal serum, and C-reactive protein and serum amyloid P are deficient in neonatal serum [88]. When treated with BRS venom human endothelial cells were found to bind polymorphonuclear cells (PMNs) and activate the release of granules [89].

Clinical effects of venom

The natural course and histology of BRS envenomation has been well studied in animal models. When rabbits were bitten by BRSs, the skin immediately developed hyperemia and within one hour became dusky. No blister was noted and histology at this stage revealed focal aggregations of leukocytes in the dermis with evidence of blood sludging in capillaries. The lesions continued to enlarge and become necrotic over the next 24 hours with histology showing thrombosis of capillary channels and evident necrosis extending through the fascia. By 144 hours (6 days), the zone of necrosis was well demarcated and histology showed necrosis with surrounding inflammatory reaction and granulation tissue at the periphery. By 288 hours (12 days), the eschar was well developed and showed histologic evidence of separation at the margins. At 30 days there was a dense scar with an absence of hair follicles and skin appendages [90]. The extent of dermal inflammation appeared to correlate with the physical diffusion of venom [91]. Polymorphonuclear leukocytes were implicated clearly in the pathogenesis of BRS venom, because rabbits made neutropenic with nitrogen mustard were much less susceptible to toxicity [92].

Dermonecrotic activity of extracted, purified BRS venom was found to be dose dependent in the rabbit, with lesion size proportional to the amount of venom injected (10–40 µg/kg) [77,93,94]. At doses of 60 µg/kg, rabbits developed pulmonary edema and died [94]. The typical lesion became erythematous, warm, and edematous within 12 hours after injection and formed a characteristic central purple papule that developed central necrosis 24 hours afterward. Histologic examination of the lesions showed vascular thrombosis and intense PMN infiltration [94]. Autopsy of the rabbits that died showed interstitial edema and leukocyte infiltration [95].

Guinea pigs administered twice the median lethal dose of BRS venom developed dyspnea, hemoptysis, and chest wall retractions at 6 hours, and became lethargic and developed bloody diarrhea before dying approximately 24 hours after envenomation. Hematologic studies revealed an initial decrease in the white blood cell count followed by a progressive increase, and a progressive decline in platelet count. Serum complement levels were decreased significantly compared with controls (451 $\pm$ 134 CH$_{50}$ units versus $835 \pm 134 \, CH_{50}$ units, $P < .05$). Autopsy revealed diffuse hemorrhage and vessel thrombosis of lungs, liver, mesentery, and kidneys, with petechial hemorrhages throughout the bowel. Guinea pigs made deficient in complement by treatment with zymosan were resistant to BRS venom [95].

Diagnostic testing

Diagnosis remains difficult at best, with no specific test available to ensure that a lesion is attributable to the bite of a BRS. Passive hemagglutinin inhibition has been reported to test for the presence of BRS venom with a sensitivity of 90% as long as 3 days after envenomation in guinea pigs [96]. The test involves incubation of the subject's wound exudate to a prepared antiserum and then exposure of the mixture to venom-coated O-negative red blood cells. Exudate containing BRS venom causes the red blood cells to settle to the bottom of the test tube. The calculated amount of venom protein to produce a positive result was 0.0037 µg/mL (natural bites in this study injected 5–23 µg of venom) [97].

A lymphocyte transformation test using adsorbed venom protein was found to detect previous exposure to loxosceles venom in a small series of patients [98].

ELISA has been developed to detect antigens from *L intermedia* in Brazil with some prospective validation in hospitalized patients [99]. *L reclusa* ELISA has been developed and found to be specific for BRS venom at low venom levels, although cross-reactivity to other nonloxosceles spider venoms was found at higher levels [100]. In a rabbit model, this assay detected venom up to 7 days after injection [101]. A venom-specific enzyme immunoassay derived from *L deserta* has been used clinically to detect spider venom in a dermal biopsy and hair from a patient 4 days after the development of a skin lesion [102].

Treatment

Animal research has helped us to determine the efficacy of various treatments with experimentally induced envenomations. We must be aware, however, of the inherent limitations in attempting to apply the animal data to humans. Many animal studies use venom preincubated with the treatment agent, or apply the treatment agent either pre-envenomation or shortly afterward, which does not approximate a true clinical scenario. In addition, there is significant variability among animal species in their susceptibility to BRS envenomation. The current mainstay of therapy is supportive care. Even in the rare case of a confirmed bite, treatment should be expectant. Despite multiple trials, early surgical excision [62,94,103,104], electric shock [105], steroids [93–95,104,106], hyperbaric oxygen therapy [38,107–110], colchicine [106], antihistamines [106], vasodilator drugs [111], anticoagulants [94,104,112], prophylactic antibiotics [103], and dapsone [93,104,106,109] remain unproven therapies for BRS envenomation. All have variable degrees of risk. The only treatment modality that consistently has shown success in animal studies of loxosceles envenomation is specific antivenin; however, the treatment seems to be most beneficial either pre-envenomation or shortly thereafter (within 1 hour) [77,93,94,104,112,113]. Intradermal specific antiloxosceles Fab fragments also have been found to attenuate the BRS lesion size up to 4 hours postenvenomation [114]. The potential value of these therapies is limited by the fact that only 10% of people bitten present in the first 12 hours [115] and that antivenin and specific Fab fragments are not available commercially. Furthermore, given the inaccuracy of the brown recluse bite diagnosis, much better documentation of the cause would be required before assuming a risk of administration. For that reason, a reliable test for BRS bite would be useful, but is unavailable at present.

Summary

The bite of the BRS continues to pose a diagnostic and therapeutic challenge. The animal data reveal sphingomyelinase D to be the most important portion of venom and implicate serum factors (such as complement, C reactive protein, and leukocytes) as important cofactors for producing disease. Diagnosis remains difficult at best, with no easily available test to ensure a lesion is attributable to the bite of a BRS. Misdiagnosis of other treatable causes of necrotic skin lesions as BRS bites has presented a challenge also. Treatment of a confirmed brown recluse bite primarily is supportive with appropriate wound care.

Animal studies and the few confirmed human cases have documented that the bite of the brown recluse is much less common than the medical and scientific communities have believed. The data also demonstrate that the bite of the recluse more often than not causes a mild wound, although it can produce a necrotic lesion. There also is support for the rare occurrence of hemolysis. Death reports involving *L reclusa* remain circumstantial. In recent years, Vetter and colleagues [5,116,117] repeatedly have underscored the need for confirmed bites as the evidential basis for our understanding of the spider and its medical significance. Given more than a century of questionable case reports, the medical community must limit BRS envenomation data to well-documented cases and not use the endpoint (ie, lesion or condition) to establish a cause retrospectively.

References

[1] Caveness W. Insect bite complicated by fever. Nashville J Med Surg 1982;10:333.
[2] Schmaus L. Case of arachnoidism (spider bite). JAMA 1929;92:1265–6.

[3] Atkins J, Wingo C, Sodeman W. Probable cause of necrotic spider bite in the midwest. Science 1957;126:73.

[4] Gertsch W, Muliak S. *Loxosceles reclusus*. Bull Am Mus Nat Hist 1940;77:317.

[5] Swanson D, Vetter R. Bites of brown recluse spiders and suspected necrotic arachnidism. N Engl J Med 2005;352:700–7.

[6] Sandidge JS. Arachnology: scavenging by brown recluse spiders. Nature 2003;426:6.

[7] Vetter R, Barger D. An infestation of 2,055 brown recluse spiders (*Araneae: Sicariidae*) and no envenomations in a Kansas home: implications for bite diagnoses in nonendemic areas. J Med Entomol 2002;39:948–51.

[8] Wasserman GS, Anderson PC. Loxoscelism and necrotic arachnidism. J Toxicol Clin Toxicol 1983;21:451–72.

[9] Anderson PC. Missouri brown recluse spider: a review and update. Mo Med 1998;95: 318–22.

[10] Rees R, Campbell D, Rieger E, et al. The diagnosis and treatment of brown recluse spider bites. Ann Emerg Med 1987;16:945–9.

[11] Chu JY, Rush CT, O'Connor DM. Hemolytic anemia following brown spider (*Loxosceles reclusa*) bite. Clin Toxicol 1978;12:531–4.

[12] Dillaha C, Jansen G, Honeycutt W, et al. North American loxoscelism. JAMA 1964;188: 153–6.

[13] Eichner ER. Spider bite hemolytic anemia: positive Coombs' test, erythrophagocytosis, and leukoerythroblastic smear. Am J Clin Path 1984;81:683–7.

[14] Gotten H, MacGowan JJ. Blackwater fever (Hemoglobinuria) caused by a spider. JAMA 1940;113:1547.

[15] Madrigal GC, Ercolani RL, Wenzl JE. Toxicity from a bite of the brown spider (*Loxosceles reclusus*): skin necrosis, hemolytic anemia, and hemoglobinuria in a nine-year-old child. Clin Pediatr (Phila) 1972;11:641–4.

[16] Minton S, Olson C. A case of spider bite with severe hemolytic reaction. An Pediatr (Barc) 1964;33:283–4.

[17] Murray LM, Seger DL. Hemolytic anemia following a presumptive brown recluse spider bite. J Toxicol Clin Toxicol 1994;32:451–6.

[18] Novak R, Kuman A, Thompson E, et al. Severe systemic toxicity from a spider bite in a six-year-old boy. J Tenn Med Assoc 1979;(Feb):109–11.

[19] Rose NJ. Report of fatality: spider bite (*Loxosceles*). IMJ Ill Med J 1970;137:339.

[20] Silcox MM, Miller L. The brown recluse spider: a sometimes fatal bite. J Emerg Nurs 1992; 18:101–3.

[21] Taylor EH, Denny WF. Hemolysis, renal failure and death, presumed secondary to bite of brown recluse spider. South Med J 1966;59:1209–11.

[22] Vorse H, Seccareccio P, Woodruff K, et al. Disseminated intravascular coagulopathy following fatal brown spider bite (necrotic arachnidism). J Pediatr 1972;80:1035–7.

[23] Wasserman G, Mydler T, Sharma V. Brown recluse spider envenomation as a cause of hemolysis and hemoglobinuria. Vet Hum Toxicol 1991;33:359.

[24] Williams ST, Khare VK, Johnston GA, et al. Severe intravascular hemolysis associated with brown recluse spider envenomation: a report of two cases and review of the literature. Am J ClinPath 1995;104:463–7.

[25] Lessenden C, Zimmer L. Brown spider bites: a survey of the current problem. J Kans Med Soc 1960;61:371–85.

[26] Nicholson J, Nicholson B. Hemolytic anemia from brown spider bite: Necrotic arachnidism. J Okla State Med Assoc 1962;55:234–6.

[27] Riley H, McLean W, Start A, et al. Brown spider bite with severe hemolytic phenomena. J Okla State Med Assoc 1964;57:218–23.

[28] Litovitz TL, Felberg L, Soloway RA, et al. 1994 annual report of the American Association of Poison Control Centers Toxic Exposure Surveillance System. Am J Emerg Med 1995;13: 551–97.

[29] Litovitz TL, Klein-Schwartz W, White S, et al. 1999 annual report of the American Association of Poison Control Centers Toxic Exposure Surveillance System. Am J Emerg Med 2000;18:517–74.

[30] Litovitz TL, Schmitz BF, Holm KC. 1988 annual report of the American Association of Poison Control Centers National Data Collection System. Am J Emerg Med 1989;7: 495–545.

[31] Litovitz TL, Schmitz BF, Matyunas N, et al. 1987 annual report of the American Association of Poison Control Centers National Data Collection System. Am J of Emerg Med 1988;6:479–515.

[32] Veltri JC, Litovitz TL. 1983 Annual report of the American Association of Poison Control Centers National Data Collection System. Am J Emerg Med 1984;2:420–43.

[33] Watson WA, Litovitz TL, Klein-Schwartz W, et al. 2003 Annual report of the American Association of Poison Control Centers Toxic Exposure Surveillance System. Am J Emerg Med 2004;22:335–404.

[34] Watson WA, Litovitz TL, Rodgers GC Jr, et al. 2004 Annual report of the American Association of Poison Control Centers Toxic Exposure Surveillance System. Am J Emerg Med 2005;23:589–666.

[35] Bernstein B, Ehrlich F. Brown recluse spider bites. J Emerg Med 1986;4:457–62.

[36] Brady W, DeBehnke D, Crosby D. Dermatological emergencies. Am J Emerg Med 1994;12: 217–37.

[37] Dreizen S, McCredie KB, Bodey GP, et al. Necrotizing dermatitis in patients receiving cancer chemotherapy. Postgrad Med 1987;81:263–71.

[38] Maynor ML, Moon RE, Klitzman B, et al. Brown recluse spider envenomation: a prospective trial of hyperbaric oxygen therapy. Acad Emerg Med 1997;4:184–92.

[39] Rosenstein ED, Kramer N. Lyme disease misdiagnosed as a brown recluse spider bite. Ann Intern Med 1987;106:782.

[40] Wasserman GS. Wound care of spider and snake envenomations. Ann Emerg Med 1988;17: 1331–5.

[41] Young VL, Pin P. The brown recluse spider bite. Ann Plast Surg 1988;20:447–52.

[42] Arnold RE. Brown recluse spider bites: five cases with a review of the literature. JACEP 1976;5:262–4.

[43] Berger RS. The unremarkable brown recluse spider bite. JAMA 1973;225:1109–11.

[44] Bey TA, Walter FG, Lober W, et al. Loxosceles arizonica bite associated with shock. Ann Emerg Med 1997;30:701–3.

[45] Borkan J, Gross E, Lubin Y, et al. An outbreak of venomous spider bites in a citrus grove. Am J Trop Med Hyg 1995;52:228–30.

[46] Broughton G 2nd. Management of the brown recluse spider bite to the glans penis. Mil Med 1996;161:627–9.

[47] Clowers TD. Wound assessment of the Loxosceles reclusa spider bite. J Emerg Nurs 1996; 22:283–7.

[48] DeLozier JB, Reaves L, King LE Jr, et al. Brown recluse spider bites of the upper extremity. South Med J 1988;81:181–4.

[49] Edwards JJ, Anderson RL, Wood JR. Loxoscelism of the eyelids. Arch Ophthalmol 1980; 98:1997–2000.

[50] Goto CS, Abramo TJ, Ginsburg CM. Upper airway obstruction caused by brown recluse spider envenomization of the neck. Am J Emerg Med 1996;14:660–2.

[51] Gross AS, Wilson DC, King LE Jr. Persistent segmental cutaneous anesthesia after a brown recluse spider bite. South Med J 1990;83:1321–3.

[52] Hampton Taylor M, Olive A. Brown recluse spider bite. NCMJ 1972;33:421–4.

[53] Hansen R, Russell F. Dapsone use for Loxosceles envenomation treatment. Vet Hum Toxicol 1984;26:260.

[54] Hardman JT, Beck ML, Hardman PK, et al. Incompatibility associated with the bite of a brown recluse spider (Loxosceles reclusa). Transfusion 1983;23:233–6.

[55] Hillis TJ, Grant-Kels JM, Jacoby LM. Presumed arachnidism: a case report (in Connecticut). Int J Dermatol 1986;25:44–8.

[56] Hollabaugh RS, Fernandes ET. Management of the brown recluse spider bite. J Pediatr Surg 1989;24:126–7.

[57] Hoover EL, Williams W, Koger L, et al. Pseudoepitheliomatous hyperplasia and pyoderma gangrenosum after a brown recluse spider bite. S Med J 1990;83:243–6.

[58] Ingber A, Trattner A, Cleper R, et al. Morbidity of brown recluse spider bites: clinical picture, treatment and prognosis. Acta Derm Veneriol 1991;71:337–40.

[59] King LE, Rees R. Dapsone treatment of a brown recluse bite. JAMA 1983;250:648.

[60] Leung LK, Davis R. Life-threatening hemolysis following a brown recluse spider bite. J Tenn Med Assoc 1995;88:396–7.

[61] Masters E. Images in clinical medicine: loxoscelism. N Engl J Med 1998;339:379.

[62] Rees RS, Altenbern DP, Lynch JB, et al. Brown recluse spider bites a comparison of early surgical excision versus dapsone and delayed surgical excision. Ann Surg 1985;202: 659–63.

[63] Rees RS, Fields JP, King LE Jr. Do brown recluse spider bites induce pyoderma gangrenosum? South Med J 1985;78:283–7.

[64] Ruelle AL, Sowell ME, Derk FF, et al. Multiple brown recluse spider envenomation. J Am Podiatr Med Assoc 1996;86:174–6.

[65] Sauer GC. Transverse myelitis and paralysis from a brown recluse spider bite. Mo Med 1975;72:603–4.

[66] Schenone H, Prats F. Arachnidism by *Loxosceles laeta*. Arch Dermatol 1961;83:139–42.

[67] Schuman SH, Caldwell ST. 1990 South Carolina Physician Survey of tick, spider and fire ant morbidity. J South Carolina Med Assoc 1991;87:429–32.

[68] Svendsen FJ. Treatment of clinically diagnosed brown recluse spider bites with hyperbaric oxygen: a clinical observation. J Ark Med Soc 1986;83:199–204.

[69] Wesley RE, Ballinger WH, Close LW, et al. Dapsone in the treatment of presumed brown recluse spider bite of the eyelid. Ophthalmic Surg 1985;16. p. 115, 116–7, 120.

[70] Wille RC, Morrow JD. Case report: dapsone hypersensitivity syndrome associated with treatment of the bite of a brown recluse spider. Am J Med Sci 1988;296:270–1.

[71] Wright SW, Wrenn KD, Murray L, et al. Clinical presentation and outcome of brown recluse spider bite. Ann Emerg Med 1997;30:28–32.

[72] Yiannias JA, Winkelmann RK. Persistent painful plaque due to a brown recluse spider bite. Cutis 1992;50:273–5.

[73] Young RA. Thrombocytopenia associated with brown recluse spider bite. J Emerg Med 1994;12:389.

[74] Morgan PN. Preliminary studies on venom from the brown recluse spider *Loxosceles reclusa*. Toxicon 1969;6:161–5.

[75] Forrester LJ, Barrett JT, Campbell BJ. Red blood cell lysis induced by the venom of the brown recluse spider: the role of sphingomyelinase D. Arch Biochem Biophys 1978;187: 355–65.

[76] Kurpiewski G, Forrester LJ, Barrett JT, et al. Platelet aggregation and sphingomyelinase D activity of a purified toxin from the venom of *Loxosceles reclusa*. Biochim Biophys Acta 1981;678:467–76.

[77] Rees RS, Nanney LB, Yates RA, et al. Interaction of brown recluse spider venom on cell membranes: the inciting mechanism? J Invest Derm 1984;83:270–5.

[78] Rees RS, Gates C, Timmons S, et al. Plasma components are required for platelet activation by the toxin of *Loxosceles reclusa*. Toxicon 1988;26:1035–45.

[79] Tambourgi DV, Magnoli FC, van den Berg CW, et al. Sphingomyelinases in the venom of the spider *Loxosceles intermedia* are responsible for both dermonecrosis and complement-dependent hemolysis. Biochem Biophys Res Commun 1998;251:366–73.

[80] Tambourgi DV, Magnoli FC, Von Eickstedt VR, et al. Incorporation of a 35-kilodalton purified protein from Loxosceles intermedia spider venom transforms human erythrocytes

into activators of autologous complement alternative pathway. J Immunol 1995;155: 4459–66.

[81] Van Den Berg CW, De Andrade RM, Magnoli FC, et al. Loxosceles spider venom induces metalloproteinase mediated cleavage of MCP/CD46 and MHCI and induces protection against C-mediated lysis. Immunol 2002;106:102–10.

[82] Merchant ML, Hinton JF, Geren CR. Sphingomyelinase D activity of brown recluse spider (*Loxosceles reclusa*) venom as studied by 31P-NMR: effects on the time-course of sphingomyelin hydrolysis. Toxicon 1998;36:537–45.

[83] Babcock JL, Suber RL, Frith CH, et al. Systemic effect in mice of venom apparatus extract and toxin from the brown recluse spider (*Loxosceles reclusa*). Toxicon 1981;19:463–71.

[84] Hufford DC, Morgan PN. C-reactive protein as a mediator in the lysis of human erythrocytes sensitized by brown recluse spider venom. Proc Soc Exp Biol Med 1981;167:493–7.

[85] Futrell JM, Morgan PN, Su SP, et al. Location of brown recluse venom attachment sites on human erythrocytes by the ferritin-labeled antibody technique. Am J Pathol 1979;95: 675–82.

[86] Gebel HM, Campbell BJ, Barrett JT. Chemotactic activity of venom from the brown recluse spider (*Loxoscelles reclusa*). Toxicon 1979;17:55–60.

[87] Morgan BB, Morgan PN, Bowling RE. Lysis of human erythrocytes by venom from the brown recluse spider, *Loxosceles reclusa*. Toxicon 1978;16:85–8.

[88] Gates CA, Rees RS. Serum amyloid P component: its role in platelet activation stimulated by sphingomyelinase D purified from the venom of the brown recluse spider (*Loxosceles reclusa*). Toxicon 1990;28:1303–15.

[89] Patel KD, Modur V, Zimmerman GA, et al. The necrotic venom of the brown recluse spider induces dysregulated endothelial cell-dependent neutrophil activation: differential induction of GM-CSF, IL-8, and E-selectin expression. J Clin Invest 1994;94:631–42.

[90] Butz WC, Stacy LD, Heryford NN. Arachnidism in rabbits. Necrotic lesions due to the brown recluse spider. Arch Pathol Lab Med 1971;91:97–100.

[91] Gomez HF, Greenfield DM, Miller MJ, et al. Direct correlation between diffusion of *Loxosceles reclusa* venom and extent of dermal inflammation. Acad Emerg Med 2001;8:309–14.

[92] Smith CW, Micks DW. The role of polymorphonuclear leukocytes in the lesion caused by the venom of the brown spider, *Loxosceles reclusa*. Lab Invest 1970;22:90–3.

[93] Cole HP 3rd, Wesley RE, King LE Jr. Brown recluse spider envenomation of the eyelid: an animal model. Ophthal Plast Reconstr Surg 1995;11:153–64.

[94] Rees RS, King LE. Management of the brown recluse spider bite. J Pediatr Surg 1989; 24:147.

[95] Rees RS, O'Leary JP, King LE Jr. The pathogenesis of systemic loxoscelism following brown recluse spider bites. J Surg Res 1983;35:1–10.

[96] Barrett SM, Romine-Jenkins M, Blick KE. Passive hemagglutination inhibition test for diagnosis of brown recluse spider bite envenomation. Clin Chem 1993;39:2104–7.

[97] Finke JH, Campbell BJ, Barrett JT. Serodiagnostic test for *Loxosceles reclusa* bites. Clin Toxicol 1974;7:375–82.

[98] Berger RS, Millikan LE, Conway F. An in vitro test for *Loxosceles reclusa* spider bites. Toxicon 1973;11:465–70.

[99] Chavez-Olortegui C, Zanetti VC, Ferreira AP, et al. ELISA for the detection of venom antigens in experimental and clinical envenoming by *Loxosceles intermedia* spiders. Toxicon 1998;36:563–9.

[100] Gomez HF, Krywko DM, Stoecker WV. A new assay for the detection of *Loxosceles* species (brown recluse) spider venom. Ann Emerg Med 2002;39:469–74.

[101] Krywko DM, Gomez HF. Detection of *Loxosceles* species venom in dermal lesions: a comparison of 4 venom recovery methods. Ann Emerg Med 2002;39:475–80.

[102] Miller MJ, Gomez HF, Snider RJ, et al. Detection of *Loxosceles* venom in lesional hair shafts and skin: application of a specific immunoassay to identify dermonecrotic arachnidism. Am J Emerg Med 2000;18:626–8.

[103] Jansen GT, Morgan PN, McQueen JN, et al. The brown recluse spider bite: controlled evaluation of treatment using the white rabbit as an animal model. S Med J 1971;64:1194–202.

[104] Rees R, Shack RB, Withers E, et al. Management of the brown recluse spider bite. Plast Reconstr Surg 1981;68:768–73.

[105] Barrett SM, Romine-Jenkins M, Fisher DE. Dapsone or electric shock therapy of brown recluse spider envenomation? Ann Emerg Med 1994;24:21–5.

[106] Elston DM, Miller SD, Young RJ 3rd, et al. Comparison of colchicine, dapsone, triamcinolone, and diphenhydramine therapy for the treatment of brown recluse spider envenomation: a double-blind, controlled study in a rabbit model. Arch Dermatol 2005;141:595–7.

[107] Hobbs GD, Anderson AR, Greene TJ, et al. Comparison of hyperbaric oxygen and dapsone therapy for loxosceles envenomation. Acad Emer Med 1996;3:758–61.

[108] Merchant ML, Hinton JF, Geren CR. Effect of hyperbaric oxygen on sphingomyelinase D activity of brown recluse spider (*Loxosceles reclusa*) venom as studied by 31P nuclear magnetic resonance spectroscopy. Am J Trop Med Hyg 1997;56:335–8.

[109] Phillips S, Kohn M, Baker D, et al. Therapy of brown spider envenomation: a controlled trial of hyperbaric oxygen, dapsone, and cyproheptadine. Ann Emerg Med 1995;25:363–8.

[110] Strain GM, Snider TG, Tedford BL, et al. Hyperbaric oxygen effects on brown recluse spider (*Loxosceles reclusa*) envenomation in rabbits. Toxicon 1991;29:989–96.

[111] Lowry BP, Bradfield JF, Carroll RG, et al. A controlled trial of topical nitroglycerin in a New Zealand white rabbit model of brown recluse spider envenomation. Ann Emerg Med 2001;37:161–5.

[112] Elgert KD, Ross MA, Campbell BJ, et al. Immunological studies of Brown recluse spider venom. Infect Immun 1974;10:1412–9.

[113] Beckwith ML, Babcock JL, Geren CR. Effects of antiserum on the systemic response in mice caused by a component isolated from an extract of the brown recluse spider (*Loxosceles reclusa*) venom apparatus. Toxicon 1980;18:663–6.

[114] Gomez HF, Miller MJ, Trachy JW, et al. Intradermal anti-*Loxosceles* Fab fragments attenuate dermonecrotic arachnidism. Acad Emerg Med 1999;6:1195–202.

[115] Hogan CJ, Barbaro KC, Winkel K. Loxoscelism: old obstacles, new directions. Ann Emerg Med 2004;44:608–24.

[116] Vetter R. Identifying and misidentifying the brown recluse spider. Dermatol Online J 1999;5:7.

[117] Vetter R, Bush S. Reports of presumptive brown recluse spider bites reinforce improbable diagnosis in regions of North America where the spider is not endemic. Clin Infect Dis 2002; 35:442–5.

ELSEVIER
SAUNDERS

CLINICS IN
LABORATORY
MEDICINE

Clin Lab Med 26 (2006) 227–241

Hepatotoxicity Associated with Herbal Products

R. Brent Furbee, MD, FACMT[a],
Kevin S. Barlotta, MD[b], Melrose Kanku Allen, MD[b],
Christopher P. Holstege, MD[c,d,e],*

[a]*Indiana Poison Center, Department of Emergency Medicine, Indiana University
School of Medicine, Room AG373, 1701 North Senate Boulevard,
Indianapolis, IN 46206, USA*
[b]*Department of Emergency Medicine, University of Virginia, P.O. Box 800774,
Charlottesville, VA 22908-0774, USA*
[c]*Division of Medical Toxicology, University of Virginia, P.O. Box 800774,
Charlottesville, VA 22908-0774, USA*
[d]*Blue Ridge Poison Center, P.O. Box 800774, Charlottesville, VA 22908, USA*
[e]*Department of Emergency Medicine & Pediatrics, University of Virginia,
P.O. Box 800774, Charlottesville, VA 22908-0774, USA*

A significant number of herbal products have been associated with hepatotoxicity. Unlike pharmaceutic products that undergo clinical trials before release to the public, herbal products have no preapproval evaluation time period in which liver injury may be identified. The association of hepatic injury with an herbal product is recognized only after numerous patients have contracted disease. This problem is confounded by the fact that less than 1% of the adverse events associated with dietary supplements are reported to the US Food and Drug Administration (FDA) [1]. Attribution of liver injury to a specific herbal product may be difficult. There are few clinical or laboratory manifestations that specifically suggest that liver injury is the result of a specific herbal. The most important clue often is the temporal relationship between initiation of the herbal product and the appearance of liver injury, and of equal importance is the resolution of the injury following withdrawal of the herbal product [2].

* Corresponding author. Blue Ridge Poison Center, P.O. Box 800774, Charlottesville, VA 22908.
    E-mail address: ch2xf@virginia.edu (C.P. Holstege).

0272-2712/06/$ - see front matter © 2006 Elsevier Inc. All rights reserved.
doi:10.1016/j.cll.2006.02.005
labmed.theclinics.com

Several factors may contribute to the hepatotoxic effects of herbal preparations. Foragers frequently misidentify plants, sometimes collecting toxic species. Seasonal variation of plant composition occurs; therefore the dosing of the biologic compounds received varies from product to product depending on the time of harvest and the part of the plant ingested. Common names often are applied to several different plants, confusing identification. Herbal preparations often contain multiple plant products or other compounds that may contribute to the hepatotoxicity [3]. Many herbal preparations used in North America are taken in addition to pharmaceutic products, and potential drug interactions may occur that have previously not been recognized. Contamination of products also has been reported. For example, Adachi and colleagues [4] reported 12 cases of N-nitroso-fenfluramine contamination of two popular herbal preparations in Japan, resulting in one liver transplant and one death.

Most of the medical literature addressing this problem exists in the form of case reports. There are few case control or cohort studies. For that reason, determination of relative toxicity is based on the number and strength of such reports. There are numerous herbal products that have been associated with hepatotoxicity (Box 1). This article reviews some of the herbal products more commonly associated with hepatotoxicity.

Box 1. Herbal products with reported hepatotoxicity

American Skullcap (*Scutellaria laterifolia*)
Cascara Sagrada (*Rhamnus purshiana*)
Chaparral (*Larrea*)
Comfrey (*Symphytum*)
Dog's tail (*Heliotropium angiospermum*)
Germander (*Teucrium chamaedrys*)
Greater celandine (*Chelidonium majus*)
Impila (*Callilepis laureola*)
Jin Bu Huan (*Stephania sinica*)
Kava (*Piper methysticum*)
Ma Huang (*Ephedra*)
Margosa oil (*Melia azadirachta*)
Mistletoe (*Phoradendron serotinum*)
Pennyroyal (*Mentha pulegium* or *Hedeoma*)
Rattlebox (*Crotalaria*)
Sassafras Oil (*Sassafras*)
Senecio (*Senecio aconitifolius*)
Senna (*Cassia acutifolia*)
Valerian (*Valeriana officinalis*)
White Chameleon (*Atractylis gummifera*)

Pyrrolizidine alkaloids

The hepatotoxic effects of the pyrrolizidine alkaloids (PAs) are well documented. Early reports began in 1920 when Wilmont and Robertson [5] described five patients with acute hepatic failure. The investigators noted that several families in South Africa were struck by this disease, which resembled similar conditions in livestock. This finding suggested that a dietary exposure was occurring. It had been demonstrated that *Senecio ilicifolius* and *S burchelli* ingestion were responsible for such symptoms in cattle, and on further inspection those plants were found to contaminate poorly winnowed wheat. In 1951, Selzer and Parker [6] reported unique clinical features of 12 patients and six autopsy results in Cape Town, South Africa. They described rapid onset of ascites, hepatomegaly, nausea, and vomiting coupled with autopsy findings consistent with Chiari's syndrome. In 1954, Bras and colleagues [7] reported comparable cases from Jamaica loosely linked with the consumption of bush tea. Similar reports subsequently arose from Egypt, India [8], Afghanistan [9], Great Britain [10], and the United States [11–14]. By the 1980s, the PAs contained within these plants had been identified as the cause. These plants come from the genera Senecio, Crotalaria, Heliotropium, and Symphytum [15]. PAs had contaminated herbal teas, flour, and cereals.

PAs are distributed widely and found in approximately 3% of the world's plants. Approximately 300 compounds with similar structures have been identified and their toxicity varies widely. The basic structure of PAs is the necine base, as shown in Fig. 1. Toxicity is determined by alterations of that base. Characteristics that result in enhancement of toxicity include

Double bond of the 1,2 position of the unsaturated necine base
Esterification of hydroxyls at 7 and 9
Branched carbon chain in the ester side chains

The PAs are metabolized by way of three pathways. They are hydrolyzed to form necine bases then either oxidized to form innocuous N-oxides or hydroxylated and dehydrated by way of cytochrome p450 (3A4 and 2B6) to

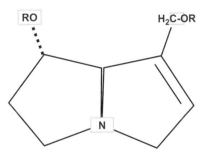

Fig. 1. Pyrrolizidine alkaloid structure.

form pyrroles [16]. Pyrroles act as alkylating agents capable of inducing hepatocellular injury. Compounds capable of inducing 3A4 metabolism, such
as phenobarbital, can increase pyrrole production, whereas 3A4 blockers reduce it. Pyrroles damage the sinusoidal endothelium causing the extravasation of red blood cells into the space of Disse. As a result, reticulin fibers are
generated in the lumen of central and sublobular veins obstructing venous
flow and causing hepatic congestion that ultimately results in hepatic necrosis [16]. The resultant clinical presentation is that of abdominal pain, hepatomegaly, and ascites.

Animal studies have demonstrated genotoxicity, including DNA binding,
cross-linking, mutagenicity, and carcinogenicity. Carcinogenicity has yet to
be demonstrated in humans.

Infants appear to be most susceptible to PA-induced toxicity. The acute
syndrome presents with abdominal pain and sudden-onset ascites. Cirrhosis
and portal hypertension also may occur. Death reportedly occurs in approximately 20% of acute cases, though the exact prevalence is not known [17].
A chronic form of toxicity also has been reported that begins with weakness
and diarrhea. Portal hypertension also may occur and can progress to
esophageal varices, encephalopathy, and death. The overall mortality of
both syndromes is 40% [16,18,19]. PAs also have been shown to cause
a veno-occlusive pulmonary disease in animals, but that has not been reported in humans with PA exposure [20].

Diagnosis usually is established by liver biopsy. Detection of PAs by high
performance liquid chromatography or gas chromatograph-mass spectroscopy is of little clinical value. Aspartate aminotransaminase, gamma-glutamyltransferase, and bilirubin frequently are elevated, but not always [21].

The treatment of PA toxicity essentially is the same as treatment of veno-
occlusive liver disease. Supportive care is focused on limiting exposure to
hepatotoxins and nephrotoxins while reducing sodium and fluid load. Reversal of coagulopathy and reduction of ascites with paracentesis are also
important. N-acetylcysteine has been used successfully in animals, but its
benefit is not proven in humans [16]. Defibrotide has been shown to modulate endothelial cell injury without increasing hemorrhage [22]. Patients presenting with multiorgan failure have a poor prognosis [23].

Liver transplant is an option. In those able to undergo the procedure,
about 30% experience clinical improvement [23]. Transjugular intrahepatic
portosystemic shunts have been of benefit in veno-occlusive disease and may
be a consideration in appropriate candidates [24].

At autopsy, the liver commonly demonstrates a fine granular cirrhosis
with a nutmeg appearance secondary to chronic passive congestion. Small
and medium-sized branches of the hepatic vein commonly show wall thick-
ening, but larger veins often are spared. Affected vessels are surrounded by
fibrosis. There often is coalescence and marked widening of sinusoids in central lobular areas. Obliteration of hepatic vein radicals has been remarkable
in some cases. Central veins often are unrecognizable. There are varying

amounts of subendothelial swelling with concentric swelling of the intima that begins with fibrin formation, then reticulin, collagen, and elastic tissue, and finally irregular swelling suggesting organized thrombus. Fibrosis begins in nonportal areas, but progresses to portal areas in the final stages [7,9].

Germander

Germander *(Teucrium chamaedrys)* has been advocated for the treatment of gout, obesity, diabetes mellitus, diarrhea, and fever. In 1986, France approved the marketing of the use of Germander. By 1992, several reports of hepatitis had surfaced in connection with its use [25,26]. Most cases involved women taking the product for weight loss in doses of 600 to 1600 mg per day for 2 or more months. Acute cholestatic hepatitis was the most common presentation with some patients developing cirrhosis. Those who did not develop cirrhosis recovered on discontinuation of the drug. Germander initially was not identified as the hepatotoxin until a patient who was accidentally re-exposed developed hepatitis [17]. In a subsequent series, 12 of 26 patients re-exposed to Germander redeveloped evidence of hepatitis [27]. Other *Teucrium* species also have been associated with hepatitis and liver failure [27–29].

Teucrium species contain glycosides, saponins, and flavonoids. Furano neoclerodane diterpenoids, namely teucrin A and teuchamaedryn A, however, are considered the responsible toxic components. Other diterpenoids also have been discovered. By way of oxidation by CYP3A4, the furan ring of these diterpenoids is converted to an epoxide that can react with CYP3A and epoxide hydrolase. Animal studies have indicated that the epoxide also can change mitochondrial permeability, activate caspase, and increase apoptosis. The epoxide can decrease hepatocyte glutathione. This activity results in plasma membrane blebs, DNA fragmentation, and cell apoptosis. Further study has indicated that glutathione depletion increased hepatocyte damage, whereas glutathione replacement decreased it. An immune cause also has been suggested. When the epoxide binds to epoxide hydrolase on the surface of the hepatocytes, autoantibody formation may lead to an immune response resulting in cell death [30].

Clinically, case reports have described a gradual onset of malaise, anorexia, and jaundice similar to acute hepatitis. Patients usually seek medical attention after noting change in skin or urine color. Elevation of conjugated bilirubin, aspartate aminotransferase, alanine aminotransferase, gamma-glutamyltransferase, and alkaline phosphatase are common. Antinuclear antibodies, antimitochondrial antibodies, and anti-smooth muscle antibodies have been reported positive [28,29]. *T spp* have been identified by gas chromatography-mass spectrometry [31] and high performance liquid chromatography [32]. Biopsies demonstrated hepatocyte necrosis and polymorphonuclear and mononuclear infiltration of the centrilobular area. Inflammatory cells were identified in the portal tracts [25].

Treatment is supportive and most cases have resolution of hepatitis after discontinuation of the supplement. Patients should be warned against its resumption.

Chaparral

Chaparral *(Larrea tridentata)* commonly is called creosote bush or greasewood. It is a desert shrub ubiquitous in the Southwest. Because it has a woody stem it technically is not an herb but commonly is regarded as one. Chaparral, made from the leaves of *L tridentata*, has been advocated for the treatment of colds, infertility, rheumatism, arthritis, diabetes, gallstones, kidney stones, and snake bites. It also is recommended as an antioxidant. Currently it is sold as a tablet or salve.

Sheikh and colleagues [33] in 1997 reviewed 13 case reports of hepatotoxicity that had occurred since 1990. They found that onset of symptoms ranged from 3 to 52 weeks from the onset of use. Although most clinical effects had resolved by 17 weeks following cessation of use, four patients progressed to cirrhosis with two requiring liver transplantation. Other cases have been reported [34,35], including one in which rechallenge resulted in return of hepatic injury [35]. In that case, the patient presented with jaundice, malaise, and elevation of transaminases and bilirubin. Her use of chaparral was unknown at that time. She had taken chaparral for 8 weeks before her first presentation, was off the compound during hospitalization, but began taking it again on discharge. She returned for readmission after 11 days of twice daily dosing [35]. The authors were criticized, however, because they failed to confirm that the causative agent in question was in fact *L tridentata*.

The mechanism of hepatotoxicity is not known definitively; however, one component has gained significant study. Nordihydroguaiaretic acid (NDGA) is a lignan that has been identified as hepatotoxin in mice. It is found in the leaves and bark of *L tridentata* and constitutes up to 10% by dry weight. It seems to be detoxified by glucuronidation. NDGA is an antioxidant. In low doses it inhibits lipoxygenase pathways and at higher concentrations it also inhibits cyclo-oxygenase pathways. It is a cytochrome p450 inhibitor in rats. One hypothesis is that at high concentrations capable of cyclo-oxygenase inhibition NDGA could favor proinflammatory mediators leading to hepatotoxicity [36].

The possibility of an immune-mediated event is particularly inviting because hepatitis only occurs rarely. The onset seems to require 2 or more months of therapeutic dosing but is variable. Though cessation of chaparral usually leads to resolution, rechallenge causes a much more rapid relapse [35].

Most reports document patients presenting with fatigue, dark urine, jaundice, right upper quadrant abdominal pain, nausea, and diarrhea. Some patients develop weight loss, pruritus, anorexia, and fever [33]. A few progress to severe hepatitis and hepatic failure [36]. Renal failure has been reported in a patient requiring liver transplant [36]. It is difficult to determine if this has a direct link to the ingestion of chaparral. Cystic renal disease has been reported in rats and one case with renal cell carcinoma has been reported in a chronic chaparral user [37]. Laboratory testing demonstrates an increase in alkaline phosphatase, alanine aminotransferase, aspartate aminotransferase, total bilirubin, gamma-glutamyltransferase, and prothrombin time. Albumin may be decreased [33,36]. Biopsy shows hepatitis with lobular collapse, nodular regeneration, mixed portal inflammation, and bile duct proliferation [36]. Treatment is supportive following withdrawal from the exposure.

Impila and white chameleon

Impila, a product from *Callilepis laureola,* is used for stomach problems, impotence, cough, and tapeworm infestations. Its use primarily occurs in Africa, especially among the Zulu. Its toxicity has been recognized since the early 1900s but its use has continued to the present day. It is estimated that 1500 people die yearly in a single South African province as a result of impila toxicity [38]; however, this may be an overestimation [39]. The plant, a member of the Compositae family, is related to the daisy and sunflower. Its tuberous root is the source of impila. It is dried and pulverized. The powder is then boiled in water and taken orally or as an enema. Toxicity may be dose dependent. Despite numerous cases of hepatotoxicity and death, it continues to be a popular herbal preparation. Deaths more commonly occur in children less than 10 years old. In patients with severe toxicity, the death rate is estimated to be 63% in the first 24 hours and 91% overall.

White chameleon, Mediterranean thistle, or Daad, is made from *Atractylis gummifera,* a low-growing thistle. Its toxicity was first described in the mid-1800s [40]. About 100 cases have been reported since. *A gummifera* has toxicity similar to that of *C laureola*. Carboxyatractyloside (CATR) and atractyloside (ATR) have been extracted from the plant.

CATR is a glycoside found in the tuber. It decomposes to ATR. The latter has been found in other plants of Africa, Europe, Asia, and South America, including the Mediterranean thistle (*A gummifera*). Another ATR-containing plant, *Xanthium strumarium*, or cocklebur, is known to cause central lobular necrosis in livestock and recently has been reported to cause hepatic damage, renal toxicity, and death in humans [41]. *X strumarium* is a common plant in the United States, with worldwide distribution.

CATR and ATR inhibit the transport of ADP across the mitochondrial membrane reducing ATP production and leading to cell death. As a result of CATR and ATR activity, mitochondrial permeability transition pores open causing the release of cytochrome c and other proteins from the intermembranous space into the cytoplasm. This phenomenon contributes to condensation of chromatin and formation of ladder DNA associated with apoptosis. Nephrotoxicity has been linked with ATR, but not CATR. ATR may also destroy tubulin, interfering with microtubule construction necessary for mitosis [42].

Onset of clinical findings reportedly is abrupt, with vomiting, abdominal pain, and diarrhea. Hepatic and renal failure lead to profound hypoglycemia, encephalopathy, convulsions, and frequently death.

Wainwright and Schonland [43] reported that the liver appeared pale and yellow without signs of congestion with sharp demarcation of centrilobular, punctate areas of congestion giving it a speckled appearance. The weight of the liver was reduced in 50% of cases, but renal weight was increased in 70%. The kidney demonstrated evidence of tubular necrosis involving convoluted tubules and loops of Henle. There were hyaline, granular, and red cell casts in the tubules. Interstitial edema and tubulovenous aneurysms occasionally were seen [43]. Although no specific therapy exists, there has been interest in the development of Fab-specific fragments [44,45].

Margosa oil

Margosa oil is extracted from the seeds of the neem tree (*Azadirachta indica*) commonly found in India, Pakistan, and the West Indies. Its fruit is toxic. It is used as a therapy for various skin diseases and otitis. Although intended for topical use, it is sometimes given orally and has been reported to cause a Reye-like syndrome in humans [46–48] and animals [49].

Although the mechanism of toxicity has not been defined clearly, it seems that margosa oil targets mitochondria by uncoupling oxidative phosphorylation and reducing ATP production [50].

In reports of childhood exposure, the amount of ingestion varied from a few drops to 12 mL on 2 successive days. Vomiting, loss of consciousness, and convulsions were reported. Transaminases were mildly elevated [46,48,50]. One child died [48]. Autopsy revealed hepatic edema without necrosis or inflammation. Cerebral edema was present. Electron micrographs demonstrated fatty vacuolation of hepatocytes with increased peroxisomes, flocculation of mitochondria, and marked proliferation of smooth endoplasmic reticulum.

Treatment is supportive. There is some evidence that carnitine and glucose may be of benefit [51].

Kava

Kava (*Piper methysticum*) is a perennial plant that has been used by South Pacific Islanders for centuries as part of spiritual services and as a ceremonial intoxicating beverage [52]. Kava has been advocated as a sedative, anxiolytic, anesthetic, muscle relaxant, and anticonvulsant [53–55]. Numerous reports have arisen demonstrating a relationship between kava ingestion and liver toxicity [56–58]. In November of 2001, European country regulatory authorities placed restrictions on the sale of herbal products containing kava [59]. The United Kingdom and Canada have banned kava sales [60,61]. In the United States, kava still is used by many health enthusiasts, despite warnings issued by the FDA regarding its safety [59,62,63].

Kava extract's bioactivity most likely is because of the presence of kavalactones (also known as kava pyrones). Numerous kavalactones have been isolated and include yangonin, desmethoxyyangonin, kavain, dihydrokavain, methysticin, and dihydromethysticin [64]. Peak plasma levels of kavalactones occur within 2 hours of ingestion; elimination of the parent compound and the metabolites occurs in the urine and feces, and their elimination half-life is approximately 9 hours.

Kava-induced hepatotoxicity possibly is related to the extraction method of kavalactones from the roots of the plants [65]. The traditional kava extracts are prepared by maceration of the roots in a water and coconut milk solution [54]. Commercial extracts commonly use either an ethanol, methanol, or an acetone as extraction solvents. It has been hypothesized that the Pacific extraction methods may remove more toxic components from the plant and contain less kavalactones [52,55]. In one study the traditional water-extraction product contained approximately 30% kavalactones, whereas the acetone-extraction product contained up to 70% kavalactones. Lower levels of kavalactones and higher variations were observed in tea bags from water extraction as compared with methanol extraction [64]. Other studies have documented that there is little difference between aqueous and acetonic and ethanolic extract content [66]. Some products have synthetic kavain added to increase the biologic activity of the extract and thus may increase further the potential for toxicity [67].

The definitive mechanism of liver injury associated with kava consumption is not known and may involve a metabolic and or an allergenic idiosyncrasy. There have been several hypotheses as to the cause of hepatotoxicity associated with kava consumption. First, kavalactones inhibit cytochrome P450 activity. Significant inhibition of CYP1A2, 2C9/19, 2D6, 3A4, and 4A9/11 has been demonstrated under experimental conditions [61,68]. It is hypothesized that those of European decent may be at more risk for inhibition because of the 7% to 9% incidence of CYP2D6 deficiency in such groups. This deficiency is rare in the South Pacific and may be one reason for the lack of reported toxicity in this population [69]. Case reports of kava-induced liver dysfunction have not demonstrated CYP2D6-poor metabolizer status [70]. Second, kavalactones inhibit cyclooxygenase enzymes (COX-1 and COX-2) [71]. COX-2 serves an important hepato-protective function and COX inhibition may contribute to the risk for kava-induced liver injury [72]. Third, kava induces glutathione depletion [67]. It has been hypothesized that kava has the potential to saturate enzymatic detoxification pathways that use glutathione and therefore place undue stress on the liver [61]. Kava products with high content of kavalactones have the potential to deplete glutathione stores markedly.

In native South Pacific kava consumers, gamma-glutamyltransferase levels have been found to be elevated, but no cases of acute liver injury have been identified [70,73]. The gamma-glutamyltransferase elevation is reversible and returns to baseline within 2 weeks of kava discontinuation [74]. This increased activity of gamma-glutamyltransferase in heavy kava consumers in the presence of normal or minimally elevated transaminases is probably not a sign of liver injury but rather reflects an induction of CYP450 enzymes [70].

Two patients, aged 59 and 55, presented with acute hepatitis associated with consumption of traditional aqueous kava extract [70]. Both patients presented with jaundice, elevated liver transferases, and elevated total bilirubin, with one patient also presenting with a prolonged thromboplastin time and eosinophilia. Symptoms developed 4 to 5 weeks after starting to drink kava with laboratory values normalizing within 3 months of ceasing kava consumption.

A 14-year-old girl developed fulminant hepatic failure requiring liver transplantation following ingestion of a kava-containing product for 4 months. No other causes of liver failure could be found. The patient's liver biopsy before transplant demonstrated hepatocellular necrosis consistent with chemical hepatitis [75]. In another report, a 39-year-old woman presented with a history of elevated liver enzyme levels following chronic ingestion of kava. One week after discontinuation of all medications, the patient's transaminases normalized. Two weeks after rechallenge with kava, her liver enzyme levels again became elevated. A liver biopsy revealed acute necrotizing hepatitis. Kava was again discontinued and the patient's transaminase levels returned to normal [76].

In a retrospective review of published (n = 7) and unpublished (n = 29) cases of kava-associated hepatotoxicity reported to the German Federal Institute for Drugs and Medical Devices between 1990 and 2002, the most frequent liver injuries were hepatic necrosis (n = 16), cholestatic hepatitis (n = 7), and lobular hepatitis (n = 1). Fulminant hepatic failure was reported in nine patients, three of whom eventually died. Of the nine patients with fulminant hepatic failure, eight underwent liver transplantation [58].

Pennyroyal

Pennyroyal oil is an herbal product that has been purported to treat upper respiratory tract and ear infections, induce abortions, and act as an insect repellent [77–79]. Although these claims are suspect, pennyroyal oil's inherent toxicity is not. The pure oil is derived from the *Mentha pulegium* and *Hedeoma pulegoides* plant species. It is available readily commercially and has a characteristic mint-like odor [78].

Pennyroyal's primary chemical component, pulegone, is metabolized by the liver using the cytochrome P450 system to menthofuran, a directly hepatotoxic metabolite [80]. Furthermore, in a manner apparently independent of menthofuran, pulegone causes depletion of glutathione stores [81]. Without adequate glutathione stores menthofuran and other toxic metabolites increase in concentration and hepatotoxicity is accentuated [77,80–83]. Subsequently, patients who ingest pennyroyal oil may develop hypoglycemia, elevated liver function tests, hyperbilirubinemia, hyperammonemia, and an elevated anion gap metabolic acidosis. Other clinical effects that may develop include nausea, vomiting, abdominal pain, gastrointestinal bleeding, renal failure, pulmonary edema, coagulopathy, disseminated intravascular coagulation, dizziness, weakness, syncope, mental status changes, and seizures [77,82,83].

In some reports of pennyroyal oil toxicity, small doses have resulted in serious toxicity with one source reporting as little as 10 to 15 mL of pure pennyroyal oil causing death [77]. There are reports describing coma and seizures with doses as low as one teaspoon (5 mL).

Animal studies have demonstrated pennyroyal-induced cellular necrosis in the centrilobular regions of the liver [80]. Pennyroyal-induced hepatitis, hepatocellular necrosis, and hepatic failure requiring transplant have been reported by multiple authors [77,82]. Bakerink and colleagues [83] reported the presence of hypoglycemia and elevated liver enzymes in two infant boys, an 8-week-old and a 6-month-old, following pennyroyal oil poisoning. The autopsy of the 8-week-old boy revealed confluent hepatocellular necrosis.

Treatment of pennyroyal oil toxicity begins with good supportive care. Prompt administration of N-acetylcysteine has been advocated to reduce the degree of liver injury [77].

Summary

A significant number of herbal products have been associated with hepatotoxicity. There are few clinical or laboratory manifestations that suggest specifically that liver injury is the result of a specific herbal. Compounding this difficulty is that the patient may have liver disease from another cause, may be taking other potentially hepatotoxic products, or may be taking a contaminated herbal product. Clinicians should consider herbal products in the differential diagnosis when evaluating patients with new-onset hepatotoxicity.

References

[1] Walker A. The relationship between voluntary notification and material risk in dietary supplement safety. In: Administration UFaD, editor. FDA docket 00N–1200; 2000.
[2] Maddrey WC. Drug-induced hepatotoxicity: 2005. J Clin Gastroenterol 2005;39(4, Suppl 2): S83–9.
[3] Thomsen M, Vitetta L, Schmidt M, et al. Fatal fulminant hepatic failure induced by a natural therapy containing kava. Med J Aust 2004;180(4):198–9 [author reply: 9].

[4] Adachi M, Saito H, Kobayashi H, et al. Hepatic injury in 12 patients taking the herbal weight loss aids Chaso or Onshido. Ann Intern Med 2003;139(6):488–92.

[5] Wilmont F, Robertson G. Senecio disease or cirrhosis of the liver due to senecio poisoning. Lancet 1920;II:848.

[6] Selzer G, Parker RG. Senecio poisoning exhibiting as Chiari's syndrome: a report on twelve cases. Am J Pathol 1951;27(5):885–907.

[7] Bras G, Jelliffe DB, Stuart KL. Veno-occlusive disease of liver with nonportal type of cirrhosis, occurring in Jamaica. AMA Arch Pathol 1954;57(4):285–300.

[8] Tandon BN, Tandon HD, Tandon RK, et al. An epidemic of veno-occlusive disease of liver in central India. Lancet 1976;2(7980):271–2.

[9] Mohabbat O, Younos MS, Merzad AA, et al. An outbreak of hepatic veno-occlusive disease in north-western Afghanistan. Lancet 1976;2(7980):269–71.

[10] Weston CF, Cooper BT, Davies JD, et al. Veno-occlusive disease of the liver secondary to ingestion of comfrey. Br Med J (Clin Res Ed) 1987;295(6591):183.

[11] Bach N, Thung SN, Schaffner F. Comfrey herb tea-induced hepatic veno-occlusive disease. Am J Med 1989;87(1):97–9.

[12] Fox DW, Hart MC, Bergeson PS, et al. Pyrrolizidine (Senecio) intoxication mimicking Reye syndrome. J Pediatr 1978;93(6):980–2.

[13] Ridker PM, Ohkuma S, McDermott WV, et al. Hepatic venocclusive disease associated with the consumption of pyrrolizidine-containing dietary supplements. Gastroenterology 1985; 88(4):1050–4.

[14] Stillman AS, Huxtable R, Consroe P, et al. Hepatic veno-occlusive disease due to pyrrolizidine (Senecio) poisoning in Arizona. Gastroenterology 1977;73(2):349–52.

[15] Stickel F, Seitz HK. The efficacy and safety of comfrey. Public Health Nutr 2000;3(4A): 501–8.

[16] Chojkier M. Hepatic sinusoidal-obstruction syndrome: toxicity of pyrrolizidine alkaloids. J Hepatol 2003;39(3):437–46.

[17] Stickel F, Egerer G, Seitz HK. Hepatotoxicity of botanicals. Public Health Nutr 2000;3(2): 113–24.

[18] Steenkamp V, Stewart MJ, Zuckerman M. Clinical and analytical aspects of pyrrolizidine poisoning caused by South African traditional medicines. Ther Drug Monit 2000;22(3): 302–6.

[19] Fishman AP. Dietary pulmonary hypertension. Circ Res 1974;35(5):657–60.

[20] Kay JM. Dietary pulmonary hypertension. Thorax 1994;49(Suppl):S33–8.

[21] Rode D. Comfrey toxicity revisited. Trends Pharmacol Sci 2002;23(11):497–9.

[22] Corbacioglu S, Greil J, Peters C, et al. Defibrotide in the treatment of children with veno-occlusive disease (VOD): a retrospective multicentre study demonstrates therapeutic efficacy upon early intervention. Bone Marrow Transplant 2004;33(2):189–95.

[23] Wadleigh M, Ho V, Momtaz P, et al. Hepatic veno-occlusive disease: pathogenesis, diagnosis and treatment. Curr Opin Hematol 2003;10(6):451–62.

[24] Senzolo M, Cholongitas E, Patch D, et al. TIPS for veno-occlusive disease: is the contraindication real? Hepatology 2005;42(1):240–1 [author reply: 1].

[25] Larrey D, Vial T, Pauwels A, et al. Hepatitis after germander (Teucrium chamaedrys) administration: another instance of herbal medicine hepatotoxicity. Ann Intern Med 1992;117(2): 129–32.

[26] Mostefa-Kara N, Pauwels A, Pines E, et al. Fatal hepatitis after herbal tea. Lancet 1992; 340(8820):674.

[27] Castot A, Larrey D. [Hepatitis observed during a treatment with a drug or tea containing Wild Germander. Evaluation of 26 cases reported to the Regional Centers of Pharmacovigilance]. Gastroenterol Clin Biol 1992;16(12):916–22.

[28] Dourakis SP, Papanikolaou IS, Tzemanakis EN, et al. Acute hepatitis associated with herb (Teucrium capitatum L.) administration. Eur J Gastroenterol Hepatol 2002;14(6): 693–5.

[29] Polymeros D, Kamberoglou D, Tzias V. Acute cholestatic hepatitis caused by *Teucrium po-lium* (golden germander) with transient appearance of antimitochondrial antibody. J Clin Gastroenterol 2002;34(1):100–1.

[30] Zhou S, Koh HL, Gao Y, et al. Herbal bioactivation: the good, the bad and the ugly. Life Sci 2004;74(8):935–68.

[31] Cavaleiro C, Salgueiro LR, Miguel MG, et al. Analysis by gas chromatography-mass spectrometry of the volatile components of *Teucrium lusitanicum* and *Teucrium algarbiensis*. J Chromatogr A 2004;1033(1):187–90.

[32] Bosisio E, Giavarini F, Dell'Agli M, et al. Analysis by high-performance liquid chromatography of teucrin A in beverages flavoured with an extract of *Teucrium chamaedrys L*. Food Addit Contam 2004;21(5):407–14.

[33] Sheikh NM, Philen RM, Love LA. Chaparral-associated hepatotoxicity. Arch Intern Med 1997;157(8):913–9.

[34] Batchelor WB, Heathcote J, Wanless IR. Chaparral-induced hepatic injury. Am J Gastroenterol 1995;90(5):831–3.

[35] Kauma H, Koskela R, Makisalo H, et al. Toxic acute hepatitis and hepatic fibrosis after consumption of chaparral tablets. Scand J Gastroenterol 2004;39(11):1168–71.

[36] Gordon DW, Rosenthal G, Hart J, et al. Chaparral ingestion. The broadening spectrum of liver injury caused by herbal medications. JAMA 1995;273(6):489–90.

[37] Smith AY, Feddersen RM, Gardner KD Jr, et al. Cystic renal cell carcinoma and acquired renal cystic disease associated with consumption of chaparral tea: a case report. J Urol 1994; 152(6 Pt 1):2089–91.

[38] Popat A, Shear NH, Malkiewicz I, et al. The toxicity of *Callilepis laureola*, a South African traditional herbal medicine. Clin Biochem 2001;34(3):229–36.

[39] du Plooy WJ, Jobson MR. Regarding "the toxicity of Callilepis laureola, a South African traditional herbal medicine". Clin Biochem 2002;35(3):179 [author reply 80].

[40] Gay J. Sur les proprietes toxiques des racines du Carlina gummifera. Bull Soc Bot de France 1858:692–4.

[41] Turgut M, Alhan CC, Gurgoze M, et al. Carboxyatractyloside poisoning in humans. Ann Trop Paediatr 2005;25(2):125–34.

[42] Stewart MJ, Steenkamp V. The biochemistry and toxicity of atractyloside: a review. Ther Drug Monit 2000;22(6):641–9.

[43] Wainwright J, Schonland MM. Toxic hepatitis in black patients in natal. S Afr Med J 1977; 51(17):571–3.

[44] Daniele C, Dahamna S, Firuzi O, et al. *Atractylis gummifera L*. poisoning: an ethnopharmacological review. J Ethnopharmacol 2005;97(2):175–81.

[45] Eddleston M, Persson H. Acute plant poisoning and antitoxin antibodies. J Toxicol Clin Toxicol 2003;41(3):309–15.

[46] Lai SM, Lim KW, Cheng HK. Margosa oil poisoning as a cause of toxic encephalopathy. Singapore Med J 1990;31(5):463–5.

[47] Sinniah D, Baskaran G. Margosa oil poisoning as a cause of Reye's syndrome. Lancet 1981; 1(8218):487–9.

[48] Sinniah D, Baskaran G, Looi LM, et al. Reye-like syndrome due to margosa oil poisoning: report of a case with postmortem findings. Am J Gastroenterol 1982;77(3):158–61.

[49] Sinniah R, Sinniah D, Chia LS, et al. Animal model of margosa oil ingestion with Reye-like syndrome: pathogenesis of microvesicular fatty liver. J Pathol 1989;159(3):255–64.

[50] Koga Y, Yoshida I, Kimura A, et al. Inhibition of mitochondrial functions by margosa oil: possible implications in the pathogenesis of Reye's syndrome. Pediatr Res 1987;22(2):184–7.

[51] Sinniah D, Sinniah R, Baskaran G, et al. Evaluation of the possible role of glucose, carnitine, coenzyme Q10 and steroids in the treatment of Reye's syndrome using the margosa oil animal model. Acta Paediatr Jpn 1990;32(4):462–8.

[52] Cote CS, Kor C, Cohen J, et al. Composition and biological activity of traditional and commercial kava extracts. Biochem Biophys Res Commun 2004;322(1):147–52.

[53] Singh YN, Singh NN. Therapeutic potential of kava in the treatment of anxiety disorders. CNS Drugs 2002;16(11):731–43.

[54] Bilia AR, Gallon S, Vincieri FF. Kava-kava and anxiety: growing knowledge about the efficacy and safety. Life Sci 2002;70(22):2581–97.

[55] Moulds RF, Malani J. Kava: herbal panacea or liver poison? Med J Aust 2003;178(9):451–3.

[56] Escher M, Desmeules J, Giostra E, et al. Hepatitis associated with Kava, a herbal remedy for anxiety. BMJ 2001;322(7279):139.

[57] Russmann S, Lauterburg BH, Helbling A. Kava hepatotoxicity. Ann Intern Med 2001; 135(1):68–9.

[58] Stickel F, Baumuller HM, Seitz K, et al. Hepatitis induced by Kava (Piper methysticum rhizoma). J Hepatol 2003;39(1):62–7.

[59] Mills E, Singh R, Ross C, et al. Sale of kava extract in some health food stores. CMAJ 2003; 169(11):1158–9.

[60] Health Canada advises against kava. Treatmentupdate 2002;14(2):5–6.

[61] Clouatre DL. Kava kava: examining new reports of toxicity. Toxicol Lett 2004;150(1):85–96.

[62] Kava and severe liver injury. FDA Consum 2002;36(3):4.

[63] Hepatic toxicity possibly associated with kava-containing products: United States, Germany, and Switzerland, 1999–2002. MMWR Morb Mortal Wkly Rep 2002;51(47): 1065–7.

[64] Hu L, Jhoo JW, Ang CY, et al. Determination of six kavalactones in dietary supplements and selected functional foods containing Piper methysticum by isocratic liquid chromatography with internal standard. J AOAC Int 2005;88(1):16–25.

[65] Whitton PA, Lau A, Salisbury A, et al. Kava lactones and the kava-kava controversy. Phytochemistry 2003;64(3):673–9.

[66] Loew D, Franz G. Quality aspects of traditional and industrial Kava-extracts. Phytomedicine 2003;10(6–7):610–2.

[67] Denham A, McIntyre M, Whitehouse J. Kava—the unfolding story: report on a work-in-progress. J Altern Complement Med 2002;8(3):237–63.

[68] Russmann S, Lauterburg BH, Barguil Y, et al. Traditional aqueous kava extracts inhibit cytochrome P450 1A2 in humans: protective effect against environmental carcinogens? Clin Pharmacol Ther 2005;77(5):453–4.

[69] Poolsup N, Li Wan Po A, et al. Pharmacogenetics and psychopharmacotherapy. J Clin Pharm Ther 2000;25(3):197–220.

[70] Russmann S, Barguil Y, Cabalion P, et al. Hepatic injury due to traditional aqueous extracts of kava root in New Caledonia. Eur J Gastroenterol Hepatol 2003;15(9):1033–6.

[71] Wu D, Yu L, Nair MG, et al. Cyclooxygenase enzyme inhibitory compounds with antioxidant activities from Piper methysticum (kava kava) roots. Phytomedicine 2002;9(1):41–7.

[72] Reilly TP, Brady JN, Marchick MR, et al. A protective role for cyclooxygenase-2 in drug-induced liver injury in mice. Chem Res Toxicol 2001;14(12):1620–8.

[73] Mathews JD, Riley MD, Fejo L, et al. Effects of the heavy usage of kava on physical health: summary of a pilot survey in an aboriginal community. Med J Aust 1988;148(11):548–55.

[74] Clough AR, Bailie RS, Currie B. Liver function test abnormalities in users of aqueous kava extracts. J Toxicol Clin Toxicol 2003;41(6):821–9.

[75] Humberston CL, Akhtar J, Krenzelok EP. Acute hepatitis induced by kava kava. J Toxicol Clin Toxicol 2003;41(2):109–13.

[76] Strahl S, Ehret V, Dahm HH, et al. [Necrotizing hepatitis after taking herbal remedies]. Dtsch Med Wochenschr 1998;123(47):1410–4.

[77] Anderson IB, Mullen WH, Meeker JE, et al. Pennyroyal toxicity: measurement of toxic metabolite levels in two cases and review of the literature. Ann Intern Med 1996;124(8):726–34.

[78] Mack RB. Boldly they rode... into the mouth of hell." Pennyroyal oil toxicity. N C Med J 1997;58(6):456–7.

[79] Sudekum M, Poppenga RH, Raju N, et al. Pennyroyal oil toxicosis in a dog. J Am Vet Med Assoc 1992;200(6):817–8.

[80] Gordon WP, Forte AJ, McMurtry RJ, et al. Hepatotoxicity and pulmonary toxicity of pennyroyal oil and its constituent terpenes in the mouse. Toxicol Appl Pharmacol 1982;65(3): 413–24.
[81] Thomassen D, Slattery JT, Nelson SD. Contribution of menthofuran to the hepatotoxicity of pulegone: assessment based on matched area under the curve and on matched time course. J Pharmacol Exp Ther 1988;244(3):825–9.
[82] Sullivan JB Jr, Rumack BH, Thomas H Jr, et al. Pennyroyal oil poisoning and hepatotoxicity. JAMA 1979;242(26):2873–4.
[83] Bakerink JA, Gospe SM Jr, Dimand RJ, Eldridge MW. Multiple organ failure after ingestion of pennyroyal oil from herbal tea in two infants. Pediatrics 1996;98(5):944–7.

ELSEVIER
SAUNDERS

CLINICS IN
LABORATORY
MEDICINE

Clin Lab Med 26 (2006) 243–253

Criminal Poisoning: Munchausen by Proxy

Christopher P. Holstege, MD[a,b,c,*],
Stephen G. Dobmeier, RN, BSN, CSPI[b]

[a]Division of Medical Toxicology, University of Virginia, P.O. Box 800774, Charlottesville,
VA 22908, USA
[b]Blue Ridge Poison Center, University of Virginia Health System, P.O. Box 800774,
Charlottesville, VA 22908, USA
[c]Department of Emergency Medicine and Pediatrics, University of Virginia, P.O. Box 800774,
Charlottesville, VA 22908, USA

The diagnosis and subsequent prosecution of Munchausen by proxy (MBP) cases requires the collaborative teamwork of health care teams, laboratory personnel, law enforcement, and social services. Poisoning occurs in a significant number of the MBP cases with a diverse variety of agents used. To aid laboratory professionals in determining the appropriate toxicology tests to perform in such criminal cases, health care professionals must focus their testing requests on substances that correspond to the victim's signs, symptoms, and ancillary test values. This article reviews MBP, with particular focus on poisoning agents that have been used in past reported cases.

History and definitions

Munchausen syndrome was first described by British physician Richard Asher in 1951 [1]. It is a psychiatric disorder that causes an individual to self-inflict injury or illness or to fabricate symptoms of physical or mental illness to receive medical care or hospitalization. Categorized as a factitious disorder in which the physical or psychological symptoms are under voluntary control, Munchausen syndrome seems to be motivated by a need to assume the role of a patient. Unlike malingering, there is not a clear external secondary gain (eg, money) in Munchausen syndrome. The term

* Corresponding author. Blue Ridge Poison Center, University of Virginia Health System, P.O. Box 800774, Charlottesville, VA.

E-mail address: ch2xf@virginia.edu (C.P. Holstege).

Munchausen was derived from Baron Karl Friederich von Munchausen, an eighteenth century German military man known for his dramatic and untruthful tall tales [2].

MBP was first described in 1977 by Sir Roy Meadow [3]. MBP is also known as Polle's syndrome, after Baron von Munchausen's only child Polle, who died mysteriously at 1 year of age [4,5]. MBP is defined as the intentional production or feigning of physical or psychological signs or symptoms in another person who is under the individual's care for the purpose of indirectly assuming the sick role. MBP has also been called factitious disorder by proxy, fabricated disorder by proxy, and Meadow's syndrome [6,7]. MBP most often is noted in the context of children, but cases have also been reported in adults [8]. MBP in children is considered child abuse and must be reported to the authorities in accordance with mandatory child abuse reporting laws [9].

MBP is distinctly different from somatoform disorder and malingering by proxy. In somatoform disorder, the signs and symptoms are real to the person afflicted and not produced under voluntary control; they are not simulated intentionally or created. In malingering by proxy, guardians coach their children to misbehave or fake disabilities to obtain an external incentive, such as supplemental security income payments. If the fabrication of an illness includes repeated hospitalization or treatment, MBP association also may occur [10].

Epidemiology

Accurate epidemiologic data pertaining to MBP are unavailable. Deception is an integral part of factitious disorders; therefore this behavior certainly is underreported [11]. An additional problem in determining prevalence is that the diagnosis criteria for MBP are not consistent. In available reports, the incidence of MBP has been noted to be 2 cases per 100,000 in children younger than 1 year of age and 0.5 cases per 100,000 in children younger than 16 years of age [12,13]. MBP is not unique to Western society, but has been reported in multiple countries and cultures [14].

Siblings of MBP victims often are affected [15–19]. In one study, 30% of the siblings of MBP victims were either poisoned or otherwise abused, with numerous siblings of MBP victims having died of uncertain causes [20]. In another review of 117 cases of MBP, 10 deaths of siblings of MBP victims were reported to occur under unusual circumstances [21]. Sudden infant death syndrome has been diagnosed in several siblings of MBP victims [22,23]. In previously reported cases of multiple sibling involvement of MBP, the siblings were affected sequentially and not simultaneously [24].

In MBP, the offender can either simulate or produce an illness. With simulation, an offender fakes an illness by verbally presenting an untrue history for a nonexistent illness or condition. For example, a caregiver can give a false history that the child had a seizure and describe in detail a grand mal convulsion that in fact did not occur. By production, the offender actually induces a pathologic condition in the MBP victim. For example, a caregiver could administer camphor to a child, causing that child to develop seizures. In one study MBP offenders actually produced illness in 70% of cases [21].

The mean time taken to make the correct diagnosis from initial presentation is 7 months in cases referred to child protection agencies and 23 months in cases not referred [25]. Mortality rates in MBP victims have been estimated at 10%, but the true rates of mortality are unknown [21,26]. Of the methods used, poisoning accounted for 34% of the MBP cases in one series. The most common presenting signs for MBP are bleeding (44%), seizures (42%), central nervous system depression (19%), apnea (15%), diarrhea (11%), vomiting (10%), and fever (10%) [12].

MBP victim

Most reported victims of MBP have been less than 5 years of age, with a mean age of 20 months [13]. MBP victims are divided nearly evenly between boys (47%) and girls (53%) [13]. The MBP victims tend to be dependent, display separation anxiety, be immature, have a symbiotic relationship with the offender, use alternative communication options, passively tolerate medical procedures, present with multiple symptoms, and fail to thrive (Box 1) [25]. The documentation of the resolution of signs and symptoms when the perpetrating caregiver is separated from the victim should raise the possibility of MBP as the cause.

MBP offender

The responsible caregivers have been described as "Great Pretenders" [9]. They are more commonly white, upper class, and educated, though all segments of the population are represented. Most of the offenders are the victim's mother, with men responsible for less than 5% of cases [13,25]. Studies have documented that 27% to 50% of the MBP offenders have some form of health care training [15,26,27]. The perpetrators tend to be calm, welcome painful medical tests, give extensive praise to medical staff, be knowledgeable about the victim's illness, shelter the victims, and have a high degree of attentiveness (see Box 1) [12,28]. The offender's personality can vary, however, and individuals also have been described as "poorly educated, single, antagonistic to nursing staff and physicians, and hardly an ideal mother" [29]. Fathers tend to be separated physically from the family or detached and unaware of the poisoning [30].

Box 1. Characteristics commonly found in MBP offenders and victims

Profile of MBP offender
Biologic mother
Extensive praise to medical staff
High degree of attentiveness
Calm despite severity of child's illness
Shelters the victim
Knowledgeable about the victim's illness
Some degree of medical education
History of similar illness as the child
Communication with the victim through methods other than
    speech
Welcomes painful medical tests and procedures without question

Traits of MBP victim
Dependent
Displays separation anxiety
Immature
Symbiotic relationship with caregiver
Views offender as ideal parent
Passively tolerates medical procedures
Excessive school absence
Not involved in normal social activities
Failure to thrive
Illness corresponds with presence of caregiver
Illness resolves with close surveillance

Poisons used in past MBP

Numerous agents have been used to poison children in cases of MBP. In a case series of 128 children with MBP, 40 (35%) were poisoned with 38 different toxins used, and 7 children received more than one poison [13]. Of poisons used, 71% were prescribed drugs. The most common drugs used in this study were anticonvulsants and opiates. A partial listing of specific agents reported in MBP investigations in the medical literature can be found in Box 2.

Criminal poisoning is a diagnostic challenge, and MBP cases are no exception. Initial visits of MBP victims to health care providers are unlikely to raise the diagnosis of MBP as a possibility. By the time the diagnosis of MBP is being entertained, testing of urine or blood may be of limited value because the agent used to poison may no longer be detected. To narrow the class of agents that may be responsible in a criminal poisoning case such as MBP, it is imperative that the health care workers fully review the

---

Box 2. Specific agents used to poison children in MBP cases as reported in the medical literature

Paregoric [51]
Antidepressants [13,52–55]
Barbiturates [17,56,57]
Caustics [58,59]
Rat poison [60]
Salt [13,17,58]
Insulin [8,28,31,34,51,61,62]
Methaqualone [17]
Benzodiazepines [13,63,64]
Ipecac [29,30,35–37]
Antihistamines [13,24]
Bethanecol [51]
Salicylates [64]
Bleach [13]
Antipsychotics [5,51,65–67]
Clonidine [67,68]
Arsenic [49]
Frusemide [17,69]
Glucose [70]
Acetaminophen [13]
Opioids [13,64]
Sulfonylureas [33,34,71]
Laxatives [51,72,73]
Carbon monoxide [13]
Anticonvulsants [13,42]

---

presenting symptoms, signs, laboratory values, and other ancillary tests. This review aids the toxicology laboratory personnel in choosing the correct panel of tests. For example, a child presenting with frequent visits of altered mental status or seizures and found to be solely hypoglycemic with no other findings should be tested for either exogenous insulin or oral hypoglycemic administration. The triad findings of hypoglycemia, elevated insulin, and suppressed c-peptide should raise the concern for potential exogenous insulin administration [31,32]. The administration of oral hypoglycemic agents of the sulfonylurea class, on the other hand, can mimic an insulinoma, with the MBP victim having hypoglycemia, elevated insulin, and elevated c-peptide [32,33]. Pancreatectomy has been reported in cases of MBP in which the diagnosis of sulfonylurea poisoning was not entertained [34]. Specific laboratory analysis for oral hypoglycemic agents should be performed in suspected cases [32].

As another example, syrup of ipecac is one of the most common reported toxins used in published MBP cases [29,30,35–37]. Syrup of ipecac currently is available as a nonprescription product in many countries, including the United States. It is prepared from the dried rhizome and roots of the *Cephaelis ipecacuanha* or *C acuminata* plant, which contain the alkaloids emetine and cephaeline. These alkaloids are potent emetics inducing vomiting by direct local gastrointestinal effects and central nervous system actions at the chemoreceptor trigger zone. Emesis following syrup of ipecac ingestion typically occurs within 20 minutes of ingestion and persists for 30 to 120 minutes. Children who are administered ipecac in MBP cases are often misdiagnosed as having gastrointestinal reflux. Chronic administration of ipecac in MBP cases may result in gastrointestinal bleeding, electrolyte abnormalities, and skeletal and cardiac myopathy [38]. Cardiomyopathy has been reported as the cause of death in such cases [39]. Emetine causes impaired myocardial cellular respiration, carbohydrate metabolism, and protein synthesis causing a progression to myofibrillar degeneration and myocytolysis [39]. Emetine and cephaeline serum levels peak within 1 hour after ingestion and are undetectable within 6 hours [40]. Emetine and cephaeline are detected in the urine within 40 minutes and may be detectable in the urine for several weeks after ingestion [30,39,40]. Children who present with repetitive emesis that resolves in a supervised setting and who have an elevated creatine phosphokinase, proximal muscle weakness, or evidence of cardiomyopathy, should have ipecac toxicity included on their differential diagnosis [30].

Laboratory testing

Routine urine or serum toxicology screens are of limited value for detecting a poison that may be contributing to an MBP victim's signs and symptoms. Most screening tests check for a small number of common agents, with numerous false negative and positive results possible. Most hospitals use commercially available urine immunoassays for drugs of abuse that can detect a combination of common drugs, such as amphetamines, barbiturates, benzodiazepines, cannabinoids, cocaine derivatives, and opioids [41]. As noted in Box 2, many of the agents that have been reported in MBP cases are not tested for on routine toxicology screens. To narrow the differential, it is imperative that the patient's case be closely reviewed to determine the class of agent that is consistent with the victim's signs, symptoms, routine laboratory values, and ancillary tests such as an electrocardiogram.

Pharmacokinetic modeling

The application of pharmacokinetic models may assist in diagnosing a case of MBP. For example, Mahesh and colleagues [42] described a

4-year-old child who presented to health care facilities on multiple occasions with altered mental status and seizures. Abuse had been suspected, but urine drug screens had revealed only the presence of the medications he was prescribed: phenytoin and carbamazepine. During his hospital admissions the serum levels of these anticonvulsants demonstrated extreme fluctuations, from subtherapeutic to toxic, without recorded dose changes. The mother of the child in this case contended that her child had abnormal drug metabolism. Evaluation of the child's pharmacokinetics by a clinical pharmacologist documented a normal serum half-life thereby suggesting surreptitious dosing and leading to a confession by the mother that she had been administrating additional doses of the drugs.

Findings that may be associated with criminal cases of MBP in which the victim's prescribed drugs are used include: (1) discrepancies between history and drug levels, (2) abnormal pharmacokinetics despite appropriate dosing, (3) resolution of abnormal pharmacokinetics when the victim is under close supervision of health care providers and the MBP perpetrator is removed from the victim [42]. The application of common therapeutic drug monitoring techniques may assist the health care team in diagnosing MBP. To accurately use clinical pharmacokinetic methods, the health care team must keep a precise record of the dose size, timing of drug administration, and exact time at which serum drug levels are obtained. With these data, fundamental pharmacologic equations can be used to determine expectant drug concentrations. Because all this information is readily available in the hospital setting, the use of pharmacokinetics can represent a simple, inexpensive, and accurate way to identify objectively the child poisoned in MBP cases.

MBP investigation

There are numerous warning signs that may provide health care workers clues that a patient is an MBP victim, especially in cases in which there is recurrent illness that cannot be explained, discrepancies between clinical findings and history are noted, symptoms occur only when the suspected perpetrator is present, and a family history of sudden or unexplained infant death has occurred (see Box 1) [27,28]. The diagnosis and management of an MBP case is complex. Kathryn Artingstall's book [9] summarizes these difficulties by stating: "The complexities involved in MBP case compilation necessitates a union of forces within the legal, medical, social/protective service, and law enforcement professions. There is no other type of investigation that requires an understanding and protocol between agencies to the degree required in MBP investigations" [9]. Documentation must be objective, accurate, detailed, and legible. Actual pertinent quotations of the suspected perpetrator should be documented. The child's signs and symptoms should be documented fully and clearly both in the presence and in the absence of the suspected caregiver. Hospital covert video surveillance of caregivers suspected of MBP should be considered, using appropriate protocols [43–46]. Appropriate hospital administration and child protective services should be contacted at the time a case of MBP is suspected. Laboratory testing should be focused and laboratory personnel should be in open communication with the health care team to decide the most appropriate battery of toxicologic testing.

Future for MBP victims

There are few studies examining the long-term impact on children who have been victims of MBP. It is likely that many of the victims are never identified or are lost to follow-up. Children have been reported to demonstrate significant psychological difficulties later in life, including conversion symptoms, fabrications, poor school attendance, diminished ability to concentrate, and emotional and behavioral problems [47,48]. The childhood problems of MBP victims have been reported to persist into adulthood, especially posttraumatic stress symptoms [49]. Victims described struggling to avoid playing the victim role, difficulty maintaining relationships, and insecurity. These victims had difficulty separating fantasy from reality, especially in relation to illness and need for medical treatment [49,50].

Summary

Health care personnel should consider the diagnostic possibility of MBP in their practices, especially in cases fitting the patterns described in this article. In suspected cases of poisoning, clinicians should attempt to narrow the testing to agents that correspond to the presenting clinical data. If assistance is needed in detecting a suspected toxin, clinical toxicology consultation should be sought.

References

[1] Asher R. Munchausens Syndrome. Lancet 1951;I:339–41.
[2] Souid AK, Keith DV, Cunningham AS. Munchausen syndrome by proxy. Clin Pediatr (Phila) 1998;37(8):497–503.
[3] Meadow R. Munchausen syndrome by proxy. The hinterland of child abuse. Lancet 1977; 2(8033):343–5.
[4] Casavant MJ. Polle's syndrome (Munchausen by proxy). Pediatr Emerg Care 1995;11(4): 264.
[5] Verity CM, Winckworth C, Burman D, et al. Polle syndrome: children of Munchausen. BMJ 1979;2(6187):422–3.
[6] AmericanPsychiatricAssociation. Diagnostic and statistical manual of mental disorders (DSM)-IV-TR). 4th edition. Washington DC: American Psychiatric Association; 2000.
[7] Schreier H. Munchausen by proxy. Curr Probl Pediatr Adolesc Health Care 2004;34(3): 126–43.

[8] Ben-Chetrit E, Melmed RN. Recurrent hypoglycaemia in multiple myeloma: a case of Munchausen syndrome by proxy in an elderly patient. J Intern Med 1998;244(2): 175–8.

[9] Artingstall K. Practical aspects of munchausen by proxy and munchausen syndrome investigation. Boca Raton: CRC Press LLC; 1999.

[10] Feldman MD. Munchausen by proxy and malingering by proxy. Psychosomatics 2004;45(4): 365–6.

[11] Wise MG, Ford CV. Factitious disorders. Prim Care 1999;26(2):315–26.

[12] Sharif I. Munchausen syndrome by proxy. Pediatr Rev 2004;25(6):215–6.

[13] McClure RJ, Davis PM, Meadow SR, et al. Epidemiology of Munchausen syndrome by proxy, non-accidental poisoning, and non-accidental suffocation. Arch Dis Child 1996; 75(1):57–61.

[14] Feldman MD, Brown RM. Munchausen by Proxy in an international context. Child Abuse Negl 2002;26(5):509–24.

[15] Alexander R, Smith W, Stevenson R. Serial Munchausen syndrome by proxy. Pediatrics 1990;86(4):581–5.

[16] Meadow R. Non-accidental salt poisoning. Arch Dis Child 1993;68(4):448–52.

[17] Rogers DW, Bentovim A, Tripp JH. Nonaccidental poisoning: the elusive diagnosis. Arch Dis Child 1981;56(2):156–7.

[18] Fleisher D, Ament ME. Diarrhea, red diapers, and child abuse: clinical alertness needed for recognition; clinical skill needed for success in management. Clin Pediatr (Phila) 1977;16(9): 820–4.

[19] Hvizdala EV, Gellady AM. Intentional poisoning of two siblings by prescription drugs. An unusual form of child abuse. Clin Pediatr (Phila) 1978;17(6):480–2.

[20] Bools CN, Neale BA, Meadow SR. Co-morbidity associated with fabricated illness (Munchausen syndrome by proxy). Arch Dis Child 1992;67(1):77–9.

[21] Rosenberg DA. Web of deceit: a literature review of Munchausen syndrome by proxy. Child Abuse Negl 1987;11(4):547–63.

[22] Lyall EG, Stirling HF, Crofton PM, et al. Albuminuric growth failure. A case of Munchausen syndrome by proxy. Acta Paediatr 1992;81(4):373–6.

[23] Hickson GB, Altemeier WA, Martin ED, et al. Parental administration of chemical agents: a cause of apparent life-threatening events. Pediatrics 1989;83(5):772–6.

[24] Arnold SM, Arnholz D, Garyfallou GT, et al. Two siblings poisoned with diphenhydramine: a case of factitious disorder by proxy. Ann Emerg Med 1998;32(2):256–9.

[25] Denny SJ, Grant CC, Pinnock R. Epidemiology of Munchausen syndrome by proxy in New Zealand. J Paediatr Child Health 2001;37(3):240–3.

[26] Meadow R. Munchausen syndrome by proxy. Arch Dis Child 1982;57(2):92–8.

[27] Thomas K. Munchausen syndrome by proxy: identification and diagnosis. J Pediatr Nurs 2003;18(3):174–80.

[28] Zylstra RG, Miller KE, Stephens WE. Munchausen syndrome by proxy: a clinical vignette. Prim Care Companion J Clin Psychiatry 2000;2(2):42–4.

[29] Colletti RB, Wasserman RC. Recurrent infantile vomiting due to intentional ipecac poisoning. J Pediatr Gastroenterol Nutr 1989;8(3):394–6.

[30] Sutphen JL, Saulsbury FT. Intentional ipecac poisoning: Munchausen syndrome by proxy. Pediatrics 1988;82(3 Pt 2):453–6.

[31] Kaminer Y, Robbins DR. Insulin misuse: a review of an overlooked psychiatric problem. Psychosomatics 1989;30(1):19–24.

[32] Marks V, Teale JD. Hypoglycemia: factitious and felonious. Endocrinol Metab Clin North Am 1999;28(3):579–601.

[33] Owen L, Ellis M, Shield J. Deliberate sulphonylurea poisoning mimicking hyperinsulinaemia of infancy. Arch Dis Child 2000;82(5):392–3.

[34] Giurgea I, Ulinski T, Touati G, et al. Factitious hyperinsulinism leading to pancreatectomy: severe forms of Munchausen syndrome by proxy. Pediatrics 2005;116(1):e145–8.

[35] Feldman KW, Christopher DM, Opheim KB. Munchausen syndrome/bulimia by proxy: ipecac as a toxin in child abuse. Child Abuse Negl 1989;13(2):257–61.

[36] Bader AA, Kerzner B. Ipecac toxicity in "Munchausen syndrome by proxy". Ther Drug Monit 1999;21(2):259–60.

[37] Cooper CP, Kamath KR. A toddler with persistent vomiting and diarrhoea. Eur J Pediatr 1998;157(9):775–6.

[38] Manno BR, Manno JE. Toxicology of ipecac: a review. Clin Toxicol 1977;10(2):221–42.

[39] Schneider DJ, Perez A, Knilamus TE, et al. Clinical and pathologic aspects of cardiomyopathy from ipecac administration in Munchausen's syndrome by proxy. Pediatrics 1996; 97(6 Pt 1):902–6.

[40] Yamashita M, Yamashita M, Azuma J. Urinary excretion of ipecac alkaloids in human volunteers. Vet Hum Toxicol 2002;44(5):257–9.

[41] Osterhoudt KC. A toddler with recurrent episodes of unresponsiveness. Pediatr Emerg Care 2004;20(3):195–7.

[42] Mahesh VK, Stern HP, Kearns GL, et al. Application of pharmacokinetics in the diagnosis of chemical abuse in Munchausen syndrome by proxy. Clin Pediatr (Phila) 1988;27(5):243–6.

[43] Bauer KA. Covert video surveillance of parents suspected of child abuse: the British experience and alternative approaches. Theor Med Bioeth 2004;25(4):311–27.

[44] Hall DE, Eubanks L, Meyyazhagan LS, et al. Evaluation of covert video surveillance in the diagnosis of Munchausen syndrome by proxy: lessons from 41 cases. Pediatrics 2000;105(6): 1305–12.

[45] Chandra P, Shankar AM. Detecting fabricated or induced illness in children: are we ready for covert video surveillance? BMJ 2005;331(7525):1144.

[46] Lewis W. Detecting fabricated or induced illness in children: covert video surveillance can protect children and parents if rules are clear. BMJ 2005;331(7525):1144.

[47] McGuire TL, Feldman KW. Psychologic morbidity of children subjected to Munchausen syndrome by proxy. Pediatrics 1989;83(2):289–92.

[48] Bools CN, Neale BA, Meadow SR. Follow up of victims of fabricated illness (Munchausen syndrome by proxy). Arch Dis Child 1993;69(6):625–30.

[49] Libow JA. Munchausen by proxy victims in adulthood: a first look. Child Abuse Negl 1995; 19(9):1131–42.

[50] Bryk M, Siegel PT. My mother caused my illness: the story of a survivor of Munchausen by proxy syndrome. Pediatrics 1997;100(1):1–7.

[51] Mehl AL, Coble L, Johnson S. Munchausen syndrome by proxy: a family affair. Child Abuse Negl 1990;14(4):577–85.

[52] Winrow AP. Amitriptyline-associated seizures in a toddler with Munchausen-by-proxy. Pediatr Emerg Care 1999;15(6):462–3.

[53] Mullins ME, Cristofani CB, Warden CR, et al. Amitriptyline-associated seizures in a toddler with Munchausen-by-proxy. Pediatr Emerg Care 1999;15(3):202–5.

[54] Watson JB, Davies JM, Hunter JL. Nonaccidental poisoning in childhood. Arch Dis Child 1979;54(2):143–4.

[55] Manikoth P, Subramanyan R, Menon S, et al. A child with cardiac arrhythmia and convulsions. Lancet 1999;354(9195):2046.

[56] Lorber J. Unexplained episodes of coma in a two-year-old. Lancet 1978;2(8087):472–3.

[57] Lorber J, Reckless JP, Watson JB. Nonaccidental poisoning: the elusive diagnosis. Arch Dis Child 1980;55(8):643–7.

[58] Friedman EM. Caustic ingestions and foreign body aspirations: an overlooked form of child abuse. Ann Otol Rhinol Laryngol 1987;96(6):709–12.

[59] Baskin DE, Stein F, Coats DK, Paysse EA. Recurrent conjunctivitis as a presentation of Munchausen syndrome by proxy. Ophthalmology 2003;110(8):1582–4.

[60] Babcock J, Hartman K, Pedersen A, et al. Rodenticide-induced coagulopathy in a young child. A case of Munchausen syndrome by proxy. Am J Pediatr Hematol Oncol 1993; 15(1):126–30.

[61] Bappal B, George M, Nair R, et al. Factitious hypoglycemia: a tale from the Arab world. Pediatrics 2001;107(1):180–1.
[62] Edidin DV, Farrell EE, Gould VE. Factitious hyperinsulinemic hypoglycemia in infancy: diagnostic pitfalls. Clin Pediatr (Phila) 2000;39(2):117–9.
[63] Vennemann B, Perdekamp MG, Weinmann W, et al. A case of Munchausen syndrome by proxy with subsequent suicide of the mother. Forensic Sci Int 2005;153:1–5.
[64] Schreier H, Ricci LR. Follow-up of a case of Munchausen by proxy syndrome. J Am Acad Child Adolesc Psychiatry 2002;41(12):1395–6.
[65] Shnaps Y, Frand M, Rotem Y, et al. The chemically abused child. Pediatrics 1981;68(1): 119–21.
[66] Burman D, Stevens D. Munchausen family. Lancet 1977;2(8035):456.
[67] Bartsch C, Risse M, Schutz H, et al. Munchausen syndrome by proxy (MSBP): an extreme form of child abuse with a special forensic challenge. Forensic Sci Int 2003;137(2–3):147–51.
[68] Tessa C, Mascalchi M, Matteucci L, et al. Permanent brain damage following acute clonidine poisoning in Munchausen by proxy. Neuropediatrics 2001;32(2):90–2.
[69] D'Avanzo M, Santinelli R, Tolone C, et al. Concealed administration of frusemide simulating Bartter syndrome in a 4.5-year-old boy. Pediatr Nephrol 1995;9(6):749–50.
[70] McSweeney JJ, Hoffman RP. Munchausen's syndrome by proxy mistaken for IDDM. Diabetes Care 1991;14(10):928–9.
[71] Aranibar H, Cerda M. Hypoglycemic seizure in Munchausen-by-proxy syndrome. Pediatr Emerg Care 2005;21(6):378–9.
[72] Fenton AC, Wailoo MP, Tanner MS. Severe failure to thrive and diarrhoea caused by laxative abuse. Arch Dis Child 1988;63(8):978–9.
[73] Yonge O, Haase M. Munchausen syndrome and Munchausen syndrome by proxy in a student nurse. Nurse Educ 2004;29(4):166–9.

ELSEVIER
SAUNDERS

CLINICS IN
LABORATORY
MEDICINE

Clin Lab Med 26 (2006) 255–273

Criminal Poisoning: Medical Murderers

R. Brent Furbee, MD, FACMT

Department of Emergency Medicine, Indiana University School of Medicine, Room AG373,
1701 North Senate Boulevard, Indianapolis, IN 46206, USA

The possibility of homicide occurring at the hands of health care providers is unthinkable to most people. That is particularly true of those of us in the medical profession. Ironically, the failure of health care workers to consider a coworker as a murderer has caused delays in the recognition of those deaths as homicides and subsequently delayed the termination of further murders. There is a paucity of medical literature on this subject. When patient homicide is discovered, individuals and institutions are reticent to document it for fear of damage to their reputations and increased exposure to litigation. Although such events appear to be rare, it is safe to assume that more homicides occur than are known, and many more occur than are reported in the medical literature. In fact, the major source for such information is to be found in books and electronic media about serial killers. As a result, it must be noted that this article often reflects undocumented details of specific incidents. For the health care professional, the purpose of this article is to heighten awareness and to demonstrate that there are definite patterns to the personalities and methods in these events. Six past medical serial killers have been chosen for review to highlight those patterns and methods.

Donald Harvey

Donald Harvey's career as a murderer began in May of 1970 in London, Kentucky at a small hospital where he worked as an orderly [1,2]. In a videotape developed by the International Association for Hospital Security for medical, security, and law enforcement personnel, he spoke at length about his victims and methods [2]. Harvey selected patients with poor communication skills and those who had little family interaction. In most cases he targeted elderly patients with chronic disease who had been hospitalized for extended periods.

E-mail address: bfurbee@clarian.org

labmed.theclinics.com

Harvey's early victims frequently were smothered or had their ventilation otherwise impaired. Among those victims was an elderly man who had splashed him with urine. In retaliation, Harvey inserted a 22 F catheter in the patient's bladder and threaded a straightened coat hanger through it, puncturing the man's bladder and pushing it the full length. Although the patient complained to a nurse that he had been abused by Harvey, his complaints were ignored. He died of peritonitis. Harvey used arsenic and found it to be an effective though somewhat unpredictable poison. Knowing that elderly patients are more likely to eat sweets, he added arsenic to their desserts. The resulting illness was a nonspecific gastroenteritis. Progression to death was gradual, requiring repeatedly administered small, sublethal doses. He also injected methanol, floor stripper, and adhesive remover intravenously and intramuscularly. Details of the clinical course of patients following these injections are sparse. He did note that decubiti and hemorrhoids were useful sites of injection because of the difficulty in detection at autopsy. Harvey claims to have used cyanide on several occasions. Like arsenic, he obtained it from laboratory supplies. He learned that with the exception of one doctor and one nurse many people at the hospital could not detect the notorious cyanide almond odor, a finding that has likewise been demonstrated in the medical literature [3,4]. On one occasion after a patient had been killed with an injection of cyanide the physician believed he smelled the odor but was dissuaded by Harvey's suggestion that instead it was the odor of vanilla in the patient's dessert.

Harvey found two times of day to be the most advantageous for carrying out his assaults. Change of shift tended to either group nursing personnel around the nurses' station and away from the patients' rooms, or if nurses made walking rounds he could enter patient rooms behind the nurses where he was undetected. Mealtimes also provided him with cover. On most floors half of the nursing staff would go to the cafeteria leaving only half the team to monitor the patients.

As an additional safeguard, Harvey developed a rudimentary alarm system. He closed the door to the patient's room, because most personnel knock before entering. A wastebasket was placed immediately behind the door so that the person entering would overturn it and then stop to right and reposition it. He drew curtains around the beds to obstruct the view and used laundry hampers and bedside tables to further obstruct the approach to the bedside where he was located. Finally, he bunched bedside curtains to obscure the point of entry.

The author and others [5] note that during the course of the interview, Donald Harvey appeared to relish the opportunity to educate his listeners. At times he appeared to embellish his statements, such as noting that he killed some of his victims simply by turning down the flow of their nasal cannula oxygen. All told, he claims to have murdered more than 70 people.

As a final note, Harvey stated he was cooperating to prevent such events from happening in the future. When asked if he would kill again given the chance, he stated, "If I was still working in a hospital and had not been caught, yes" [2].

Kristen Gilbert

In March of 1989, Kristen Gilbert took her first job as a registered nurse at the 197 bed Veterans' Administration Medical Center (VAMC) in Leeds, Massachusetts [6,7]. Not long after, she began to be associated with unexpected sudden deaths in her patients or those on her floor. Months later, a VAMC physician also noted that Gilbert was associated with a disturbing number of unexpected deaths. He eventually asked her supervisor to avoid assigning her to care for his patients. Though fellow nurses initially did not share his concern, Gilbert became known as the Angel of Death. In 1991, while reviewing death records, a VAMC clerk noted that a single name, Gilbert's, was associated with a most deaths on the Ward C intensive care unit where she worked. In a year, the deaths on her shift were triple the number on any other ward. Of the 31 deaths occurring between 1990 and 1991, she had discovered 22 and had initiated 50% of the codes, many times more than any of her coworkers. The clerk approached her nursing supervisor but reportedly was told to stop making false accusations. The supervisor later denied any recollection of that conversation.

By the beginning of 1996, Kristen Gilbert's name was on 75% of the codes and 50% of the deaths occurring on Ward C since her employment in 1989. Even as the rate of codes increased, the Medical Emergency Committee, responsible for reviewing such events, did not appear to be alarmed. Her coworkers, on the other hand, had increasing suspicion. Concerned that Gilbert might be injecting patients with epinephrine, a coworker monitored the vials stocked on the floor. Following an unexpected code she found three epinephrine vials missing. Knowing that epinephrine injections used in codes are usually given in preloaded syringes, she realized that the missing vials should not have been used in the resuscitation. When she found the empty ampules in the trash following the code she realized they may have been used to precipitate the arrest. Guilt-ridden, three of Gilbert's coworkers finally approached their supervisor. As a result, an investigation was begun after 7 years.

Gilbert eventually was convicted of three counts of first degree murder, one count of second-degree murder, and two counts of attempted murder. She was sentenced to life in prison. During the course of her activity she had used epinephrine, ketamine, and acepromazine to harm or kill patients.

Genene Jones

A licensed vocational nurse (LVN), Genene Jones seemed bright, interested, and well read compared with others at her level of training [8,9].

She had lost her first job at San Antonio's Methodist Hospital allegedly for exceeding her authority. After losing a second job she came to the Pediatric Intensive Care Unit (PICU) of the Bexar County Medical Center in October of 1978. Early on, she exhibited bizarre behavior when a child died. Her orientation nurse described her behavior as berserk. She sat at the bedside and sobbed for half an hour, later developing an almost ritualistic response to deaths on the unit.

Genene had few friends and definite enemies. The nurses and residents who followed her orders and advice were favored, but those who did not defer to her were held in contempt and frequently derided to others on the unit. She began to make predictions about the children who were going to die, and when they did her crying vigils at the bedside and processions to the morgue became more bizarre. She committed several medication errors and at times refused to give medicines to children that she, an LVN, believed were not indicated. Amazingly, she was not fired.

In September of 1981, after the death of two children on Genene's shift, two coworkers had seen enough. There were too many deaths occurring. Because physicians and residents tend to rotate through and many of the nurses either came in and out from other units or were temporary workers, few people actually had a complete overview of what was occurring. Convinced Jones was connected to the increasing arrests in the unit, they collected data from the PICU's statistical log. Over the ensuing 6 months they compiled a chart of the deaths between January 1, 1981 and March 17, 1982. Several had occurred in children following innocuous surgical procedures and many had inexplicable causes. They found that in those 15 months, there had been 43 deaths. Genene Jones's assigned patients constituted 22 of them and she had been present for a total of 29. Because many of the children had multiple cardiac or respiratory arrests, the percentage at which Jones was present drew further concern. Cardiopulmonary arrests were occurring almost entirely on the 3:00 to 11:00 shift, when Genene worked. The coworkers went to the nursing administrator with their complaint but were rebuffed. Several days and two more deaths passed, but nothing changed. They took their concerns to the medical director of the PICU who seemed appropriately concerned. The medical director notified the director of pediatrics and at the latter's recommendation began reviewing the deaths for the preceding 6 months.

One physician became convinced that the recent spate of coagulopathies occurring in patients was related to overmedication with heparin. He questioned Jones as to the concentration she used when flushing heparin locks. Her response was 1000 times the proper dose. The medical director ordered that heparin dosing was to be witnessed by a second person thereafter. But Jones's patients continued to die.

In November of 1982, Genene took a month of medical leave. During that time, not a single code blue occurred. The medical director of the PICU was concerned, though his chart review did not show direct evidence of Jones causing arrests. He was dealing with one of the ironies of detecting serial killers in hospitals: The killer is often the person who writes the note detailing pre-arrest events. The numbers troubled the medical director, however, especially in the face of a code-free period in Genene's absence. Within a week of her return, the codes began again.

What should have been the beginning of the end for Genene occurred when a child admitted to the unit for treatment of pneumonia mysteriously developed recurrent episodes of bleeding. With the child near death, a pediatric attending decided to give protamine empirically on the assumption that the hemorrhage was because of a heparin overdose. The bleeding stopped. The doctor ordered that the child be moved from the PICU and cared for only by nurses that he selected. As a result of his demands, the director of pediatrics initiated an internal investigation. He asked the director of nursing to talk with personnel in the PICU, and he planned to do a chart review.

In the meantime, a 4-month-old child was admitted to the unit following open-heart surgery. Initially he had respiratory problems but began to improve. When Jones took over his care on the next shift, she complained to the child's physician that he was not responding appropriately and needed a CT scan. The physician declined, stating that the problem was not neurologic. Later that day while coworkers were busy with another patient Jones approached a neurologist not involved in her patient's care. She assured him that the child was stable enough for a scan. In an attempt to help the PICU staff already engaged in a code, the neurologist ordered the scan. Jones accompanied the child to radiology where he arrested and died. The chief of cardiovascular surgery went to the director of pediatrics and was told an investigation was underway. Unimpressed, he threatened to stop admitting postoperative patients to the PICU. An emergency meeting of key administrators was convened. They decided that a panel of outside medical experts should review the charts and decide if further action would be warranted. Respected physicians from the United States and Canada were brought together but in the end they could not find sufficient evidence of homicide to act. The hospital decided to restrict the PICU nursing staff to registered nurses only, thereby preventing Genene Jones from working in that unit.

Eventually, Jones called a former resident whom she had befriended at the medical center. Kathleen Holland, a pediatrician, was setting up a practice in the small town of Kerrville Texas, about 60 miles northwest of San Antonio. Holland hired Jones to work in her clinic. The clinic opened on September 16, 1982. The following day, during a visit for cold symptoms, an 8-month-old child suffered a respiratory arrest. She recovered and her parents were thankful for the quick action of the clinic nurse, Genene Jones. During a checkup 9 months later the child suffered a second respiratory arrest and died. Her death occurred immediately after she received an injection by Genene. A missing vial of succinylcholine provided an important clue as to the cause of the nine respiratory arrests that occurred in the Kerrville pediatric clinic. That child's death would eventually bring Genene Jones to court where in two separate cases she was sentenced to a total of 159 years. She is eligible for parole in 2009.

Michael Swango

Michael Swango graduated valedictorian of his Quincy, Illinois high school class [10,11]. He had always had a preoccupation with violence. He graduated college with a 3.89 grade point average and entered the Southern Illinois University School of Medicine in 1979 where he worked as an emergency medical technician (EMT) during his medical school tenure. Swango's unusual behavior began to draw attention when he was assigned to work on the hospital wards. Five patients died mysteriously while under his care. Classmates joked that if they wanted a patient to die they would assign them to Double-O-Swango, a reference to the James Bond 007 license to kill.

In 1982 while on an obstetrics and gynecology rotation, the chief resident discovered Swango was leaving his duties to work as an EMT and was falsifying data on patients' records. She reported him to the medical school administration. To avoid expulsion, he hired an attorney and in a compromise agreed to repeat the rotation and complete his training. Although reportedly receiving a disparaging Dean's letter from his medical school, Swango was offered a general surgery internship and neurosurgical residency at Ohio State University.

The known murders appear to have begun in February of 1984 when a nursing student and a patient witnessed Swango injecting another patient's IV line a few minutes before she suffered a cardiac arrest, which she survived. The patient later wrote, "Someone gave me some medicine in my IV and paralyzed all of me, lungs, heart, and speech" [10]. She described Swango as the person, but he denied having been near her room. Several suspicious deaths occurred, prompting nurses to share their concerns about Swango with the nursing director, who then took them to the program director of neurosurgery. Their concerns reportedly did not impress the program director, but eventually Swango was suspended and an investigation begun. The investigation was performed by the program director in consultation with the hospital attorney and the dean of the College of Medicine. Swango was reinstated and allowed to finish his internship but not offered a position in the neurosurgical residency. Later, in response to scathing criticism including an ABC News report, two former Ohio State University officials reportedly conceded that more should have been done [12].

Swango returned to Illinois and resumed work as an EMT at Adams County Ambulance Corps. His paramedic coworkers saw him as somewhat bizarre but tolerated what they believed were idiosyncrasies because of his extensive medical knowledge. That attitude began to change after they experienced a series of episodes of sudden onset abdominal pain, nausea, vomiting, and dizziness. The paramedics decided to set a trap. They left a pitcher of iced tea in a room where Swango would be alone. They retrieved the tea and had it tested. Swango had been adding arsenic obtained from Terro Ant Killer to his coworkers' beverages. Swango was eventually tried for seven counts of aggravated battery. He was convicted and sentenced to 5 years in prison, but paroled after 2-1/2 years.

Following his release, Swango found work as a laboratory technician at a coal company. His past had been forgotten to the extent that when several employees fell ill he was not suspected. In 1992, after sending numerous applications for employment as a physician, he was offered an internal medicine residency position in Sioux Falls, South Dakota. He and his girlfriend, a nurse, moved there and initially he performed his duties as a resident without known incident. Two events lead his residency director to discover his true past: an application to the American Medical Association triggered a background check that revealed his past conviction, and a rerun of an ABC television program was seen regarding his poisoning conviction in Illinois. Swango subsequently was expelled from the residency. Shortly thereafter his girlfriend died of a gunshot wound to the chest, believed to be self-inflicted. By June of 1993, Swango again gained admission to a residency program. This time he moved to New York for training in psychiatry at the State University of New York (SUNY), Stony Brook Medical School. Shortly after starting his clinical duties, at least five patients died unexpectedly and mysteriously under his care. He had added do not resuscitate orders to all of their charts. Swango was dismissed in October of 1993 when SUNY received word that he had falsified his application and that it included a pseudonym. SUNY conducted its own internal investigation concluding no harm had come to any patients. SUNY did, however, send out letters to medical school deans and contacted the Federal Bureau of Investigations (FBI), who subsequently opened an investigation.

Shortly after, Michael Swango abruptly disappeared. He made his way to Zimbabwe and began medical work at a mission. Again, patients began to die unexpectedly. A few, however, survived to describe being injected by the doctor and within moments suffering paralysis. Eventually, nurses demanded that the chief administrator notify police. A search of Swango's residence revealed multiple drugs and liquid-filled syringes. Swango fled to Zambia and Europe but after a year returned to the United States where he was promptly arrested on charges of fraud. With Swango in jail, the FBI accelerated its investigation. He eventually was sentenced to life without possibility of parole for the murders of three of the Stony Brook patients.

It seems that Swango had used several poisons over the years but most frequently used arsenic to contaminate food or injected potassium chloride. It seems that some of his victims suffered temporary paralysis and recovered to identify him as the perpetrator. Others died quickly. As in the Majors case described below, patient complaints were ignored. (See later discussion of Orville Lynn Majors.)

Efren Saldivar

In the late 1980s, Efren Saldivar was hired as a respiratory therapist at Glendale Adventist Medical Center [13,14]. He was considered competent and knowledgeable of pharmaceuticals and computers. He was assigned to night shift work where he had little supervision. Over time, coworkers began to note that when discussions of patients who needed to die were held, the patients promptly died. Saldivar began to be the common denominator of those deaths. It was not until April of 1997 that one of Saldivar's coworkers reported concerns that he may be injecting patients and killing them. The coworker admittedly did not like Efren, so his complaint was suspect. In one of the few published medical reports detailing a health care serial killer, Andresen and colleagues stated, "In 1998, one staff member finally reported to hospital administrators the suspicion that an unusual number of deaths were occurring at night and on the floors where the subject worked. An internal hospital review was performed, and it was concluded that no data were statistically correlated to any unusual patient deaths at the facility" [13].

A coworker of Saldivar's had made a casual comment to a bar patron about his activity in the hospital. The patron in turn attempted to blackmail the hospital. He had little information but recognized Efren's name. The hospital notified the police. In a bizarre twist, Saldivar admitted to police investigators that he had injected patients to prevent them from suffering. He acknowledged about 50 such acts but later recanted. He also implicated some of his coworkers. Efren's employment was terminated on March 13, 1998. Investigators doggedly pursued physical evidence to support their belief that he was a serial killer. More than 1000 deaths that had occurred during the 8 years Saldivar had been employed were reviewed. The investigators narrowed that list to 20 of the most recent suspicious deaths. Brian Andersen and coworkers at Lawrence Livermore Forensic Science Center in Oakland California were able to demonstrate elevated pancuronium bromide levels in some of the patients [13].

In March of 2002, Saldivar pleaded guilty to six counts of murder and one of attempted murder. He was sentenced to life in prison without parole. It is unclear what agents he used, but in addition to pancuronium bromide, morphine and succinylcholine had been discovered in his locker by coworkers. It seems that at least one coworker was complicit in the murders. Ursula Anderson was given immunity to prosecution for her testimony that she had provided pancuronium bromide to Saldivar with knowledge of his intent to inject patients.

Charles Cullen

Charles Cullen gives us perhaps the best example of how easily a serial killer can drift from institution to institution without detection [6,15]. For

16 years he worked at 10 hospitals in Pennsylvania and New Jersey. He confessed to 30 to 40 murders that he characterized as an attempt to help the victims, but examination of the cases suggests other motives.

By 1992, Cullen was working the night shift in a Pennsylvania hospital. By working nights in the intensive care unit he was in a setting most conducive for killing, with fewer coworkers and sicker patients. In 1993, a patient's son complained to physicians and nurses that a male nurse had given his mother an injection that clearly had not been ordered. He even identified Cullen, but his complaints were ignored. The patient was released the next day and died that afternoon of a suspected myocardial infarction. Her son told the county prosecutor's office that she had been murdered, prompting an autopsy. A generic urine drug screen was negative; however, she was not tested for the presence of digoxin, Cullen's favored poison. He moved to other hospitals where there were several instances of his administering unordered medicines, but these events were never formally documented or communicated to the next employer.

In August of 2002, Cullen's coworkers at St. Luke's Hospital had found procainamide and nitroprusside vials with discarded syringes on a ward where they were not approved for use. The nurses increasingly had been suspicious of Cullen and were concerned that he might be harming patients. In an unusual action they decided to bypass hospital administrators and go straight to the police. Ironically, the police ultimately found nothing for which they could charge him. Two jobs later Cullen was working at Somerset Medical Center in Somerville New Jersey. The computer tracking system for the pharmacy there revealed he had requisitioned unordered drugs for patients who were not assigned to him. One patient died of a myocardial infarction because of digoxin administration. An outside investigator suggested deliberate poisoning but that theory was resisted by the hospital in favor of the assertion that she had been poisoned by herbal tea.

A few weeks later, another patient who had not been under Cullen's care also died. The cause of death was initially believed to be myocardial infarction, but an autopsy revealed digoxin, a drug that was not ordered for the decedent. When a medical toxicologist from the New Jersey Poison Center opined that the hospital had a poisoner, they resisted again. Cullen continued to work while one patient sustained an insulin overdose and a second died of precipitous hypoglycemia. On October 31, Somerset Medical Center fired Cullen for lying on his job application. Following investigation, police arrested him on December 12. He was charged with the murder of Father Florian Gall. Found guilty, he was sentenced to life without parole.

Orville Lynn Majors

A licensed practical nurse (LPN), Lynn Majors joined the Vermillion County Hospital (VCH) staff in the fall of 1993. VCH was a small rural but modern hospital with a dedicated staff. As with most small towns, the

members of the hospital staff knew each other well. When the four-bed critical care unit had patients, Majors would be assigned there to help with a registered nurse (RN) as his supervisor. When the unit was empty, he usually
was assigned to pass medications on the medical floor. The admission rate
in that ICU consistently had been close to 350 patients annually, with about
27 deaths. In 1993 the rate increased almost imperceptibly, but by the spring
of 1994 a climb in those numbers began to draw attention. Rumors reportedly began to circulate that Majors was associated with that increase. By
summer of 1994, the increase in ICU cardiopulmonary arrests was noted
clearly, and in July the death rate in the ICU began to accelerate. There
are conflicting stories as to when the hospital administration became aware
and what steps were taken, but in early 1995 the nursing director of the
ICU completed a survey comparing the deaths in the ICU for 1993 to
1994 with employee time cards. What she found was of grave concern. Of
the 147 deaths in the VCH ICU between May of 1993 and December of
1994, 130 occurred when Lynn Majors was working. In March, VCH officials
notified the Indiana State Police of their concerns. Majors was placed on
leave and eventually fired. Thus began the largest criminal investigation in
Indiana's history. It would last 4 years and cost more than 2 million dollars.

The Indiana State Police assembled an independent medical investigative
team that consisted of an emergency physician, an RN, two pathologists,
two intensivists, a medical toxicologist, a cardiac electrophysiologist, a cardiac pathologist, and an epidemiologist. For the next 2 years, charts were
reviewed on all patients who had died during the time period in question.
The thrust of the investigation was to answer two questions for each case:
(1) Was the death consistent with the patient's clinical course? (2) If not,
was there a person or persons who appeared to be associated with the
deaths?

Within a few weeks their review showed that deaths in the ICU commonly followed one of three patterns.

- Sudden onset of hypertension followed by circulatory collapse and cardiac arrest
- Sudden loss of consciousness followed by oxygen desaturation, then
  dysrhythmia
- Unheralded terminal dysrhythmia with wide complex tachycardia, then
  asystole

Among the investigative team members it generally was held that more
than 100 of the cases appeared suspicious. Majors was in close proximity
when death occurred in nearly all of the cases. Eventually, seven cases
were selected for trial. Although many more cases were suspected murders,
the prosecution team decided that presenting a large number of cases would
tend to be confusing to witnesses and the jury.

The investigators determined that Majors had killed the most victims
with potassium chloride. Electrocardiogram findings of QRS widening,

P wave changes and sine wave patterns were documented frequently. A search of Majors' van revealed eight vials of potassium chloride, two syringes of epinephrine, and three vials of injectable nitroglycerin. Investigators believe that if Majors worked on the medicine floor he would inject patients with epinephrine intravenously causing a hypertensive crisis and eventually ventricular tachycardia. He would then initiate a code and almost invariably lidocaine would be ordered as part of the resuscitation effort. It is speculated that Majors would then add potassium to the lidocaine infusion or inject potassium directly into the intravenous line. The patient would be moved from the floor to the ICU and Majors would be moved with the patient to staff the area with an RN. In the ICU, he would inject the recruited patient with more intravenous potassium. Amazingly, on one occasion there were three simultaneous cardiac resuscitations in progress in the four-bed ICU. Majors had discovered all three. As with Genene Jones, when Majors took a vacation, the deaths stopped.

Some family members described unusual behavior on Majors' part. In one case he was working with the intravenous fluid bags at the time a family member entered to visit the patient. Majors literally ran from the room almost knocking down the patient's wife. He sat down at the nurses' station and stared into the patient's room. Moments later, the patient gasped and fell back on the bed, unconscious and cyanotic. Though the patient survived the initial resuscitation, the nurse's notes state that he died hours later after suffering a respiratory arrest while on the ventilator!

For all of the resuscitations, only one set of electrolytes was documented. The potassium was 6.8 mEq/L. Probably because the patients were older and no one suspected anything other than natural causes, routine laboratory work, drug screens, and autopsies were almost never done. As a result of the work of the Indiana State Police investigative team, Majors was arrested on December 29, 1997.

In October of 1999, Orville Lynn Majors was sentenced to 180 years is prison for six of the seven murders for which he was tried. Like other serial killers, he had several dedicated supporters, many of whom saw him as a scapegoat. Certain compelling statistics were not allowed to be presented by the prosecution, however. During the investigation, an intense epidemiologic study of VCH was performed. Time cards, vacation dates, and time and date of deaths were reviewed in a blinded fashion. The conclusion of the study by Stephen Lamm, MD, of Washington DC was that the mortality was of "epidemic proportions" from July to December 1994. "Increased mortality occurred in the Intensive Care Unit...One intensive care nurse was uniquely and strongly associated with that mortality...No other service or service provider shows any association that even approximates in magnitude that of the ICU nurse" [16].

The Lamm study concluded: "The likelihood of someone dying in the Intensive Care Unit was 42.96 times greater than it would be if he were not working" [16]. Graphs relating time worked to deaths were also excluded, leading one police investigator to remark that if the jury had been allowed to see those charts, the trial would have been over in half a day.

The common threads

The poisoners

In most reported cases, the perpetrators are narcissistic. Although they occasionally claim to be euthanizing patients to end their pain, closer scrutiny indicates that there is secondary gain in the form of excitement or a feeling of superiority. Genene Jones, an LVN, frequently performed tasks for which only RNs were qualified. Investigators in the Orville Lynn Majors case speculated that he appeared to try to pass himself as a physician, commonly wearing surgical scrubs and no name tag indicating he was an LPN. Donald Harvey characterized it as follows, "I controlled other people's lives, whether they lived or died. I had that power to control. After I didn't get caught for the first fifteen, I thought it was my right. I appointed myself judge, prosecutor and jury. So I played God" [17].

Another striking characteristic is that the poisoners frequently polarized their coworkers, having a few staunch supporters and an equal number of detractors. Often they appeared to be more knowledgeable than others at their level of training, and in most cases assumed tasks or roles greater than their capability. They curried favor with their supervisors, providing a shield for their activity and leading to deflection of criticism as jealousy by their coworkers. A surprising number of serial killers are suspected by coworkers. In general, it is the nursing staff that recognizes the problem first. In many cases physicians and nursing and hospital administrators are so difficult to convince that more deaths occur even after the killer has been identified.

Men are overrepresented among serial killers in the health care system, making up only 7% of all nurses but accounting for 33% of the murderers [18].

Surreptitious behavior often is noted by coworkers or family members. It is remarkable that killers have exhibited bizarre behavior that is noted only in retrospect. Equally impressive is the number of times that lethal injections are made with families present, but the connections between the injection and death are not made.

One of the most frequently asked questions regarding these people is, "Why did they do it?" M. William Phelps, in his account of Kristen Gilbert, *Perfect Poison*, states, "Adults don't wake up and decide to become serial killers; they are wired at some point—usually during childhood—so that they might later cultivate a malevolence and perpetrate crimes based on what they have been taught" [7].

The victims

For serial killers to operate in a health care setting, selection of victims is important. The very old or very young are most often targeted because they are unable to communicate. In some cases, the victims may even recognize the perpetrator but are unable to verbalize their fears. Sadly, even when they can, their complaints are disregarded as delusions. In the Majors case, a patient even told his family that a nurse was trying to kill him and that if the family did not take him from the hospital that evening, he would not survive until morning. The family disregarded his concerns and the patient was killed during the night.

When deaths are sudden and unexpected they should raise concern. This especially is true when multiple deaths have occurred. Several things appear to shelter the serial killer in this setting, but the greatest among them is the near refusal to accept that such a heinous thing could occur by a person known to others. For that reason, these deaths often are accepted as natural and not murders. That is particularly true among the elderly. In fact, a common defense for health care serial killers is that the patient was old and sick so death was anticipated. Furthermore, the likelihood of an autopsy being ordered on an 80-year-old patient is much lower than in the young. Even elderly patients almost always have a clinical course that declines before death. Health care workers would do well to ask themselves how many times they have lost patients when death actually was a complete surprise.

The method

Potassium chloride has been a popular drug among serial killers because it is readily available and quick acting. Because of postmortem redistribution, the serum concentration increases rapidly after death. An elevated postmortem potassium concentration is a common finding and of no predictive value in the determination of the pre-mortem level. In recent years efforts have been made by hospitals to avoid accidental administration of potassium chloride. Though seldom reported in medical literature, potassium overdose and death has been a concern in the health care setting [19]. When given surreptitiously, it is unlikely to be treated successfully in resuscitation attempts unless electrolytes are measured. Often overlooked is neuromuscular paralysis that occurs as a result of potassium administration.

Neuromuscular paralytic agents are available in the hospital setting and are not controlled substances. They have rapid onset and appear to induce coma. Patients who survive the exposure, however, frequently can identify the assailant (if they are believed). Laboratory detection is possible but not available rapidly in most hospitals. Kerskes and colleagues [20] described the use of high-performance liquid chromatography-electrospray ionization mass spectrometry for the detection of quaternary nitrogen muscle relaxants such as pancuronium and rocuronium.

Because of its use in homicidal poisoning, the detection of succinylcholine has been the subject of much study. Gao and coworkers [21] were able to detect succinylcholine to a concentration of 0.250 µg/ml in human plasma, but concentrations may be significantly less than those in postmortem specimens. They applied their method in a patient receiving 1 mg/kg as an IV bolus. The initial plasma concentration of 25.33 μg/ml declined to 0.11 μg/ml in 3 minutes. By 4 minutes, it was undetectable. In postmortem specimens, such attempts at obtaining levels would be of little use.

In 2001 William Sybers, a Florida physician and medical examiner, was found guilty of the first-degree murder of his wife [22]. The conviction was based heavily on laboratory determination that she had been injected with succinylcholine. A method was described to identify the metabolite, succinylmonocholine, as a marker for the neuromuscular paralytic agent. The metabolite is present for a much longer period and was believed to occur only after exposure to succinylcholine and not as an endogenous compound. In February of 2003, Sybers appealed on the basis that the test for succinylmonocholine was new and not accepted as standard medical practice. His appeal won and a new trial was ordered. He subsequently agreed to a plea bargain and was sentenced to 10 years and a $500,000 fine though he continued to maintain his innocence. He was released on time served for the original conviction. In November of 2003, LeBeau and Quenzer of the FBI Laboratory in Quantico, Virginia, released results of a small study of succinylmonocholine in patients who had not been injected with succinylcholine before death. They were able to identify small concentrations of the compound in autopsy tissue from the six patients they studied. They concluded that, "succinylmonocholine is not an exclusive indicator of exposure to the parent drug, succinylcholine" [23].

Therapeutic doses of succinylcholine result in paralysis that can be managed just by supporting ventilation. Massive doses of that and other paralytic agents may have additional effects not seen at therapeutic doses. For example, larger doses may effect cardiac muscle or potassium concentrations. Prolonged paralysis has been reported [24] but there appear to be other potentially life-threatening effects from paralytic agents, such as hyperkalemia, hyperthermia, or cholinergic activity [25].

Opioids historically have been used widely to murder. These agents are found in wide variety throughout the hospital, but they are controlled. Parenteral administration may occur if the drug can be removed and replaced with water or other liquid. Many undocumented reports exist concerning health care workers who are discovered diverting opioids when patients complain of pain in the face of repeated or high dose analgesic administration. Naloxone, if given in adequate doses, reverses opioid-induced coma. Many health care providers are unaware that opiate screens typically only demonstrate the presence of morphine, codeine, or heroin, with 6-acetyl morphine used to distinguish the latter [26,27]. Oxycodone or hydrocodone occasionally causes positive opiate screens if present in high doses. Synthetic agents, such as meperidine, propoxyphene, or fentanyl derivatives, are not detected on generic opioid screens.

Sedative hypnotics such as benzodiazepines may be used, but seem to be less dependable as lethal agents. Benzodiazepines cause less profound respiratory compromise than opioids or paralytic agents. Veterinary pharmaceuticals also may be used.

Arsenic has long been used in malicious poisonings. Donald Harvey used it to kill patients and Michael Swango used it in an attack on coworkers. For serial killers it has the advantage of lacking a recognizable toxidrome. The initial symptoms are similar to gastroenteritis and the poison can be administered in small doses that have a cumulative and eventually fatal effect. It has the disadvantage of being detectable even in exhumations. In living patients, 24-hour urine specimens are the most useful to demonstrate arsenic. Elevated arsenic concentrations may be found in people who have consumed seafood, but speciation of the type of arsenic can help exclude that [28].

Cyanide allegedly was used by Donald Harvey and Michael Swango. Many other serial killers have used it in the past. Humans are capable of metabolizing small amounts of cyanide, but increasing doses cause symptoms such as altered consciousness, tachypnea, tachycardia, and acidosis. Lethal doses rapidly produce respiratory arrest [29]. There are disadvantages to its use as a lethal agent, however. It is difficult to obtain. Incorrect usage can injure the perpetrator, and it is believed that some people are capable of detecting its odor on the death of victims. The evidence for that is scant, though some authors note wide variation in humans' ability to detect the bitter almond odor [3]. Laboratory detection usually is available at reference laboratories but not in hospitals. One concern about cyanide analysis is that whole blood concentrations, although widely used, may not be as reliable as red cell or plasma cyanide concentrations. Vesey and Wilson [30] reported significant artifactual cyanide formation because acidification during the test caused cyanide production from thiocyanate. Plasma or red blood cell cyanide analysis is recommended, therefore, when cyanide poisoning is suspected [29].

Laboratory studies

Laboratory studies have a limited but critical role in the detection of health care serial killers. They also play an important role in their prosecution. A major deficiency is the inaccuracy of postmortem urine or serum concentrations in predicting pre-mortem concentrations. Several reports of postmortem redistribution of drugs demonstrate that many drugs shift from internal organs back into central circulation after death. Postmortem blood collection from large thoracic vessels or the heart may be several times higher in concentration than blood collected from the femoral or other peripheral vessels [31].

Blood chemistries also are variable. Although some electrolytes, such as sodium or chloride, decline postmortem, potassium begins to climb within an hour after death [32–35]. This information was derived from comparing postmortem electrolyte concentrations with pre-mortem concentrations obtained a short time before death.

Unfortunately, many of the specimens examined in investigations of suspected serial killings are obtained following exhumation. These materials generally are much less revealing of toxins but have some usefulness. In a review of their experience and the previous medical literature, Grellner and Glenewinkel [36] cite 40 pharmaceutical agents that have been recovered by postmortem sampling and the interval between death and testing. Neuromuscular paralytic agents are among compounds successfully recovered [37].

The institution

A chillingly consistent practice in hospitals where serial killers have operated is the slow response of administrators and physicians to involve the police. This seems to be because of a fear of litigation and potential adverse media coverage, but sadly costs more patient lives. Health care providers and administrators are neither trained nor appropriate to conduct investigations of suspected homicides.

Hospital mortality committees are required to provide surveillance of deaths that occur. Variations in mortality rates must be explored, not simply excused. There are several factors that can indicate or contribute to a potential problem.

Deaths occur around meal times
As Donald Harvey noted, that is a time when half of the nursing staff is off the unit. The remaining staff members are busy in other rooms leaving many patients unattended.

Deaths occur in 24-hour cycles (same shift)
This was noted with Kristen Gilbert and Orville Lynn Majors. In addition, vacation times often correspond to cessation of codes and deaths, as seen with Genene Jones and Lynn Majors.

Deaths do not follow glide slope
Before typical natural death a progressive decline in clinical course often predicts the outcome. This decline can be subtle in the elderly or the critically ill. Patients usually show a clinical decline in advance of terminal events, whereas murdered patients have abrupt arrests.

Poor success rates in codes
The immediate survival rate of in-hospital codes is 44% with 17% finally living to leave the hospital. Success rates appear to be lower when a serial killer is at work. In a review of 14,720 cardiac arrests in 207 hospitals, Peberdy and colleagues [38] found the most common causes were cardiac

arrhythmias, acute respiratory insufficiency, and hypotension. Resuscitation teams have to assume that they are working with the most common causes of cardiac arrest. They seldom have the time to determine and correct the cause of the arrest if an unknown toxin is at work.

Evidence of uncharted injections

Although this is a factor that is difficult to find during a routine chart review it deserves notation. In-hospital poisonings generally are administered orally or more often intravenously. Because the perpetrator usually is the person charting, injections of unordered medicines are undocumented. Discovery of needle marks, witness reports of injections, or questionable discarded medications should be checked against physicians' orders and nursing notes.

Medications frequently come from the hospital

In several cases, the hospital pharmacy or medications on the wards serve as the source for the serial killer's poison. This is because not only are the medications easy to procure but also many of these medications do not show up on routine drug screens. Serum potassium concentration begins to increase shortly after death making it an unreliable indictor of pre-mortem potassium concentration. Neuromuscular paralytic drugs, another frequent choice of agents, are not found by a drug screen and require specific testing that generally is beyond the ability of most hospital laboratories.

Although state laws prescribe certain circumstances that mandate a coroner's case, an autopsy is not necessarily performed even in those circumstances. Particularly, deaths of elderly patients are considered natural simply because of their age. As in the Major's case, out of 140 deaths none had postmortem examinations unless they were exhumed as part of the investigation. As Donald Harvey put it, "I could have been apprehended with the first one if they had done the autopsy" [2].

If a patient death is not consistent with the patient's clinical course, an autopsy is imperative. If the autopsy is not consistent with the reported medical conditions, homicide should be in the differential diagnosis. Physicians have an obligation to report concerns to the coroner's or medical examiner's office.

Patient complaints ignored

Unfortunately, this almost always is found in retrospect. Remarkably, even the victims are often unaware that they are being abused.

Employee suspicions ignored

Almost without exception, it is the killer's coworkers who discover their activity. In case after case, physicians and administrators discount reports and denigrate whistle-blowers.

Poor cross-communication among hospitals

Probably the most effective approach to this problem is better communication between hospitals and pre-employment screening to look for potential problems.

Summary

Numerous health care professionals have been found guilty of murdering their patients. These perpetrators used various poisons to kill their victims. Even though each of these murderers was unique in how he or she killed, several common characteristics have been noted regarding these cases that should heighten health care workers' and administrators' concern of potential foul play.

References

[1] Beaver W. Chilling confessions of cinncinnati's cyanide killer. New York, NY: Windsor Publishing Company; 1991. Mandelsberg R, editor. Medical murderers.

[2] In Our Midst: An interview with Donald Harvey [videotape]. Lombard, IL: Communicorp Television Productions; 1989.

[3] Gonzalez ER. Cyanide evades some noses, overpowers others. JAMA 1982;248(18):2211.

[4] Kirk RL, Stenhouse NS. Ability to smell solutions of potassium cyanide. Nature 1953; 171(4355):698–9.

[5] Newton M. The encyclopedia of serial killers. New York: Checkmark Books; 2000.

[6] Bardsley M. Angels of death: the male nurses. In: Bardsley M, editor. Crime Library: Court TV; 2005. Available at: http://www.crimelibrary.com/notorious_murders/angels/male_nurses/index.html. Accessed January 15, 2006.

[7] Phelps M. Perfect poison. New York: Kensington Publishing Corp.; 2003.

[8] Moore K, Reed D. Deadly medicine. New York: St. Martin's Press; 1988.

[9] Ramsland K. All about Genene Jones. In: Bardsley M, editor. Crime Library: Court TV; 2005. Available at: http://www.crimelibrary.com/notorious_murders/angels/genene_jones/1.html. Accessed January 18, 2006.

[10] Bardsley M. Serial killers: truly weird & shocking. In: Bardsley M, editor. Crime Library: Court TV; 2005. Available at: http://www.crimelibrary.com/serial_killers/weird/swango/index_1.html. Accessed December 20, 2005.

[11] Stewart J. Blind eye: how the medical establishment let a doctor get away with murder. New York: Simon & Schuster; 1999.

[12] Lore D. Book opens wounds OSU suffered over Swango case. Columbus Dispatch. September 14, 1999.

[13] Andresen BD, Alcaraz A, Grant PM. The application of pancuronium bromide (Pavulon) forensic analyses to tissue samples from an "Angel of Death" investigation. J Forensic Sci 2005;50(1):215–9.

[14] Ramsland K. All about Efren Saldivar. In: Bardsley M, editor. Crime Library: Court TV; 2005. Available at: http://www.crimelibrary.com/notorious_murders/angels/efren_saldivar/1.html. Accessed January 12, 2006.

[15] Mair G. Angel of death. New York: Chamberlain Brothers; 2004.

[16] Available at: http://www.courttv.com/archive/legaldocs/newsmakers/orville.html. Indiana v. Orville Lynn Majors Probable Cause Affidavit. Accessed December 23, 2005.

[17] Schechter H. The serial killer files. New York: Random House Publishing; 2003.

[18] Pyrek K. Healthcare serial killers: recognizing the red flags. Forensic Nurse Magazine. 2003: September/October. Available at: http://www.forensicnursemag.com/articles/391feat.html. Accessed January 25, 2006.

[19] Anon. Intravenous potassium predicament. Clin J Oncol Nurs 1997;1(2):45–9.

[20] Kerskes CHM, Lusthof KJ, Zweipfenning PGM, et al. The detection and identification of quaternary nitrogen muscle relaxants in biological fluids and tissues by ion-trap LC-ESI-MS. J Anal Toxicol 2002;26(1):29–34.

[21] Gao H, Roy S, Donati F, et al. Determination of succinylcholine in human plasma by high-performance liquid chromatography with electrochemical detection. J Chromatogr B Biomed Sci Appl 1998;718(1):129–34.

[22] McGraw S. Notorious murders/not guilty? The Bill Sybers case. In: Bardsley M, editor. Crime Library: Court TV; 2005. Available at: http://www.crimelibrary.com/notorious_murders/not_guilty/bill_sybers/index.html. Accessed January 22, 2006.

[23] LeBeau M, Quenzer C. Succinylmonocholine identified in negative control tissues. J Anal Toxicol 2003;27:600–1.

[24] Ohata H, Kawamura M, Taguchi Y, et al. Overdose of vecuronium during general anesthesia to an infant. Masui 2005;54(3):298–300.

[25] Otteni JC, Steib A, Pottecher T. Cardiac arrest during anesthesia and recovery period. Ann Fr Anesth Reanim 1990;9(3):195–203.

[26] Fehn J, Megges G. Detection of O6-monoacetylmorphine in urine samples by GC/MS as evidence for heroin use. J Anal Toxicol 1985;9(3):134–8.

[27] Kintz P, Jamey C, Cirimele V, et al. Evaluation of acetylcodeine as a specific marker of illicit heroin in human hair. J Anal Toxicol 1998;22(6):425–9.

[28] Nixon DE, Moyer TP. Arsenic analysis II: rapid separation and quantification of inorganic arsenic plus metabolites and arsenobetaine from urine. Clin Chem 1992;38(12):2479–83.

[29] Curry S, LoVecchio F. Hydrogen and inorganic cyanide salts. 2nd edition. Philadelphia: Lippincott Williams & Wilkins; 2001. Sullivan J, Krieger G, editors. Clinical environmental health and toxic exposures.

[30] Vesey C, Wilson J. Red cell cyanide. J Pharm Pharmacol 1978;30:20–6.

[31] Anderson W, Prouty R. Postmortem redistribution of drugs. Chicago, IL: Yearbook Medical Publishers, Inc.; 1989. Baselt R, editor. Advances in analytical toxicology.

[32] Coe JI. Postmortem chemistry: practical considerations and a review of the literature. J Forensic Sci 1974;19(1):13–32.

[33] Coe JI. Postmortem chemistries on blood with particular reference to urea nitrogen, electrolytes, and bilirubin. J Forensic Sci 1974;19(1):33–42.

[34] Coe JI. Postmortem chemistry of blood, cerebrospinal fluid, and vitreous humor. Leg Med Annu 1977;1976:55–92.

[35] Coe JI. Postmortem chemistry update: Emphasis on forensic application. Am J Forensic Med Pathol 1993;14(2):91–117.

[36] Grellner W, Glenewinkel F. Exhumations: synopsis of morphological and toxicological findings in relation to the postmortem interval. Survey on a 20-year period and review of the literature. Forensic Sci Int 1997;90(1–2):139–59.

[37] Andresen BD, Alcaraz A, Grant PM. Pancuronium bromide (Pavulon) isolation and identification in aged autopsy tissues and fluids. J Forensic Sci 2005;50(1):196–203.

[38] Peberdy M, Kaye W, Ornato J, et al. Cardiopulmonary resuscitation of adults in the hospital: a report of 14720 cardiac arrests from the National Registry of Cardiopulmonary Resuscitation. Resuscitation 2003;58(3):297–308.

ELSEVIER
SAUNDERS

Clin Lab Med 26 (2006) 275–285

CLINICS IN
LABORATORY
MEDICINE

Index

Note: Page numbers of article titles are in **bold face** type.

A

Abdominal pain, in arsine gas poisoning, 71–72

Absinthe, seizures due to, 200

Abuse, drug, **147–164**
  cocaine, **127–146**
  dextromethorphan, 157–159
  Ecstasy-related compounds, 147–153, 169–172, 189
  fentanyl, 159–161
  khat, 153–156
  salvia, 156–157
  seizures due to, 189

Abyssinian tea (khat), 153–156

Acepromazine poisoning, by health care workers, 257

Acetaminophen poisoning, **49–65**
  acute, definition of, 52
  clinical features of, 17, 49–50
  diagnosis of, 49–50
  drug metabolism in, 51–52
  epidemiology of, 49
  from Tylenol Extended Relief, 53–54
  histopathology of, 50–51
  laboratory tests in, 17–19
  metabolic acidosis in, 38
  nonacute, 54
  prognosis for, 58–60
  risk factors for, 51–52
  treatment of, 52–57

Acetoacetate, formation of, in poisoning, 40

Acetone, formation of, in poisoning, 40

Acetylcholine, excess of, seizures due to, 187

N-Acetylcysteine, for acetaminophen poisoning
  adverse reactions in, 57
  duration of, 55–56
  indications for, 52–53
  mechanism of action of, 55
  nonacute, 54
  oral versus intravenous, 56–57
  prognosis with, 58–60

with extended relief formulation, 53–54

Acetyl-para-aminophenol poisoning. *See* Acetaminophen poisoning.

Acidosis
  lactic, in poisoning, 40
  metabolic. *See* Metabolic acidosis.

Acrodynia, in mercury poisoning, 79

Activated charcoal, for poisoning, 5–8
  complications of, 7–8
  dose for, 6
  drug-related, 202
  efficacy of, 6–8
  gastric lavage with, 3–5
  isoniazid, 198
  mechanism of, 5–6
  superactivated, 6
  thallium, 77
  versus supportive care, 6–7

Adenosine, excess of, seizures due to, 187–188

African salad (khat), 153–156

Alkalis, metabolic acidosis due to, 37–38

Alopecia, in thallium poisoning, 74–75

Alpha-fetoprotein, in acetaminophen poisoning prognosis, 60

N,N-Alpha-methyltryptamine (AMT), 148–150

Amphetamines, abuse of, 150–152

AMT (N,N-alpha-methyltryptamine), 148–150

Amyl nitrite, for cyanide poisoning, 43

Amylase, in acetaminophen poisoning prognosis, 60

Anemia, in poisoning
  carbon monoxide, 100
  lead, 87–88

Changing Your Address?

Make sure your subscription changes too! When you notify us of your new address, you can help make our job easier by including an exact copy of your Clinics label number with your old address (see illustration below.) This number identifies you to our computer system and will speed the processing of your address change. Please be sure this label number accompanies your old address and your corrected address—you can send an old Clinics label with your number on it or just copy it exactly and send it to the address listed below.

We appreciate your help in our attempt to give you continuous coverage. Thank you.

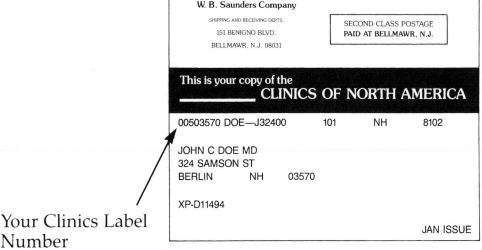

Your Clinics Label Number
Copy it exactly or send your label along with your address to:
Elsevier Periodicals Customer Service
6277 Sea Harbor Drive
Orlando, FL 32887-4800
Call Toll Free 1-800-654-2452

Please allow four to six weeks for delivery of new subscriptions and for processing address changes.